Federated Learning for Neural Disorders in Healthcare 6.0

This reference text offers a relevant and thorough examination of the overlap between neuroscience and federated learning. It explores the complexities of utilizing federated learning algorithms for MRI data analysis, demonstrating how to improve the accuracy and efficiency of diagnostic procedures. The book covers topics such as the prediction and diagnosis of Alzheimer's disease using neural networks and ensuring data privacy and security in federated learning for neural disorders.

This book:

- Provides a thorough examination of the transformative impact of federated learning on the diagnosis, treatment, and understanding of brain disorders.
- Focuses on combining federated learning with magnetic resonance imaging (MRI) data, which is a fundamental aspect of contemporary neuroimaging research.
- Examines the use of federated learning as a promising approach for collaborative data analysis in healthcare, with a focus on maintaining privacy and security.
- Explores the cutting-edge field of healthcare innovation by examining the interface of neuroscience and machine learning, with a specific focus on the breakthrough technique of federated learning.
- Offers a comprehensive understanding of how federated learning may transform patient care, covering both theoretical ideas and practical examples.

It is primarily written for graduate students and academic researchers in electrical engineering, electronics, and communication engineering, computer science and engineering, and biomedical engineering.

Future Generation Information Systems

Series editor - Bharat Bhushan

With the evolution of future generation computing systems, it becomes necessary to occasionally take stock, analyze the development of its core theoretical ideas, and adapt to radical innovations. This series will provide a platform to reflect the theoretical progress, and forge emerging theoretical avenues for the future generation information systems. The theoretical progress in the Information Systems field (IS) and the development of associated next generation theories is the need of the hour. This is because Information Technology (IT) has become increasingly infused, interconnected and intelligent in almost all context.

Industry 6.0: Technology, Practices, Challenges, and Applications
Kishor Kumar Reddy C, Srinath Doss, Lavanya Pamulaparty,
Kari J Lippert and Ruchi Doshi

Convergence of Deep Learning and Artificial Intelligence in Internet of Things
Ajay Rana, Arun Rana, Sachin Dhawan, Sharad Sharma and
Ahmed A. Elngar

Next Generation Communication Networks for Industrial Internet of Things Systems
Sundresan Perumal, Mujahid Tabassum, Moolchand Sharma and
Saju Mohanan

Artificial Intelligence and Optimizing Techniques for Smart Information System Generations
Edited by: Aleem Ali, Rajdeep Chakraborty and Nawaf R. Alharbe

Federated Learning for Neural Disorders in Healthcare 6.0

Edited by
Kishor Kumar Reddy C and Anindya Nag

CRC Press
Taylor & Francis Group
Boca Raton London New York

CRC Press is an imprint of the
Taylor & Francis Group, an **informa** business

Designed cover image: Shutterstock

First edition published 2025
by CRC Press
2385 NW Executive Center Drive, Suite 320, Boca Raton FL 33431

and by CRC Press
4 Park Square, Milton Park, Abingdon, Oxon, OX14 4RN

CRC Press is an imprint of Taylor & Francis Group, LLC

ISBN: 978-1-032-96887-2 (hbk)
ISBN: 978-1-032-96888-9 (pbk)
ISBN: 978-1-003-59108-5 (ebk)

DOI: 10.1201/9781003591085

Typeset in Sabon
by Newgen Publishing UK

Contents

Preface

The proposed book, *Advanced Federated Learning for Neural Disorders in Healthcare 6.0*, addresses the urgent need to tackle the complexities of diagnosing and managing neurological disorders. Despite significant advancements in medical technology, neurological disorders such as dementia, Alzheimer's, Parkinson's, and various mental health issues remain substantial challenges, affecting millions globally. This proposed book aims to present innovative solutions through federated learning, a distinctive architecture for collaborative data analysis that prioritizes privacy and security. Federated learning presents a solution to traditional challenges in data sharing within the healthcare industry. Federated learning enhances our understanding of intricate brain processes by decentralizing the model training and leveraging data from other universities. This proposed book will elucidate this groundbreaking concept, providing a comprehensive theoretical underpinning and practical guidance for its application in neuroscience.

Chapter 1 explores the fundamental concepts of federated learning, its process and its architecture for healthcare applications. Additionally, this chapter discusses the different use cases of federated learning in healthcare applications and the various functions involved in solving healthcare problems. Finally, the key challenges of federated learning implementation are also explained in this chapter.

Chapter 2 explores the neural disorders that constitute a huge and significant global health challenge, involving millions of people around the world with impairments ranging from Alzheimer's and Parkinson's diseases to autism and TBI. Such disorders have serious consequences, often resulting in cognition loss, reduced quality of life, and vast economic burdens on healthcare systems. With the development of healthcare 6.0, powered by AI, IoT, and Big Data, there is a complete overhaul in the diagnosis, treatment, and management of neural disorders.

In Chapter 3, we delve into the emerging landscape of Explainable AI (XAI) in healthcare. We examine the pressing need for transparency and accountability in AI-driven healthcare systems, highlighting how XAI methodologies can enhance trust and improve patient outcomes. This chapter provides an overview of popular XAI methods such as LIME, SHAP, and Integrated Gradients, exploring their applications across various healthcare domains including radiology and personalized medicine. Additionally, we discuss ethical considerations and the importance of interdisciplinary collaboration to ensure the responsible deployment of XAI in clinical settings. The insights offered here aim to inform the future of ethical AI in healthcare.

Chapter 4 provides an overview of the intersection of neuroscience and artificial intelligence, or how the intricate workings of biological neurons inspire advances in machine learning. With biological neurons and their communication through action potentials and synaptic plasticity, its full complexity offers insights into building more adaptive and efficient AI systems. ANNs make these processes extremely simple, however, and only partially achieve the full adaptability of their biological counterparts. This chapter discusses neural mechanisms like spike-timing-dependent plasticity and hierarchical processing that illustrate how such principles might be used to design more dynamic, energy-efficient AI models that bridge the gap between human cognition and computational design.

Chapter 5 explores how federated learning (FL) can be used in the optimized treatment of neural disorders like epilepsy, Alzheimer's, and Parkinson's disease by allowing multiple healthcare institutions to work together on machine learning (ML) models without sharing sensitive patient information. Federated learning preserves privacy and does not break legal requirements. The chapter describes the premise of FL, applications in health care, and a few of the challenges arising when sharing data across different institutions, including security and heterogeneity. Case studies include developments with FL that are improving diagnostics, informing and guiding personalized treatments for all patients through future ethical, legal, and regulatory considerations in FL to advance the care of neural disorders.

Chapter 6 explores neuroimaging methods using state-of-the-art imaging modalities such as fMRI, PET, SPECT, and MRI. An overview of artificial intelligence, its neural imaging algorithm, and uses. The additional dimensions will further emphasize how important neuroimaging is for diagnosis and tailored treatment. To better understand the structure, function, and dynamics of the brain as well as to diagnose, predict, and treat neurological conditions, researchers, clinicians, and students who wish to apply advanced AI methods for these purposes will find this chapter to be a valuable resource. It discusses the future directions of neuroimaging and brain data analysis.

Chapter 7 explores how AI and federated learning are reshaping cross-institutional research and treatment for neural disorders. By facilitating secure collaborations, FL allows institutions to utilize diverse datasets while maintaining patient privacy. We explore the methodologies that enhance diagnostic accuracy and personalized treatments, along with the challenges and ethical considerations involved. Ultimately, this chapter highlights the potential of these technologies to transform patient care in the field of neural disorders.

Chapter 8 explores the integration of federated learning with blockchain technology to enhance the security and reliability of data. Federated learning trains models without data sharing, and blockchain enhances security through key components such as data integrity, distribution, cryptography, and smart contracts. This content is highly beneficial for college students, researchers, and industry professionals, offering them deep insights into the field of security, helping them build knowledge on emerging secure AI-driven healthcare systems, and equipping them to address real-world challenges in data privacy and secure data transfer.

Chapter 9 explores the intersection of federated learning and personalized medicine in the context of neural disorders. By enabling collaborative data analysis while preserving patient privacy, federated learning offers innovative solutions for tailoring therapies. We investigate its applications in enhancing treatment strategies and improving patient outcomes. It highlights how these advancements are poised to redefine healthcare practices in the era of personalized medicine.

Chapter 10 explores the fundamental concepts and importance of federated learning, its process, and how its architecture is suited to diagnosing schizophrenia. Additionally, this chapter also discusses how virtual reality (VR)/augmented reality (AR) is used in the therapy process through various game-based activities that are designed to measure emotional behaviors like fear, and sadness, motor activities, and also to measure the effectiveness of therapy. Finally, the integration of federated learning, and virtual reality/augmented reality for the diagnosis and therapy of schizophrenia is also explained in this chapter.

Chapter 11 discusses dementia, a serious worldwide health concern, emphasizing the value of early detection for efficient treatment and control of the disease's progression. This chapter examines the revolutionary potential of deep learning methods for dementia diagnosis, emphasizing their capacity to examine intricate datasets such as genetic data, neuroimaging, and medical records. These models can detect tiny biomarkers and patterns that are frequently missed by conventional diagnostic tools by utilizing convolutional neural networks (CNNs) and recurrent neural networks (RNNs). The chapter examines important algorithmic developments, recent deep learning applications in dementia diagnosis, and possible ethical issues. It also talks about potential future integrations of these cutting-edge models into clinical practice, to improve diagnostic precision and patient care in the fight against dementia.

Chapter 12 examines an innovative federated learning methodology for diagnosing epilepsy via EEG records, emphasizing the notable neurological alterations linked to the condition. The study distinguishes seizure signals from normal brain activity by analyzing a dataset of 500 patients, with remarkable accuracy rates of 0.997 for training and 0.9925 for testing. This research illustrates the potential of AI to better diagnostic tools while underscoring the need for data privacy, thereby facilitating the development of sophisticated real-time monitoring devices that can improve patient care and enable timely interventions.

Chapter 13 explores Alzheimer's disease (AD) and the role of MRI in Neuroimaging. Alzheimer's disease (AD) is a significant medical and social challenge, with rising prevalence and complex diagnostic processes. Neuroimaging techniques, particularly Magnetic Resonance Imaging (MRI), have revolutionized the understanding of AD progression, with traditional structural MRI (sMRI) revealing insights like hippocampal atrophy. However, advanced technologies such as Functional MRI (fMRI), Diffusion Tensor Imaging (DTI), Magnetization Transfer Imaging (MTI), and Arterial Spin Labeling (ASL) enhance early detection capabilities. This article discusses MRI's role in identifying preclinical AD and its comparison with PET and CT scans. It also highlights the potential of integrating machine learning with MRI data to improve diagnostic accuracy, aiming to contribute to early and precise detection of Alzheimer's disease.

Chapter 14 explores the utilization of convolutional neural networks (CNNs) for the identification and forecasting of brain tumors, highlighting the revolutionary influence of deep learning in medical imaging. This study utilizes CNNs to improve the precision and efficiency of brain tumor diagnosis, overcoming the shortcomings of conventional techniques that are often sluggish and prone to errors. The study employs a federated learning strategy to maintain data privacy while enabling collaborative model training among several healthcare facilities. The results indicate considerable potential in automating tum our detection, attaining elevated accuracy rates and eventually enhancing patient outcomes through prompt diagnosis and action.

About the editors

Kishor Kumar Reddy C is currently working as an associate professor in the Department of Computer Science and Engineering, Stanley College of Engineering and Technology for Women, Hyderabad, India. He has research and teaching experience of more than 13 years. He has published more than 90 research papers in national and international conferences, book chapters, and journals indexed by SCIE, Scopus and others. He has authored 2 textbooks and 12 edited books. He is a member of ISTE, CSI, IAENG, UACEE, and IACSIT.

Anindya Nag obtained an M.Sc. in Computer Science and Engineering from Khulna University in Khulna, Bangladesh, and a B.Tech. in Computer Science and Engineering from Adamas University in Kolkata, India. He is currently a lecturer in the Department of Computer Science and Engineering at the Northern University of Business and Technology in Khulna, Bangladesh. His research focuses on health informatics, medical Internet of Things, neuroscience, and machine learning. He serves as a reviewer for numerous prestigious journals and international conferences. He has authored and co-authored around 32 publications, including journal articles, conference papers, book chapters, and has co-edited five books.

Contributors

Noora Fatima Abdul Haleem
Department of Computer Science and Engineering, Stanley College of Engineering and Technology for Women, Hyderabad, Telangana, India

Sumayya Afreen
Department of Computer Science and Engineering, Stanley College of Engineering and Technology for Women, Hyderabad, Telangana, India

Syeda Sadia Ahmed
Department of Computer Science and Engineering, Stanley College of Engineering and Technology for Women, Hyderabad, Telangana, India

Nikhilesh Anand
School of Medicine, University of Texas, Edinburg, Texas, 78539, USA

Anniappan Vasuki
Department of ECE, SRM Institute of Science and Technology, Vadapalani, Chennai, India

Swagata Ashwani
Carnegie Mellon University, USA

Hina Bansal
Centre for Computational Biology and Bioinformatics, Amity Institute of Biotechnology, Amity University, Noida 201303, Uttar Pradesh, India

Boggarapu Srinivasulu
Department of IT, BVRIT HYDERABAD College of Engineering for Women, Hyderabad, India

Bonthala Prabhanjan Yadav
Department of Computer Science, Sumathi Reddy Institute of Technology for Women, Warangal, India

Hari Chandra Prasad Cheerla
Saint Louis University, Missouri, USA

Chinna Ovu Reddi Umarani
Department of Computer Science and Engineering, National Engineering College, Kovilpatti -628503, Tuticorin District, India

Dammu Venkata Ravi Kumar
Department of CSE, Aditya University, Surampalem, Andhra Pradesh, India

Srinivasa Rao Dhanikonda
Department of Artificial Intelligence and Data Science, Faculty of Science and Technology (IcfaiTech), ICFAI Foundation for Higher Education (Deemed to Be University), Hyderabad, India

Srinath Doss
Faculty of Engineering and Technology, Botho University, Botswana

Areesha Fatima
Department of Computer Science and Engineering, Stanley College of Engineering and Technology for Women, Hyderabad, India

Gundekari Anusha
Department of Artificial Intelligence and Machine Learning, Sreenidhi Institute of Science & Technology, Hyderabad, Telangana, India

Neetu Jabalia
Department of Science & Technology & Renewable Energy, Chandigarh, India

Jahangeer Naskath
Department of Computer Science and Engineering, National Engineering College, Kovilpatti -628503, Tuticorin District, India

Herat Joshi
Data Science – Team Lead, Great River Health Systems, Iowa, USA

Shenson Joseph
University of North Dakota Texas, USA

Vineetha Kaashipaka
Department of Electronics and Communications Engineering, Sreenidhi Institute of Science and Technology, Hyderabad, India

Emilija Kisic
Faculty of Information Technology, Belgrade Metropolitan University, Tadeusa Koscuska 63, 11000 Belgrade, Serbia

Nitesh Kumar
Department of Pharmacology & Toxicology, National Institute of Pharmaceutical Education and Research (NIPER), Hajipur, Vaishali-844102 Bihar, India

Avula Mahathi
Department of Computer Science and Engineering, Stanley College of Engineering and Technology for Women, India

Nandini Manickam
Department of ECE, SRM Institute of Science and Technology, Kattankulathur, Chengalpattu, India

Selvakumar Manickam
National Advanced IPv6 Center, Universiti Sains, Malaysia

Sarasa Meenakshi
Department of Pharmacy Practice, National Institute of Pharmaceutical Education and Research (NIPER), Hajipur, Vaishali-844102 Bihar, India

Ashirbad Mishra
Dept. of CSE, Pennsylvania State University, University Park, PA, USA

Mayank Mishra
National Institute of Pharmaceutical Education and Research, Hajipur, India

Krishna Murti
Department of Pharmacy Practice, National Institute of Pharmaceutical Education and Research (NIPER), Hajipur, Vaishali-844102 Bihar, India

Nagarajan Karthikeyan
Department of Computer Science and Engineering, Syed Ammal Engineering College, Ramanathapuram-623502, Tamil Nadu, India

Yash Nautiyal
Centre for Computational Biology and Bioinformatics, Amity Institute of Biotechnology, Amity University, Noida 201303, Uttar Pradesh, India

Ayesha Nuzha
Department of Computer Science and Engineering, Texas A&M University, Corpus Christi, USA

Sudev Kumar Padhi
Department of CSE, IIT Bhilai, Durg, Chhattisgarh, India

Sadhu Charan Panda
Department of Community Medicine, VSS Institute of Medical Sciences and Research, Sambalpur, Odisha, India

Alipsa Pattnaik
School of Applied Sciences, Birla Global University, Bhubaneswar, Odisha, India

Deepti Rani Pattanaik
Dept. of Statistics, Sambalpur University, Odisha, India

Monalisha Pattnaik
Dept. of Statistics, Sambalpur University, Odisha, India

Vijayakumar Ponnusamy
Department of ECE, SRM Institute of Science and Technology, Kattankulathur, Chengalpattu, India

Ved Prakash
Department of Endocrinology, Indira Gandhi institute of medical sciences (IGIMS) Sheikhpura, Patna- 800014, Bihar, India

Jagadeshwari Puttanapura
Department of Computer Science and Engineering, Stanley College of Engineering and Technology for Women, Hyderabad, India

Ravega Venkata Gandhi
Mai Nefhi College of Engineering And Technology, ASMARA, Eritrea

Sandeep Ravikanti
Visvesvaraya Technological University, Karnataka, India

Kishor Kumar Reddy C
Department of Computer Science and Engineering, Stanley College of Engineering and Technology for Women, Hyderabad, India

Thejoramnaresh Reddy Boya
Department of Computer Science & Engineering, Aurora's Technological & Research Institute, Telangana, India

Kritika Shukla
Centre for Computational Biology and Bioinformatics, Amity Institute of Biotechnology, Amity University, Noida 201303, Uttar Pradesh, India

Sushama Singh
National Institute of Pharmaceutical Education and Research, Hajipur, India

Monika Singh T
Department of Computer Science and Engineering, Stanley College of Engineering and Technology for Women, Hyderabad, India

Krishna Priya Thammana
Wright State University, Dayton, OH, USA

Lingala Thirupathi
Department of Artificial Intelligence and Machine Learning, Sreenidhi Institute of Science & Technology, Hyderabad, Telangana, India

Nemanja Zdravković
Faculty of Information Technology, Belgrade Metropolitan University, Tadeusa Koscuska 63, 11000 Belgrade, Serbia

Chapter 1

Federated learning in healthcare 6.0 paradigm, technologies and challenges

Anniappan Vasuki, Vijayakumar Ponnusamy, Emilija Kisic, and Nemanja Zdravković

1.1 INTRODUCTION

Federated Learning (FL) is a technology that permits several devices to collaboratively create a Machine Learning (ML) algorithm with the supervision of a main server without swapping their information [1]. Major domains like healthcare, finance, and others, require data privacy while using personal user data for other companies or devices. Although FL seems like a promising ML method ensuring local data privacy and protection, it is subject to attacks much like other ML models.

This chapter overviews the core concepts of FL architecture and provides a comparison of FL and ML approaches. The distinctive structure of FL for healthcare applications, different use cases that utilize the FL algorithms, FL algorithms fused with ML models, and key challenges in FL while using it for healthcare applications are discussed in detail in this chapter.

This chapter is structured as follows: In Section 1.1, the basic introduction, outline of the FL algorithm, different types of FL algorithms, and FL architecture are discussed. The role of FL in healthcare, the limitations of ML algorithms, the importance of FL in healthcare, and FL architecture for healthcare applications are explained in Section 1.2. In the next Section, 1.3, various use cases of FL in healthcare such as Electronic Health Record (EHR) management, remote monitoring, medical imaging, diagnosis of schizophrenia, and decentralized FL for healthcare networks are explained. The key challenges of FL in the healthcare domain are discussed in Section 1.4. Finally, this chapter concludes in Section 1.5 with the future scope of FL algorithms in the healthcare domain.

1.1.1 Federated learning – an outline

This section presents an outline of FL. Figure 1.1 shows the part of FL across various devices.

Federated learning has four major processes.

DOI: 10.1201/9781003591085-1

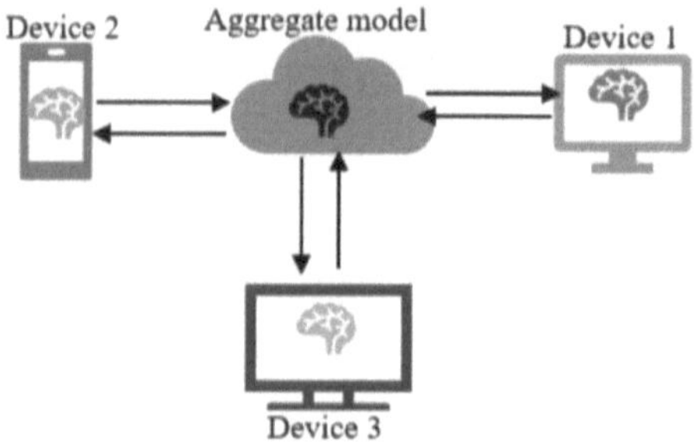

Figure 1.1 Role of FL across devices.

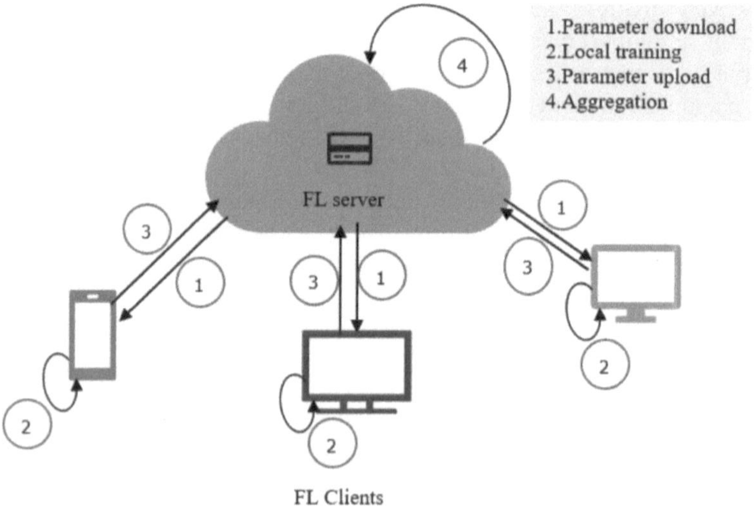

Figure 1.2 FL framework.

- Selection of client: The main server chooses the client devices randomly or based on an algorithm from a group of devices.
- Parameter Sharing: Next, parameters of the global model will be available to the local devices. This process is done by main server.
- Training of local ML model: Client begins training local ML model based on received key parameters of global model.
- Integration of local ML models: The final step involves clients sharing the local ML model parameters they have learnt with the main server, which then aggregates the local ML models it has received. The simplified framework of FL is shown in Figure 1.2.

1.1.2 Categories of federated learning

The different categories of FL are discussed in this section [2].

- Vertical FL: Vertical FL is applied to conditions where datasets with varying features are stored on each device. Vertical FL, for example, may be utilized to develop a shared ML method when two domains have different feature sets but data on the same user group.
- Horizontal FL: Horizontal FL is used for similar feature sets stored on each device. This is used in Google Keyboard, where smartphones have different training data sets but the same features.
- Transfer FL: Updating new features in the existing pre-trained model to extend the applications can be done using transfer FL.
- Cross-Silo FL: This FL category is used when the devices are fewer in number, but it is used in all levels of applications.

Cross-Device FL: This type of FL is used in an application that has a great number of gadgets. The client selection process plays an essential role in this type of FL model.

1.1.3 Generalized architecture of federated learning

The generalized architecture of FL is illustrated in Figure 1.3 [3]. The global model with a central server first selects the client devices. After that, it provides the chosen clients with the parameters of its ML model. Using the

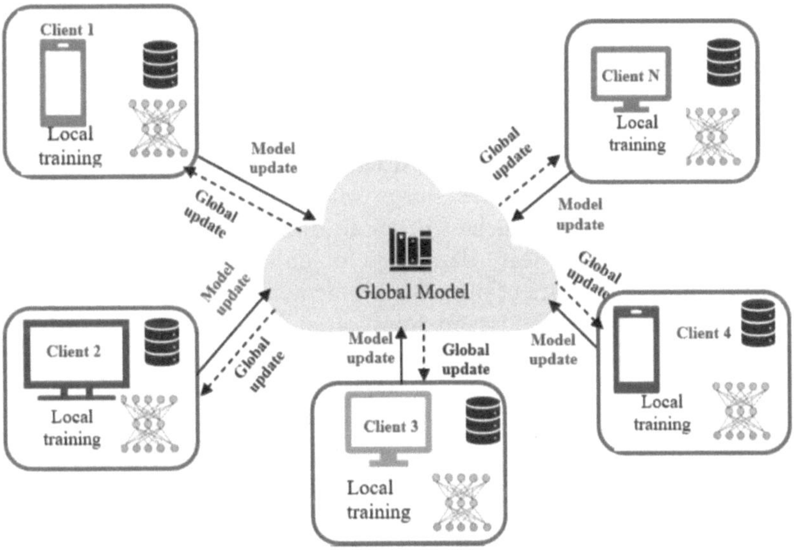

Figure 1.3 Generalized architecture of FL.

received parameters, the client devices train their local ML model. Next, the client delivers the server its trained model. In this case, the clients do not share their private data, the trained ML model alone is shared with the main server to ensure the local client's data privacy. This feature in the FL model makes it applicable in the domains that deal with sensitive data. Healthcare is one such domain that mostly deals with sensitive data. The next section, 1.2, discusses FL's effects on the healthcare industry. The central server combines and tests the trained model after obtaining it from the local clients.

1.2 ROLE OF FEDERATED LEARNING IN HEALTHCARE

Technological enhancement in computing devices provides wide accessibility of EHR in the healthcare domain [4]. These records, which contain data, make it possible to extract enormous amounts of knowledge. Extracting knowledge enhances numerous aspects of healthcare by using ML-based data analysis techniques. By using ML techniques to evaluate EHR records, procedures and treatments can be made safer and more effective for patients, improving care quality in the process.

This section discusses the limitations of ML in healthcare and explores the essentials of FL in the healthcare sector.

1.2.1 Limitations of machine learning model in healthcare

In the past several years, the healthcare sector has made substantial use of artificial intelligence (ai) and deep learning technology to analyze digital medical data from EHRs in order to better understand health conditions and the course of diseases.

This facilitates medical research efforts and helps with diagnosis and evaluations. The potential for privacy breaches during data analysis is one of the primary issues with classical AI technologies. In healthcare systems, EHR data is extremely sensitive and private compared to other fields. To protect healthcare settings such as hospitals, insurance agencies require the retrieval of shared healthcare databases for data processing and examination; simply deleting patient information metadata is insufficient.

Machine learning methods commonly applied in the healthcare sector focus on examining EHR data. The specific medical records of each patient, including appointments, diagnoses, treatments, and imaging tests, are included in this data.

The EHRs were facilitated by the usage of information technology in medical institutions. These records serve as a significant source of data for a variety of analytical approaches that aim to extract knowledge to support medical practices. The current study demonstrates how deep learning techniques can derive valuable insights from EHR data, directly enhancing patient outcomes and the standard of care. For ML-based solutions to be implemented, an ML model that has been used to learn structures and bring out pertinent information from original information is necessary. To ensure that the resulting analysis approach is accurate, this training stage is essential. A huge dataset with a range of samples must be employed to guarantee the standard of the ML model. The quality of dataset annotation concerning the expected classification, sample diversity, and quantity of data items all have a direct impact on the training results. Obtaining or creating one of these datasets is frequently an expensive and time-consuming process. Several entities collect the data, deliver it to a main data storage location, and then merge the data to produce a method [5]. Therefore, the data owners may be unaware of these procedures and the ML model's possible future uses. Conventional ML procedures in the healthcare domain may violate laws in their respective domains.

Medical data sharing presents several obstacles and issues that are impeding the growth of powerful ML algorithms in the healthcare domain. Hence, a different ML model, which utilizes FL technology, is needed to analyze medical records. The following Section, 1.2.2, discusses the fundamentals of FL in the healthcare industry.

1.2.2 Importance of federated learning in healthcare

Federated learning (FL) makes it possible to train ML models locally at the local data's location, as explained in Section 1.1.1, and only gives the enquiring party access to the finished, non-reverse-engineerable model [6,7]. As a result, FL eliminates the need to expose sensitive information and private datasets to third parties, to organizations carrying out research, and to facilitate the use of data for more objectives. Every participant in the data collection receives the training algorithm from a central body that oversees the learning process. Each participant feeds the key elements of a local model, used on their private data, to the central entity.

Finally, using an aggregation technique, the central entity creates a single global model from the essential components of all local models. The following Section, 1.2.3, discusses the FL architecture for healthcare applications in detail.

1.2.3 Architecture of federated learning for healthcare applications

Figure 1.4 displays an architecture for federated analysis and learning with EHR data. which this section addresses.

This framework's main goal is to enable medical facilities like hospitals and labs to use private medical datasets for decentralized data analysis and ML research without jeopardizing patient privacy.

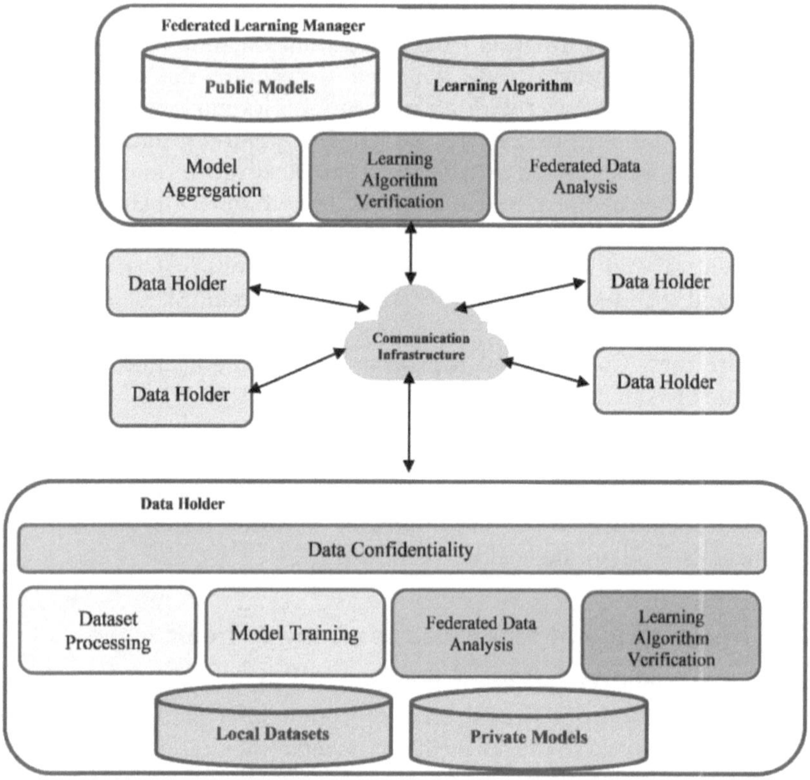

Figure 1.4 FL architecture for healthcare.

Institutions that possess data can maintain datasets that include a variety of medical data, such as prescription drug orders, imaging test results, and diagnostic outcomes. These databases contain sensitive data that is governed by legal and regulatory frameworks. Before their data can be used for potential analysis in studies, individual patients must explicitly consent to its use.

It is expected that data owners are aware that using the FL framework requires collaboration on analyses and model training that protect privacy. The organization can request that other private organizations apply analysis and learning algorithms so they can experiment with medical data. The FL framework may include additional incentive mechanisms, such as financial or regulatory ones.

The main parameters of the FL architecture are:

- **Local model:** The data owners will never willingly share information with outside parties because local datasets contain sensitive information. Additionally, the learning process collaborators may utilize several standards and data formats to save EHR data in every dataset. Data owners use their datasets to train a local model, often using the FL manager to incorporate parameters from models that other data owners have shared. These proprietary models are used for internal data analysis by the data owner or organization; they shouldn't be shared directly with other FL organizations.

- **Data confidentiality:** Sharing data amongst data holders requires protecting the privacy of analysis findings and learning model parameters. An outgoing data confidentiality module verifies that data, including analysis findings and learning models, are free of sensitive information. This module can be used to create different approaches because it is built on a zero-trust security concept. Associating institutions will share research findings and instructional strategies which may contain private information through open networks. High degrees of secrecy should be guaranteed by security measures, especially in cases when the institutions have mutual confidence in exchanging medical data.
- **Dataset processing:** The module for processing datasets includes features that allow external learning algorithms to retrieve and understand the data within local datasets. The data format used by individual private entities may require data type conversion which should be compatible with a specific learning algorithm. Based on private data, this module, which ought to be provided with a template containing the necessary data formats, should determine which conversions are suitable. The use of metadata can offer details about a dataset's properties, allowing automated systems to process the data to be compatible with learning algorithms.
- **Learning algorithm verification:** The block for verifying learning algorithms incorporates methods for examining algorithms obtained from external sources and ensuring that they do not intentionally reveal sensitive information from private datasets. Implementing such verification could involve including a "manifesto" alongside each learning algorithm, detailing the inputs and outputs. The manifesto specification can be used to verify that learning algorithms are following it.
- **Model training:** The training algorithm is executed by the model training module, which utilizes local datasets' data to produce the resulting learning models.
- **Federated data analysis:** The module for federated data analysis prioritizes handling data analysis requests that are private or remote and do not rely on learning algorithms. The analysis of federated data is especially important in medical applications as it allows

for decision-making based on a wider range of knowledge about a specific condition. To make sure that no private information is disclosed, the appropriate modules for security will authenticate externally for federated data analysis. The provision of a certain level of computational power is necessary for data holders to analyze the data and tasks reserved for training and produce the needed partial results. Therefore, a reward system is needed to legitimize this computing power. Data holders may be motivated by the opportunity to utilize the analysis results for their purposes. The benefit mentioned depends on a study delivering pertinent results to all data holders, which might not be achievable. The benefit is contingent on a study delivering the necessary information. Therefore, there is an opportunity for additional advancement of incentive systems for involvement in FL studies, intending to compensate data holders for the expenses associated with knowledge generation.

- **Communication infrastructure:** Even in insecure networking contexts, data holders can safely share learning models and analysis outcomes thanks to the communication infrastructure. This assumption is essential because the data holder won't be in the same administrative domain and will need to communicate online.
- **Federated learning manager:** The communication network links all data custodians to the FL manager, acting as the central component that orchestrates the decentralized learning and analysis procedures. The implementation of the manager often involves a centralized component, such as a cloud instance. Nevertheless, distributed methods deliver the necessary architecture functions.
- **Model aggregation:** To create a single learning model from all public models from private businesses, the manager uses the model aggregation approach. The methods will be decided by the learning methods used by private organizations. The public entity's federated data analysis module focuses on combining data analysis findings from private companies to provide the final analysis result. Additionally, the government agency uses a verification module as part of its learning process. This module can participate in distributed analysis procedures that need agreement from all participants, as well as store and provide manifestos.
- **Public models:** The manager maintains a collection of publicly available models made with the aggregation approach. Depending on the model's objectives, the person who requested the training may receive it. Participants in the learning process can also obtain them for their benchmarking using private data or for training private models. Additionally, the public organization keeps a repository containing all of the system's analysis and learning algorithms.

1.3 USE CASES OF FEDERATED LEARNING IN HEALTHCARE

This section examines FL's varied applications and the state of technology in the healthcare industry.

1.3.1 Federated EHRs management with FL

By using AI to improve healthcare services and protect user privacy with the cooperation of various stakeholders, including patients and healthcare providers, FL can offer more dependable results for analyzing and managing EHR data intelligently [8]. In [9], an analytics management system for EHRs incorporates a collaborative learning protocol grounded in FL, emphasizing privacy and resource efficiency. This system functions through the collaboration of many hospitals and a cloud server. Each hospital uses a cloud computing-based neural network to extract specific EHR information in this configuration.

A straightforward data perturbation technique is being evaluated to change the training data to preserve model parameter privacy during FL.

This method can efficiently protect against model memorization attacks throughout the learning phase. Access to modified EHR data by attackers is possible; however, obtaining or restoring the original information presents significant challenges. In addition, a method based on FL is suggested in [10] for forecasting hospitalizations of patients with heart conditions by analyzing their past EHRs. Locally trained EHR health data uses patient smartphones and hospitals to focus on demographics like age, gender, and physical attributes. After that, the cloud server uses a global Support Vector Machine (SVM) classifier to combine the trained model parameters into a single prediction model. The objective is to forecast upcoming hospital admissions for patients with cardiac conditions to optimize hospital resource management, including the estimation of future treatment requirements, while ensuring the confidentiality of the private dataset. The use of FL in [11] aims to enhance the confidentiality of healthcare data by facilitating the distributed learning of EHR data across various hospital locations. In [12], a solution utilizing differential privacy is implemented. Local hospitals conceal local changes before sending them to the server by producing artificial noise to protect critical data.

Multilayer perceptron, SVM, and logistic regression are models used. FL utilizes these models, and the results demonstrate that differential privacy-based FL methods achieve a competitive level of accuracy compared to conventional FL approaches.

In [13], researchers examine a novel FL-based approach known as Split Neural Network (SplitNN), which involves implementing the standard FL setup linked to split learning. A deep neural network is partitioned into many segments, with every segment training done by a separate client in split learning.

The learnt data could be spread among several clients or only at one; however, none of the clients are permitted to access the data of other clients. The model is segmented into many parts, which are subsequently distributed to various clients for network training by transferring the weights of the divided layer, eliminating the necessity for sharing raw data.

In [13], to ensure that user information is kept private, A portion of the deep network is trained by each radiology client centre, and its neural parameters are sent to a central server for model aggregation.

A statistical channel-based FL algorithm is being studied by researchers to improve the training performance of EHRs in smart healthcare, as detailed in [14]. This method entails the random uploading of a limited subset of local gradients from participating hospitals to the server, emphasizing channels exhibiting the greatest variation. The model aggregation process exclusively employs neural channels exhibiting significant changes during the training loop, excluding those with minimal alterations and reduced feature representation.

A binary classification problem is established in the FL simulation to predict mortality utilizing neural networks. It performs better than conventional FL schemes in terms of training convergence rates. Furthermore, patient clustering is employed to enhance federated mortality prediction [15]. Finding patient subgroups with analogous diagnoses and geographical locations is necessary for training a neural network model to predict death based on medication variables.

A separate study focuses on reducing complexity in FL environments to predict mortality from EHRs. This is accomplished through the application of LoAdaBoost, an adaptive boosting method, to elevate the efficacy of FL in contexts involving both Independent and Identically Distributed Data (IID) and non-IID data distributions. The work [16] examines training in EHR in the context of healthcare in Florida. The study employs Recurrent Neural Networks (RNNs) to forecast preterm birth three months prior, leveraging structured datasets and uncertainty training methodologies.

Hospitals and data centres utilize blockchain technology to manage an immutable data ledger, thereby ensuring secure model communication [16]. Since the blockchain records the transmission logs and model modifications, any entities may view the FL process transparently.

1.3.2 FL for federated remote health monitoring

There has been a growing requirement for innovative strategies to transition remote healthcare administration from hospitals to home settings.

A global model can be developed utilizing distributed household data with the oversight of a server, such as a cloud server, facilitating in-home health monitoring via FL to ensure mitigation of data leakage for the local user's data [17].

The Internet of Medical Things (IoMT) device in each home, like a user's mobile phone, can utilize Convolutional Neural Networks (CNNs) to develop a personalized model. This is achieved by merging its data with a well-balanced dataset and adjusting the model gradients, which results in simultaneous updates across all homes and the cloud. The imbalanced and non-IID data issues are effectively addressed, leading to improved personalized predictions. In [18], a proposal is presented for a system designed to monitor wearable health, where smartphones work together with a cloud server to build a shared CNN model to recognize human activity, all while emphasizing the importance of privacy protection.

The use of transfer learning aims to address the discrepancy in model distribution between cloud and smartphone models and customize the training model, thereby facilitating personalization. The findings from the implementation indicate that the FL algorithm demonstrates superior accuracy, with a 5.3% enhancement in recognizing wearable activities when juxtaposed with conventional techniques.

Applications in healthcare and medicine, including disease diagnosis, fall prediction, and health monitoring, could greatly benefit from the FL scheme's extension. To keep tabs on obesity and its associated health problems, another healthcare monitoring system was created in [19] that makes use of FL. Federated natural language processing is one way to reduce data sharing in collaborative training settings by using clinical notes from many hospitals or clinics. Each facility builds a model of the patient, which is used to train a neural network to predict the procedural terminology code of the day based on the language used in the notes.

A phenotyping ML is created to train collaboratively in several places to categorize diseases into three groups: dubious, absence, and presence. In addition, [20] discusses a mobile activity monitoring method using FL to assist healthcare applications like assisted living and fall detection. The dataset used for federated NN training involves real-world human activity recognition and is spread across mobile devices. Activities like sitting, walking, standing and climbing stairs are included.

To evaluate the efficacy of medicines on patients in a dispersed healthcare system, the study detailed in [21] entails creating an FL-based health monitoring system. It is worth mentioning that every hospital has its own customized therapy effect estimator. The coordinating site's total treatment effect is ascertained through the use of a site indicator, and individual treatment effects are based on patient characteristics. These estimators can be further sub-grouped according to these criteria.

1.3.3 FL for federated medical imaging

Implementing AI-based medical data imaging, which combines data from multiple medical institutions into a single, centralized entity, is challenging because of privacy concerns. FL has demonstrated potential in facilitating extensive medical imaging applications due to its ability to facilitate learning from several source datasets without requiring the public release of data.

In [22], with the aid of a global classifier housed in the cloud, the FL method has been proposed, focussing on the resolution of disparities across clients (such as hospitals) by using a federated process to turn all clients' images into a shared image space. The above allows for the creation of a dataset of diffusion-coefficient images from multiple sources to aid in automated classification. Each company uses a Generative Adversarial Network (GAN) to create fake image datasets and change its original images into the desired image domain. This successfully addresses privacy concerns that come up with different clients.

Additionally, a suggestion for an FL model for federated brain imaging using deep neural networks (DNNs) to aid with brain cancer segmentation has been made in [23]. In this instance, a set local dataset and sufficient processing capacity are available to each shared client, such as a Magnetic Resonance Imaging (MRI) scanner, to train the DNN structure. After that, they share the weight modifications with the federated server using a model averaging technique so that they may be totalled. Even though FL can keep user data safe, it can still be hacked in ways like reconstructing training samples on the server.

Next, a technique called "differential privacy" is used to change the updates, add noise to the training process of each node, and limit the amount of data that is shared during the model exchange. In [24], an additional federated brain imaging strategy is suggested that uses MRI scans that are spread out among several colleges and medical centres. In this case, medical sites and the central server work together to make an FL model that acts like a complete system for standardizing data, fixing confusing factors, and checking the range of high-dimensional parameters that can change. The MRI datasets utilized in this investigation included 455 healthy controls, 181 people with Moderate Cognitive Impairment (MCI) that does not worsen over time, 208 people with continuous MCI, 234 people with Alzheimer's disease, and 232 people with Parkinson's disease. Covariates like age and sex were also examined in this work.

To cut down on training latency in a federated setting, an Alternating Direction Method of Multipliers (ADMM) -based method for iteration reduction is also used. Federated multi-institutional teamwork for brain tissue-based MRI analytics is an analogous method that the authors of [25] take into consideration. Approximately ten medical facilities are working together, and each one uses a neural network model to look at each brain scan picture and find areas that look like they might be having problems. A FL-based methodology is provided in [26] to help identify acute neurological symptoms, such as severe headaches or loss of consciousness, to facilitate X-ray imaging in smart healthcare.

Each organization uses the X-ray image dataset from the Radiological Society of North America to train a CNN-based DenseNet1212 model. This model can promote feature reuse, allow features to proliferate, and reduce the number of neural parameters required. Differential privacy can be improved for FL-based medical imaging with the help of a Dopamine method [27]. Patients only have faith in the hospital that is closest to them, and hospitals should not collaborate. On the other hand, servers may be truthful and inquisitive. Hospitals need to make sure that patients have the right privacy settings for each local update round to satisfy this situation. This will let the server build the world model it needs with a high level of accuracy and little data loss. To ensure that every update has the same impact on the local momentum as it does on the overall model, each hospital modifies the privacy loss calculation by adding Gaussian noise. This is done to strike a compromise between the expense of privacy and the accuracy loss.

The simulations utilize a CNN-based SqueezeNet model [28], demonstrating a classification accuracy enhancement for the real-time medical dataset. A technique for multi-institutional cooperation on MRI reconstruction is proposed in [29]. The target site's latent characteristic distribution matches the intermediate latent features that were learnt from several hospitals. An adversarial domain identifier facilitates aligning the latent space distribution in the target domain and cooperatively training local reconstruction networks at several local sites.

An adversarial domain identifier facilitates not only the cooperative training of local reconstruction networks at many local locations but also the alignment of the latent space distribution in the target domain. Each hospital silo's photo patches are utilized to integrate a CNN into a low-dimensional feature representation using autonomously segmented tissue areas. level labels as data features to train a weakly supervised learning model on its large slide picture dataset. Subsequently, the gradients are generated and submitted to the server for averaging.

Consequently, the hospital uses its large dataset of slide pictures to train a weakly supervised learning model, incorporating slide-level and patient-level labels as data features. After that, the created gradients are sent to the server so that they can be averaged. A different study in [30] suggests a FL approach for the analysis of functional magnetic resonance imaging (fMRI), in which the weight-sharing procedure is coordinated by a decentralized iterative optimization algorithm that is constructed with a randomization technique. A domain adaptation approach is developed using labelled, unlabelled, or semi-labelled image or text datasets for cross-silo learning. Furthermore, [31] illustrates the breast density classification problem solved by FL, indicating that the FL approach can exceed the performance of independent training methods by an average of 6.3%.

1.3.4 FL for diagnosis of schizophrenia

One of the most inescapable conditions nowadays is mental health, which affects people from childhood through adolescence and maturity. Maintaining our physical and mental health is essential since it influences our daily activities, including our thoughts, feelings, and behaviours.

This encompasses social, psychological, and emotional health. The way people live, eat, work, learn, and interact with others has drastically changed as a result of technological improvements. People are now less able to manage stress, emotions, and thoughts as a result, which might lead to mental illnesses. One such severe mental illness that impairs cognitive processing and is challenging to detect is schizophrenia [32]. Psychosis, severe impairment in one's ability to comprehend the world, and behavioural changes are hallmarks of schizophrenia. About 24 million people worldwide suffer from schizophrenia, and those affected are often in their late teens and early twenties. In India, the lifetime prevalence of schizophrenia spectrum disorder was 1.41%, and the present prevalence is 0.41%. There are three categories of symptoms for schizophrenia. The negative symptoms, the cognitive symptoms, and the positive or psychotic symptoms.

The psychotic symptoms are characterized by:

- Hallucination: possessing an incorrect impression of a person, thing, or occasion. detecting an untrue sensation. It involves the senses of taste, touch, smell, sound, and sight. They constantly hear strange voices and noises.
- Delusion: despite evidence to the contrary, they maintain a false belief in everything. There are several types of delusions that they may have, including paranoia, control, reference, and grandiose.
- Disorganized speech: they have trouble expressing their true opinions. People have difficulty understanding.
- Abnormal movement: like dressing unsuitably for the occasion.

The negative symptoms are characterized by:

- Blunted effect: shows less emotions

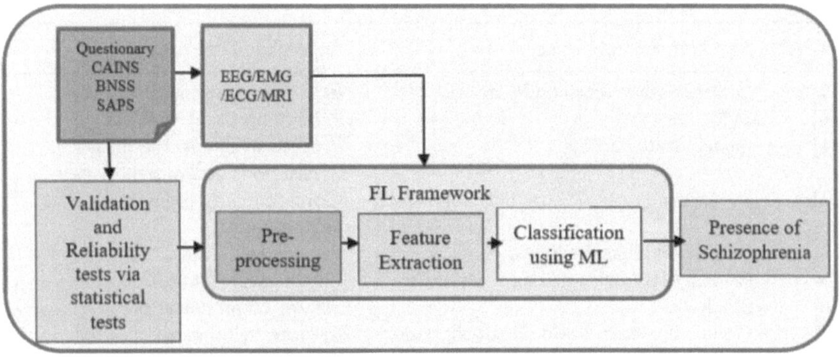

Figure 1.5 FL framework for diagnosis of schizophrenia.

- Alogia: lack of content or speech
- Anhedonia: loss of pleasure
- Asociality: fewer social interactions
- Avolition: having less motivation

The cognitive symptoms that affect day-to-day functioning are characterized by:

- Low attention
- Poor decision making
- Lack of problem-solving abilities

According to international common diseases, questionaries [37] are framed and evaluated based on the symptoms. The scale used to evaluate the responses in this case goes from 1 (minimum) to 5 (maximum). When a score is higher than moderate, it is deemed symptomatic and warrants additional research. Actigraphs and headsets are used to collect EEG data to analyze brain signals and cognitive processes. Before being fed into a neural network, these signals undergo pre-processing and normalization. Through a decentralized network connected by a number of devices, a FL framework is developed. This makes it possible to share models over the cloud and train them using local data from devices. This keeps the patient's private information private and stops it from being shared. ML algorithms [38] are used to identify the features and patterns. Concerning the presence of schizophrenia, the model performance is evaluated and classified. The FL framework for diagnosis of schizophrenia is illustrated as shown in Figure 1.5.

Table 1.1 summarizes the use cases discussed in this section.

Table 1.1 Use cases of FL in healthcare

Ref. No	*Algorithm/Framework used*	*Application/Use case*
[9]	Collaborative Learning Protocol	EHR management
[10]	SVM	Prediction using HER
[11]	Distributed learning	Prediction of adverse drug reactions and mortality rate
[12]	SVM, Perceptron & Logistics Regression	Confidentiality of HER
[13]	SplitNN	Segmentation
[14]	Stochastic Channel-Based FL	Smart healthcare
[15]	Neural Network-LoAdaBoost, RNN	Mortality prediction
[16]	Blockchain	Secure communication
[17]	Generative convolutional autoencoder	Remote healthcare
[18]	CNN	Personalized healthcare
[19]	Transfer Learning	Personalized healthcare
[20]	Phenotyping ML	Healthcare monitoring
[21]	DNN	Healthcare monitoring
[22]	GAN	Medical imaging
[23]	DNN	Brain tumour segmentation
[24]	FL framework	Multi disease prediction
[25]	ADMM	Hemorrhage detection
[26]	CNN	X-ray imaging
[27]	FL framework	Privacy in medical imaging
[28]	Deep Bayes-SqueezeNet	Classification of medical images
[29]	CNN	MRI reconstruction
[30]	Cross-silo learning	MRI reconstruction
[31]	Transfer learning	Breast density classification
[32]	FL framework	Diagnosis of schizophrenia
[33]	Distributed networking, MQTT protocol	Brain tumour segmentation

1.3.5 Decentralized federated learning for healthcare networks

Artificial intelligence (AI) is utilized in smart healthcare to analyze and learn from patient data. Conventional centralized artificial intelligence necessitates moving medical institutions' privacy-sensitive data to data centres that handle the combined information. ML models need huge and different datasets for training which is lacking in individual medical centres.

Training in data centres requires increased energy and communication resources, which may compromise privacy. A Message Queuing Telemetry Transport (MQTT) protocol (MQTT)-based real-time decentralized systems are analyzed using various FL techniques [38] in [33]. The network-based ML solutions using FL tools depend on a parameter server and distributed patterns managed by consensus are developed.

The segmentation of brain tumours is evaluated using datasets received from routine clinical workflows using an updated version of the U-NET algorithm [39].

The FL procedure is carried out on several geographically dispersed computers connected by the Internet and situated in several nations. An MQTT protocol-based distinctive network and fully distributed FL algorithms [40] are used to cooperate with the interchanging deep ML model parameters. The discussion encompasses the real-time learning process for each epoch, and recommendations for an optimal data set is incorporated into the MQTT payload, with a considered reduction in the model parameter, serialization and Quality of Service (QoS).

Classification Task:

(i) One of the most important responsibilities in medical diagnosis is tumour segmentation, which not only helps physicians and radiologists but also shortens the time they have to consider possible therapies.
(ii) Brain tumour segmentation aims to find regions of interest that capture the shape and breadth of the tumour from a sequence of MRI slices.
(iii) This is achieved by giving each pixel in the images a class label that indicates the presence, absence, and/or shape of the tumour.
(iv) To ensure appropriate segmentation labels in this context, the unique medical equipment used requires the definition of complicated processing algorithms that can handle MRI images with varying spatial resolutions, modalities, and noise levels.
    - U-NET model: The U-Net architecture consists of two primary components: the decoder, is responsible for identifying the segmentation region, and contextual information of images is extracted using an encoder. An input image is transformed into the compressed domain using different layers of the CNN model. The final segmentation from the input image is extracted using a decoder through up-sampling and concatenation operations. The structure is identical to that of the encoder.
    - MQTT protocol: The proposed system employs MQTT-compliant publish and subscribe mechanisms for sharing model elements of U-NET.
    - Aggregation and optimization: The aggregate and local model optimizations of FL process are executed using synchronous and asynchronous policies.
    - Synchronous policy: All system nodes—clients and Parameter Server (PS), if relevant—utilize a common time reference during the training process with synchronous orchestration.

As a result, the model aggregation needs to hold off until every client on the timetable has finished local model optimization. It should be noted that in fully decentralized training, the PS and client aggregation stages can be utilized in their original form.

- **Asynchronous policy:** The local models are consolidated by the clients, or PS, in the asynchronous orchestration, irrespective of their temporal proximity. Similar to this, in the asynchronous CFA algorithm implementation, a medical centre that completes its local model optimization moves straight on to the accumulation level which is independent of the completion of neighbour local model optimization.
- **Synchronous and asynchronous FL architecture:** While developing network architecture for naïve FL supported by the internet, the main challenges must be resolved. First, slower clients may be penalized for their speed (straggler effect) and require more time to train due to their retention of huge datasets (many MRI images) or inadequate computational capabilities. Second, in the event that the PS or the clients employ global model updates, they should prevent potential deadlock scenarios brought on by packet losses, i.e., low-quality links and clients that receive their model updates later than their neighbours.

Four different architectures are implemented as shown in Figure 1.6 to overcome these issues.

(i) **PS-Synchronous, Client-Synchronous**
The design shown in Figure 1.6 is in line with the suggested vanilla FL implementation. All components of the network maintain a unified temporal framework supported by the MQTT broker, during the training process [40], the PS and the clients work synchronously (S) with FL. The PS waits until each client has completed their model optimization procedures while keeping an eye on the PS weights topic on the MQTT broker. Upon the release of each client's weight, the PS is activated, and the aggregation [41] phase commences. The clients are released, and the PS reverts to a waiting state following the publication of the global model update.

(ii) **PS-Synchronous, Client-Asynchronous**
The PS follows the synchronous behaviour as observed in the above-discussed architecture PS-S/C-S. In contrast, clients do asynchronous actions: after finishing their model optimization phase, they could continue to train using local data before the PS global model is changed. In this case, they replace the local weights with the most recent global model and halt the local model optimization process.

(iii) **PS-Asynchronous, Client-Asynchronous**
Here, the clients and the PS are both asynchronous. Even though not all clients have completed their model optimization processes, the PS updates the global model every transaction per second by collecting local model weights from the MQTT broker.

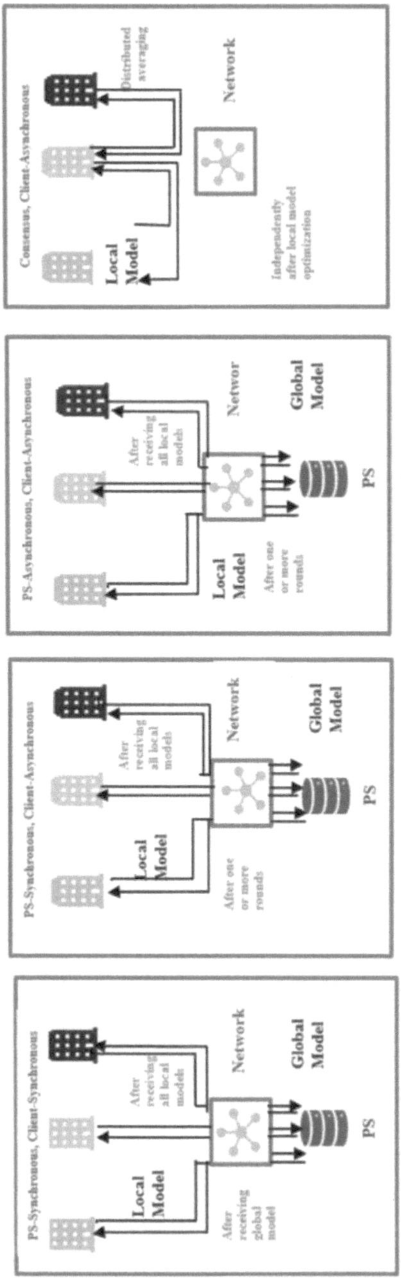

Figure 1.6 Decentralized architecture of FL.

(iv) Consensus-Driven (No PS), Client-Asynchronous
The architecture facilitates local model exchange among clients and underpins Consensus-based FL (CFL). Every client is asynchronous, and this is completely decentralized. Through direct communication of neighbourhood-specific subjects via the MQTT, the clients upload and download the most recent local model weight values.

MQTT brokers facilitate communication between networked multi nodes by acting as a channel, which may be distributed across various nations and structured according to a specified connection matrix. After completing a round, a client downloads its neighbours' weights, changes the local model using a predetermined procedure, and then posts the revised local model on its weight's topic.

1.4 CHALLENGES IN IMPLEMENTING FEDERATED LEARNING WITHIN THE HEALTHCARE SECTOR

FL is an ongoing process in which a model is continuously updated. For this reason, as things progressed, new issues and challenges emerged. The problems are available to the researchers for quick and effective resolution. Since the entire process takes place online, security and privacy are always top priorities in this industry, particularly when it comes to reliable healthcare solutions. The key challenges of FL in healthcare technologies are discussed in this section [34].

Challenges in privacy: In FL, the uploaded, locally trained model may be able to link the data back to the source, which may still be a privacy risk. The gradients, for instance, can be used to deduce the information needed to compute the gradients [35].

Personalization techniques: The intention in FL is to train models utilizing a central repository while preserving the integrity of the data sample. In order to allow users to train their models over a greater number of data samples, personalization needs to allow users to access a richer model in addition to modifying a global model for every single client. The major challenges during personalization are (i) heterogeneity of devices during computing, storage, and interaction abilities; (ii) diversification of data due to non-IID; (iii) model heterogeneity for various models in customized contexts

Communication issues: Communication is crucial to FL-enabled healthcare services because it serves as a channel between FL users and the aggregation server. Effective interaction and strategies of resource allotment significantly enhance student learning.

IoMT devices need to connect to the aggregation server more and more as the number of devices increases in order to broadcast downlink models and update uplink models. Under these circumstances, the aggregation server can select a suitable group of IoMT devices by using effective scheduling policies.

The quick and dynamic alterations in wireless links give a considerable challenge for communication. This affects the updates' quality between the aggregation server and IoMT units. Examining the effects of user dropout in addition to more reliable design objectives like outage likelihood and device availability could be one way to find a solution.

Quality of training data: Because different hospital sites have varied computational capacities and data characteristics, the training quality can be significantly reduced [36]. In this case, it is logical to implement incentive programs to motivate medical institutions to provide accurate updates to the aggregate server and make use of high-quality training data. The incentive systems are developed by using game theory and blockchain. Training requirements, including modifications to data types, learning rates, and the classification of training purposes as either classification or regression, should be established flexibly to allow FL entities, such as patients, doctors, and nurses, to easily and appropriately adjust their activities. The development of adaptive FL techniques is essential, as these changes can influence the FL design and the foundational learning models utilized by both FL users and the aggregation server.

Robustness of dataset: The distinctive datasets such as images, text, time series and audio, in addition to that different data types like heart rate, blood group and body temperature are used by different clients. Additionally, new diversified FL techniques must be evolved, enabling the central server to handle this diversity via private ensemble learning, even when collaborating parties utilize distinct models.

The study [37] presents an inference technique enabling users to manage a collection of heterogeneous models without the necessity of consolidating the data in a single location.

Security issues in FL-based smart healthcare: There exist several client-side actors who could assume the role of attackers and attempt to disrupt the model aggregation process by providing harmful or false model updates in FL-based smart healthcare systems. Serious privacy concerns, such as data leaking, would arise if an outside party were to conduct server-side attacks to get data regarding the aggregated global model. Also, while the model is being relayed from local clients to the central server, an attacker could taint feature information or change local updates during local data training.

1.5 CONCLUSION

Federated learning, a collaborative AI technique in development, has attracted great awareness because of its promise to give smart healthcare networks and applications that are scalable and enhance privacy. This chapter examines the essential principles of FL and explores the rationale behind its application in the healthcare sector. A framework for healthcare applications is discussed in a concise manner. This chapter presents recent advancements in FL across various healthcare applications. This chapter also provides a synopsis of future developments and draws attention to several interesting problems in FL-smart healthcare.

REFERENCES

[1] Priyanka Mary Mammen, "Federated Learning: Opportunities and Challenges," *arXiv preprint arXiv:2101.05428,* 2021.

[2] H. Ludwig and N. Baracaldo, Introduction to Federated Learning. In: Ludwig, H., Baracaldo, N. (eds) *Federated Learning.* Springer, Cham, 2022, https://doi.org/10.1007/978-3-030-96896-0_1.

[3] Ticao Zhang and Shiwen Mao, "An Introduction to the Federated Learning Standard," in *GetMobile: Mobile Computing and Communications,* vol. 25, no. 3, pp. 18–22, 2022, https://doi.org/10.1145/3511285.35112.

[4] Rodolfo Stoffel Antunes, Cristiano André da Costa, Arne Küderle, Imrana Abdullahi Yari and Björn Eskofier, "Federated Learning for Healthcare: Systematic Review and Architecture Proposal," in *ACM Transactions on Intelligent Systems and Technology (TIST),* vol. 13, no. 4, pp. 1–23, 2022, https://doi.org/10.1145/3501813.

[5] Neeta Rana and Hitesh Marwaha, "Role of Federated Learning in Healthcare Systems: A Survey," in *Mathematical Foundations of Computing*, vol. 7, no. 4, pp. 459–484, 2024, doi: 10.3934/mfc.2023023.

[6] Dinh C. Nguyen, Quoc-Viet Pham, Pubudu N. Pathirana, Ming Ding, Aruna Seneviratne, Zihuai Lin, Octavia Dobre and Won-Joo Hwang, "Federated Learning for Smart Healthcare: A Survey," in *ACM Computing Surveys (Csur),* vol. 55, no. 3, pp. 1–37, 2022, https://doi.org/10.1145/3501296.

[7] Jie Xu, Benjamin S. Glicksberg, Chang Su, Peter Walker, Jiang Bian, and Fei Wang, "Federated Learning for Healthcare Informatics," in *Journal of Healthcare Informatics Research,* vol. 5, pp. 1–19, 2021, https://doi.org/10.1007/s41666-020-00082-4.

[8] M. Ali, F. Naeem, M. Tariq and G. Kaddoum, "Federated Learning for Privacy Preservation in Smart Healthcare Systems: A Comprehensive Survey," in *IEEE Journal of Biomedical and Health Informatics*, vol. 27, no. 2, pp. 778–789, Feb. 2023, doi: 10.1109/JBHI.2022.3181823.

[9] M. Hao, H. Li, G. Xu, Z. Liu and Z. Chen, "Privacy-aware and Resource-saving Collaborative Learning for Healthcare in Cloud Computing," *ICC 2020 – 2020 IEEE International Conference on Communications (ICC)*, Dublin, Ireland, 2020, pp. 1–6, doi: 10.1109/ICC40277.2020.9148979.

[10] Theodora S. Brisimi, Ruidi Chen, Theofanie Mela, Alex Olshevsky, Ioannis Ch. Paschalidis and Wei Shi, "Federated Learning of Predictive Models from Federated Electronic Health Records," *International Journal of Medical Informatics*, vol. 112, no. 1, pp. 59–67, 2018, https://doi.org/10.1016/j.ijmedinf.2018.01.007.

[11] Olivia Choudhury, Aris Gkoulalas-Divanis, Theodoros Salonidis, Issa Sylla, Yoonyoung Park, Grace Hsu and Amar Das, "Differential Privacy-enabled Federated Learning for Sensitive Health Data," arXiv:1910.02578, 2020, https://doi.org/10.48550/arXiv.1910.02578.

[12] Dianbo Liu, Timothy Miller, Raheel Sayeed and Kenneth D. Mandl, "FADL: Federated-autonomous Deep Learning for Distributed Electronic Health Record," arXiv:1811.11400, 2018, https://doi.org/10.48550/arXiv.1811.11400.

[13] Praneeth Vepakomma, Otkrist Gupta, Tristan Swedish and Ramesh Raskar, "Split Learning for Health: Distributed Deep Learning without Sharing Raw Patient Data," arXiv:1812.00564, 2018, https://doi.org/10.48550/arXiv.1812.00564.

[14] Rulin Shao, Hongyu He, Hui Liu and Dianbo Liu, "1Stochastic Channel-based Federated Learning for Medical Data Privacy-preserving," arXiv:1910.11160, 2019, https://doi.org/10.48550/arXiv.1910.11160.

[15] Li Huang, Andrew L. Shea, Huining Qian, Aditya Masurkar, Hao Deng and Dianbo Liu, "Patient Clustering Improves Efficiency of Federated Machine Learning to Predict Mortality and Hospital Stay Time Using Distributed Electronic Medical Records," in *Journal of Biomedical Informatics*, vol. 99, no. 1, p. 103291, 2019, https://doi.org/10.1016/j.jbi.2019.103291.

[16] D. C. Nguyen, P. N. Pathirana, M. Ding and A. Seneviratne, "Blockchain and Edge Computing for Decentralized EMRs Sharing in Federated Healthcare," *GLOBECOM 2020–2020 IEEE Global Communications Conference*, Taipei, Taiwan, 2020, pp. 1–6, doi: 10.1109/GLOBECOM42002.2020.9347951.

[17] Q. Wu, X. Chen, Z. Zhou and J. Zhang, "FedHome: Cloud-Edge Based Personalized Federated Learning for In-Home Health Monitoring," in *IEEE Transactions on Mobile Computing*, vol. 21, no. 8, pp. 2818–2832, 1 Aug. 2022, doi: 10.1109/TMC.2020.3045266.

[18] Y. Chen, X. Qin, J. Wang, C. Yu and W. Gao, "FedHealth: A Federated Transfer Learning Framework for Wearable Healthcare," in *IEEE Intelligent Systems*, vol. 35, no. 4, pp. 83–93, 1 July-Aug. 2020, doi: 10.1109/MIS.2020.2988604.

[19] Dianbo Liu, Dmitriy Dligach and Timothy Miller, "Two-stage Federated Phenotyping and Patient Representation Learning," in *Proceedings of the Association for Computational Linguistics*, vol. 2019, p. 283, 2019, doi: 10.18653/v1/W19-5030.

[20] Gautham Krishna Gudur and Satheesh K. Perepu, "Federated Learning with Heterogeneous Labels and Models for Mobile Activity Monitoring," arXiv e-prints 2020, https://doi.org/10.48550/arXiv.2012.02539.

[21] Gavini Sreelatha, C. Kishor Kumar Reddy, Marlia Mohd Hanafiah, R. MadanaMohana, "Hybrid Electro search beetle optimization based task scheduling and game theory SOA based resource allocation in multi cloud computing", in *Wiley Journal of Software: Practice and Experience*, Sept. 2024, https://doi.org/10.1002/spe.3370.

[22] Kishor Kumar Reddy, Advaitha Daduvy, R Madana Mohana, Basem Assiri, Mohammed Shauib, Sadaf Alam and Abdullah Sheneamer, "Enhancing Precision Agriculture and Land Cover Classification: A Self –Attention 3D Convolutional Neural Network Approach for Hyperspectral Image Analysis," in *IEEE Access*, 2024, doi: 10.1109/ACCESS.2024.3420089

[23] Kishor Kumar Reddy, Palakurthi Anaghaa Reddy, Himaja Janapati, Basem Assiri, Mohammed Shauib, Sadaf Alam and Abdullah Sheneamer,

"A Fine Tuned Vision Transformer (FTVT) based Enhanced Multi-Class Brain Tumor Classification using MRI Scan Imagery", in *Frontiers in Oncology Cancer Imaging and Image-directed Interventions*, August 2024, DOI: 10.3389/fonc.2024.1400341

[24] Kishor Kumar Reddy C, Aarti Rangarajan, Deepti Rangarajan, Mohammed Shuaib, Fathe Jeribi and Shadab Alam, "A Transfer Learning Approach: Early Prediction of Alzheimer's Disease on US Healthy Aging Dataset", in *MDPI Mathematics*, July 2024. https://doi.org/10.3390/math12142204

[25] Kishor Kumar Reddy C, Ritika Badam, Shauib Ahmed, "IoT Driven Accessibility:A Refreshable OCR-Braille Solution for Visually Impaired and Deaf-Blind Users through WSN", in *JETECH Elsevier*, April 2024, doi: 10.1016/j.ject.2024.04.007

[26] Xiaohang Xu, Hao Peng, Lichao Sun, Md Zakirul Alam Bhuiyan, Lianzhong Liu and Lifang He, "Fedmood: Federated learning on mobile health data for mood detection," *arXiv preprint arXiv:2102.09342,* 2021, https://doi.org/10.48550/arXiv.2012.02539.

[27] Zengqiang Yan, Jeffry Wicaksana, Zhiwei Wang, Xin Yang and Kwang-Ting Cheng, "Variation-Aware Federated Learning with Multi-Source Decentralized Medical Image Data," in *IEEE Journal of Biomedical and Health Informatics,* vol. 25, no. 7, pp. 2615–2628, 2021, doi:10.1109/JBHI.2020.3040015.

[28] W. Li, *et al.*, Privacy-Preserving Federated Brain Tumour Segmentation. In: Suk, HI., Liu, M., Yan, P., Lian, C. (eds) *Machine Learning in Medical Imaging. MLMI 2019. Lecture Notes in Computer Science*, vol 11861. Springer, Cham, 2019, https://doi.org/10.1007/978-3-030-32692-0_16.

[29] S. Silva, B. A. Gutman, E. Romero, P. M. Thompson, A. Altmann and M. Lorenzi, "Federated Learning in Distributed Medical Databases: Meta-Analysis of Large-Scale Subcortical Brain Data," in *2019 IEEE 16th International Symposium on Biomedical Imaging (ISBI 2019)*, Venice, Italy, 2019, pp. 270–274, doi: 10.1109/ISBI.2019.8759317.

[30] M. J. Sheller, B. Edwards, G. A. Reina, et al., "Federated Learning in Medicine: Facilitating Multi-institutional Collaborations without Sharing Patient Data," in *Scientific Report,* vol. 10, p. 12598, 2020, https://doi.org/10.1038/s41598-020-69250-1.

[31] Utkarsh Chandra Srivastava, Dhruv Upadhyay and Vinayak Sharma, "Intracranial Hemorrhage Detection Using Neural Network Based Methods With Federated Learning," arXiv:2005.08644, 2020, https://doi.org/10.48550/arXiv.2005.08644.

[32] Mohammad Malekzadeh, Burak Hasircioglu, Nitish Mital, Kunal Katarya, Mehmet Emre Ozfatura and Deniz Gündüz, "Dopamine: Differentially Private Federated Learning on Medical Data," arXiv–2101, 2021, https://doi.org/10.48550/arXiv.2012.02539.

[33] Ferhat Ucar and Deniz Korkmaz, "COVIDiagnosis-Net: Deep Bayes-SqueezeNet Based Diagnosis of the Coroavirus Disease 2019 (COVID-19) from X-ray Images," in *Medical Hypotheses,* vol. 140, p. 109761, 2020, https://doi.org/10.1016/j.mehy.2020.109761.

[34] D. C. Nguyen, M. Ding, P. N. Pathirana and A. Seneviratne, "Blockchain and AI-Based Solutions to Combat Coronavirus (COVID-19)-Like Epidemics: A Survey," in *IEEE Access*, vol. 9, pp. 95730–95753, 2021, doi: 10.1109/ACCESS.2021.3093633.

[35] Xiaoxiao Li, Yufeng Gu, Nicha Dvornek, Lawrence H. Staib, Pamela Ventola and James S. Duncan, "Multi-site fMRI Analysis Using Privacy-preserving Federated Learning and Domain Adaptation: ABIDE Results," in *Medical Image Analysis*, vol. 65, p. 101765, 2020, https://doi.org/10.1016/j.media.2020.101765.

[36] Holger R. Roth, Ken Chang, Praveer Singh, Nir Neumark, Wenqi Li, Vikash Gupta, Sharut Gupta, Liangqiong Qu, Alvin Ihsani and Bernardo C. Bizzo, "Federated learning for breast density classification: A real-world implementation," In *Proceedings of the Domain Adaptation and Representation Transfer, and Distributed and Collaborative Learning*. Springer, 181–191, 2020, https://doi.org/10.1007/978-3-030-60548-3_18.

[37] Mustafa Abdul Salam, Elsayed Badr, Eman Monier and Alwan Mohamed, "Schizophrenia diagnosis using optimized federated learning models," in *IJCSNS*, vol. 829, 2022, https://doi.org/10.22937/IJCSNS.2022.22.4.100.

[38] Jie Xu, Benjamin S. Glicksberg, Chang Su, Peter Walker, Jiang Bian and Fei Wang, "Federated Learning for Healthcare Informatics," in *Journal of Healthcare Informatics Research*, vol. 5, pp. 1–19, 2021, https://doi.org/10.1007/s41666-020-00082-4.

[39] K. M. J. Rahman et al., "Challenges, Applications and Design Aspects of Federated Learning: A Survey," in *IEEE Access*, vol. 9, pp. 124682–124700, 2021, doi: 10.1109/ACCESS.2021.3111118.

[40] V. A. Patel *et al.*, "Adoption of Federated Learning for Healthcare Informatics: Emerging Applications and Future Directions," in *IEEE Access*, vol. 10, pp. 90792–90826, 2022, doi: 10.1109/ACCESS.2022.3201876.

[41] Christopher A. Choquette-Choo, Natalie Dullerud, Adam Dziedzic, Yunxiang Zhang, Somesh Jha, Nicolas Papernot and Xiao Wang, "CaPC Learning: Confidential and Private Collaborative Learning," arXiv:2102.05188, 2021, https://doi.org/10.48550/arXiv.2102.05188.

Chapter 2

Evolving neural disorders in the era of healthcare 6.0

Classifications, types, and societal impact

Mayank Mishra, Sushama Singh, Sarasa Meenakshi, Ved Prakash, Nitesh Kumar, Nikhilesh Anand, and Krishna Murti

2.1 INTRODUCTION

2.1.1 Understanding neural disorders

Human illnesses are conditions that impair the normal function of specific body parts. A wide range of human problems are classified as cardiac, inheritable disease, psychological, brain, epidermis, trauma, tissue infections, and gastrointestinal problems [1]. Neurological disorders (NDs) particularly affect the brain and can disrupt functions like movement, communication, learning, and cognition. Since the brain governs nerve functions any damage or injury to the brain or nerves can be fatal and disastrous [2].

2.1.2 Prevalence

Although mortality rates from neurological diseases have decreased as medical knowledge and technology have advanced, these conditions continue to cause significant morbidity and misery. In 2016, neurological disorders accounted for 10.2% of worldwide cases, leading to 9 million deaths and 276 million years lived with disability. Early detection of these disorders could alleviate the long-term impacts of chronic and debilitating conditions [3]. The "Global Burden of Disease" study estimated that there are more than 80 million survivors of stroke worldwide, along with 43.8 million individuals affected by dementia, 45.9 million living with epilepsy, and 6.1 million diagnosed with Parkinson's disease [4–6]. These are precarious, chronic, and fatal diseases. Thus, early diagnosis is essential for better treatment outcomes [7].

2.1.3 Advances in healthcare 6.0 technology

Historically, various techniques like decision trees, random forests, and neural networks have been used to diagnose critical diseases. However, the identification of neurological diseases remains one of the most challenging problems in medical diagnosis is being able to detect. Current diagnostic

 DOI: 10.1201/9781003591085-2

technologies, such as MRI, EEG, PET, fMRI, fNIRS, CT, and SPECT, produce massive amounts of data for the identification, monitoring, and treatment of neurological disorders. Experts often conduct a manual examination of these large datasets to uncover patterns and make a diagnosis [8]. Computer aided diagnostic (CAD) systems have been developed to assist neurologists by analysing large medical data sets more efficiently. CAD algorithms, rooted in pattern recognition theories, are now an essential part of medical diagnostics [9].

2.2 INTERNET OF THINGS AND BIG DATA IN HEALTHCARE: CHARACTERISTICS AND TRANSFORMATIVE IMPACT

"Internet of Things" (IoT) was first introduced by Kevin Ashton to describe a network of physical objects capable of independently transferring data. For example, wearable technology and smart devices such as air conditioners and lights can function automatically through smartphone apps. In healthcare, IoT devices enhance the quality of care by generating vast amounts of structured and unstructured data from clinics, hospitals, laboratories, and research institutes. Big data analytics derived from IoT devices improve the therapy effectiveness of treatments and improve diagnostic accuracy for chronic conditions like cancer, diabetes, and cardiovascular diseases. The extensive data generated also contribute to research, providing insights into general health outcomes among patients. The concept of big data was first introduced in 1999 in a paper by the Association for Computing Machinery titled "Visually Exploring Gigabyte Datasets in Real Time" [10]. In 2001, Doug Laney identified four key characteristics of big data: volume (terabytes of data), variety (various types and sources), veracity (data reliability), and velocity (the speed of data processing to improved decision-making). In healthcare, big data can improve operational efficiency, advance patient care, identify health risks, enable early disease detection, offer real-time alerts, reduce treatment costs and re-admission rates, and support telemedicine and preventative care visits [11].

2.3 CLASSIFICATION OF NEURAL DISORDERS

2.3.1 Classification based on pathology

Neural disorders can be classified based on the underlying pathology, each presenting unique features and consequences. These categories include degenerative, inflammatory, vascular, neoplastic, congenital, traumatic, and metabolic disorders. Understanding these classifications helps in diagnosing and managing various neurological conditions, as outlined in Table 2.1 and Table 2.2.

Table 2.1 Types of Neurodegenerative Diseases (NDs) According to Their Pathology

Types Of Disorders	*Features*	*Examples*
Degenerative disorders	Progressive degeneration of neurons or their connections.	Alzheimer's disease Parkinson's disease Huntington's disease Amyotrophic lateral sclerosis (ALS)
Inflammatory disorders	An autoimmune response or infection usually induces nervous system inflammation.	Multiple sclerosis Encephalitis Meningitis
Vascular disorders	Strokes and aneurysms are examples of problems with brain blood flow.	Ischemic stroke Haemorrhagic stroke Cerebral aneurysm
Neoplastic disorders	Tumours are abnormal growths of tissue in the brain or spinal cord.	Brain tumours Spinal cord tumors
Congenital disorders	Conditions appear during birth, frequently as a result of genetic abnormalities or developmental issues.	Cerebral palsy Spina bifida Hydrocephalus
Traumatic brain injury (TBI)	Physical force damages the brain.	Concussions
Metabolic disorders	Abnormal metabolism or chemical reactions in the brain.	Phenylketonuria (PKU) Tay-Sachs disease Mitochondrial disorders

Table 2.2 Manifestations of Neurodegenerative Diseases (NDs) and Their Causative Factors

Manifestations	*Disorder*	*Causative factors*
Headache, vomiting, light sensation, increased thirst	Migraine (neuropsychiatric disorder)	Stress, caffeine, sensitivity to light
Facial weakness, arm weakness, speech problems	Stroke (ND)	Inactivity, smoking, obesity, high blood cholesterol, diabetes mellitus
Slurred speech, lack of muscle control, lack of bowel control	Cerebral palsy (neuropsychiatric disorder)	Low birth weights, complicated labor
Anxiety, loss of consciousness, muscle jerking	Epilepsy (neuropsychiatric disorder)	Bleeding into the brain, brain injury
Reduce appetite, weakness	Malnutrition (ND)	Nutrition deficiency, toxic food
Lack of eye contact, reduced sensitivity to pain, repetition of words	Autism (ND)	Identical twins, premature births
Headache, depression, seizures, vision problem	Multiple sclerosis (neuropsychiatric disorder)	Genetic factors, smoking, infection, low vitamin D

Table 2.2 (Cont.)

Manifestations	*Disorder*	*Causative factors*
Memory loss, loss of smell, walking problem, slow blinking	Parkinson's disease (neuropsychiatric disorder)	Exposure to pesticides, head injury, high dairy products
Blurred vision, slurred speech	Traumatic brain injury (ND)	Road accidents, falls, violence
Confusion, inappropriate use of words	Alzheimer's disease (neuropsychiatric disorder)	Lifestyle, environmental toxins, high blood pressure

2.4 TECHNOLOGICAL CLASSIFICATION IN HEALTHCARE 6.0

In 1956, the term "artificial intelligence" (AI) was coined by American computer scientist John McCarthy to describe machines that can carry out cognitive tasks such as learning and problem-solving functions traditionally linked to human intelligence. Deep learning refers to artificial neural networks capable of both supervised and unsupervised learning. In healthcare, AI is employed to examine medical data for purposes such as disease prevention, diagnosis, patient monitoring, and the development of new treatment protocols. By doing so, AI alleviates the burden on clinicians who encounter the difficulties of managing large volumes of medical information. Despite extensive research on diagnosing complex disorders, the clinical application of AI remains challenging. Epileptologists are employing wearable sensors and AI-enabled devices like iPads to diagnose and treat uncommon epilepsy conditions [12, 13]. Machine Learning (ML), a subset of AI, depends on various algorithms. Among these, random forest algorithms demonstrate greater stability in neuroimaging data, particularly when dealing with very small sample sizes and large, high-dimensional parameter spaces compared to other models. They have been highly successful in the proper classification of different types of dementia such as mild cognitive impairment [14] and ADs, as well as other disorders like psychogenic non-epileptic seizures, Parkinson's disease [15], and schizophrenia. Different techniques have been used to classify comparable illnesses, including dementia [14].

2.5 TYPES OF NEURAL DISORDERS

2.5.1 Neurodegenerative disorders

2.5.1.1 Dementia – Alzheimer's disease

Alzheimer's disease (AD) is a prevalent cause of dementia in elderly individuals. It is characterized by the deposition of beta-amyloid (Aβ) plaques outside neurons, the formation of intraneuronal fibrillar inclusions composed of abnormally phosphorylated tau protein, and the degeneration of neurons and synapses. A European population-based study reported that the prevalence of Alzheimer's disease increased progressively with age, from 0.6% in the 65 to 69 age group to 22.2% in those aged 90 years and older [16]. The clinical diagnostic criteria for Alzheimer's dementia were first articulated in 1984 but were modified in 2011 and again in 2018, incorporating biomarkers and the acknowledgment that the disease can exist at pre-symptomatic levels [17].

2.5.1.1.1 Mechanism of disease

The pathophysiology of AD remains controversial. The "amyloid-cascade hypothesis" posits that beta-amyloid buildup is central to the disease process [18, 19]. Amyloid precursor protein (APP) is a type 1 transmembrane protein synthesized by various cell types, with the central nervous system cells being the most significant contributors. APP can be cleaved through two pathways within the cell. In the non-amyloidogenic pathway, it is processed by α-secretase, resulting in the formation of sAPPα and C83. Further, it gets processed by γ-secretase which leads to its release of p3 and amyloid precursor protein intracellular domain (AICD). This step involves the cleavage of APP by β-secretase (BACE-1), resulting in the generation of sAPPβ and C99. The C99 fragment is subsequently processed by γ-secretase, leading to the release of Aβ and AICD. An excessive accumulation of Aβ results in the formation of amyloid plaques [20]. The neural mechanism of AD is given in Fig. 2.1.

2.5.1.1.2 Current medication therapies

Despite the growing number of reported cases of AD and its potential socioeconomic impacts, no treatment has yet been developed that could stop or at least hinder the progression of the disorder. So far, only six drugs received approval: aducanumab; donepezil; galantamine; rivastigmine; memantine; and memantine and donepezil combination by the US FDA [21].

I. Aducanumab – Aducanumab is a monoclonal antibody that specifically targets soluble forms of beta-amyloid fibrils and oligomers, aiding in the removal of amyloid-beta plaques. The recommended intravenous dose given over one hour every four weeks must be 10 mg/kg and at least 21 days apart. The U.S. FDA gave the green light to aducanumab in April 2021 to treat AD through amyloid plaque reduction associated with this disease [22].
II. Tacrine – The first acridine-derived cholinergic agent to be allowed by the U.S. FDA was tacrine in 1993. It is a central acetylcholinesterase inhibitor that allows increased acetylcholine levels in different regions

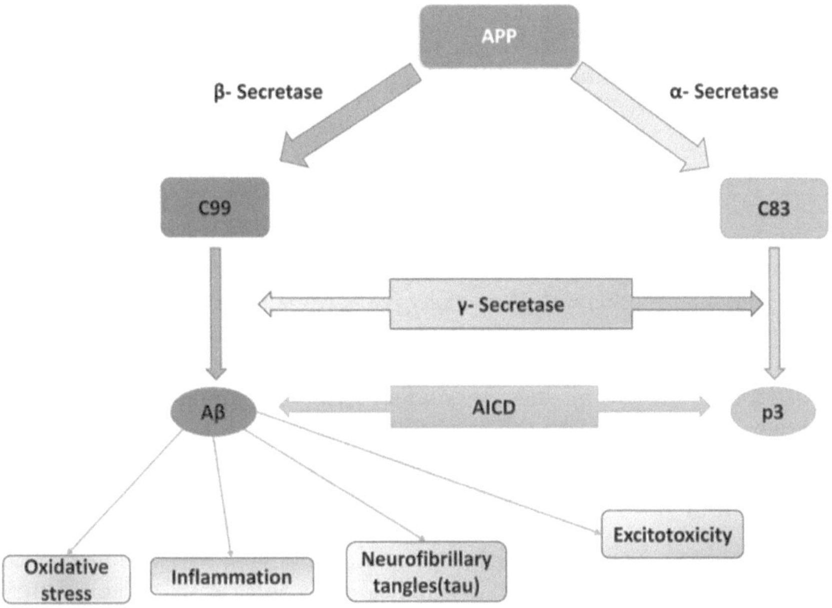

Figure 2.1 Mechanism of Alzheimer's Disease (AD).

of the brain to enhance cognition [23]. Due to enormous adverse effects, such as feeling like throwing up and vomiting, lack of appetite, and dizziness, the medication was taken off the market in 2013. It also had liver toxicity, which caused this drug to be withdrawn from the market.

III. Donepezil – Donepezil is a cholinergic agent developed from piperidine that acts as a central, reversible, non-competitive acetylcholinesterase inhibitor, affecting the breakdown of acetylcholine. By reducing glutamate-induced excitotoxicity, lowering early inflammatory cytokines, promoting a neuroprotective isoform of acetylcholinesterase, and decreasing oxidative stress, this medication can influence the severity of the disease at both the molecular and cellular levels. The drug was approved in 1996 and was the first to be administered to patients with mild to moderate AD [24, 25].

IV. Rivastigmine – This drug, approved by the FDA in 2000, was introduced in Switzerland in 1997. This is approved to heal mild to moderate AD as well as mild to severe dementia associated with PD. It binds to the anionic and stearic sites of acetylcholinesterase (ache) and butyrylcholinesterase and acts as a pseudo-irreversible inhibitor of both enzymes [26].

V. Galantamine – It serves as a tertiary isoquinoline alkaloid that suppresses acetylcholinesterase in a reversible, competitive, and selective manner. It also enhances the intrinsic activity of acetylcholine at the nicotinic receptor [27]. The FDA authorized this medication in 2001 [28].

2.5.1.1.3 Main applications of AI in AD research

AI will have many applications, but it will be limited by the availability of data, for instance, to the size of the sample and the difficulties of gathering such data. The mathematical and physical problems in modeling intricate biological systems present further obstacles since some components are still difficult to understand [29]. With big data, neuroimaging and genetics are incorporating algorithms into the studies. Also, the setting up of biobanks and the expansion of telehealth have made it possible for fluid biomarkers to develop this kind of approach to their research by integrating large amounts of clinical and neuropsychological data into their models [29–31].

I. *Neuroimaging* Neuroimaging is essential in the characterization of AD. The structural state of the brain is indicated by MRI scans, and often they are used in diagnosing neurological conditions or atrophy. This imaging technique considerably helps evaluate the progression of the disease in the assessment of cognitive decline [32–34]. Moreover, fMRI detects brain activity by observing the blood flow changes. This technique tells something about neural function and is crucial for understanding how regions in the brain are dynamically affected by AD [35, 36]. The researchers integrated the demographic data, clinical information, and CSF data using voxel-based morphometry to construct an SVM prediction model that discriminated correctly between CN and AD with an accuracy of 0.949. Their results suggested that cognitive features in patients with MCI were more predictive than structural attributes, meaning some overlap between cognitive function and brain atrophy [29].
II. *Multimodal biomarker-based studies* The introduction and use of biomarkers have changed the diagnosis and research scenario in Alzheimer's disease. Key ad biomarkers include (1) decreased levels of Aβ42 or a low Aβ42/Aβ40 ratio in cerebrospinal fluid along with evidence of amyloid deposits in the brain detected through PET imaging; (2) elevated levels of total tau (t-tau) and phosphorylated tau (p-tau), both indicating cortical neuronal loss and the presence of neurofibrillary tangles; and (3) reduced hippocampal volume as observed by MRI scans [37]. Another key component of biomarker investigations is a cognitive examination [38]. The Clinical Dementia Rating (CDR) score has proved to be very important in categorizing individuals in supervised learning models, aiding in determining a diagnosis of MCI or AD. The score is often combined with

the mini-mental state examination (MMSE) score representing cognitive function. Neuro-ophthalmological exams may provide some biomarkers because changes in the retina indicate changes in the brain during neurodegeneration [29].

III. *Conversion and progression* The primary objective of applying ML algorithms to longitudinal data related to AD is to develop predictive models that assess the risk and timing of conversion from mild cognitive impairment (MCI) to AD and to evaluate the severity of disease progression. [39–42]. Such models are time-dependent, hence making them more complex. Repeated measures design is a well-established method with statistical learning to prove results and reduce variability, but it is much harder to predict time-to-event outcomes in ML [43–45]. These challenges have been addressed through the creation of technological advancements in digitalization. For example, tracking devices can collect data externally [46], while telemedicine consultations [47], and more numerous sensors and devices installed within homes can also make data collection possible [48]. While these solutions might be very costly in the short term, they help curb indirect costs that can accumulate in the long term.

2.5.1.2 Parkinson's disease (PD)

Parkinson's disease (PD) is a prevalent progressive neurological disorder, following AD, characterized by four primary features: bradykinesia, rigidity, postural instability, and resting tremors. The incidence increases with age, moving from 41 per 100,000 in their thirties to more than 1,900 per 100,000 over the age of 80 [49]. This leads to neuropathological alterations in the brain due to the disorder. Abnormal protein aggregates, such as Lewy bodies, form within the cell bodies of affected neurons and are also accompanied by spindle- or thread-like structures called Lewy neurites. These neurites emanate from specific induction sites and progress in a topographically predictable manner throughout the nervous system [50]. The major neuropathological correlates with motor impairment due to the destruction of dopaminergic nigrostriatal neurons with Lewy bodies. However, such cytoskeletal damage may also take place in Glutamatergic, Cholinergic, GABAergic, Serotonergic, noradrenergic, and adrenergic neurons [51]. Often, symptoms of the disease are classified as either motor or non-motor. Some symptoms are exacerbated by dopaminergic medications. Overall, it is estimated that up to 80% of nigrostriatal dopaminergic neurons have been lost before there are clear manifestations of the disease [52]. In a diagnosis of Parkinson's disease, slow voluntary movements, which involve a loss of both the velocity and amplitude of repetitive movements, or bradykinesia, must be accompanied by another feature, such as muscle rigidity, resting tremor, or postural instability [53]. These patients can be suffering from a

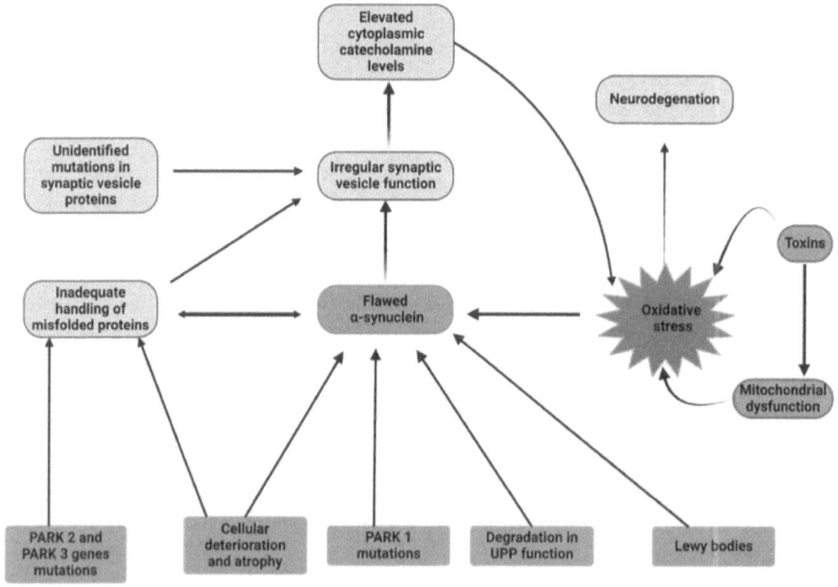

Figure 2.2 Pathophysiology of Parkinson's Disease (PD).

wide range of pre-motor symptoms, even up to ten years before the motor symptoms develop and a final diagnosis can be made for the patient suffering from Parkinson's disease [54]. Non-motor signs include autonomic function abnormalities, sleep difficulties, cognitive and mental disorders, and sensory complaints. The pathophysiology of PD is given in Fig. 2.2.

2.5.1.3 Huntington's disease (HD)

Huntington's disease (HD) is a neurodegenerative condition that begins later in life because it is inherited in an autosomal dominant manner. Actually, the disease was first identified in the medical literature as a distinct clinical entity by George Huntington not many years after he completed his medical school education in 1872 [55]. It took ten years to identify and sequence the Huntington's disease gene, with multiple efforts made in the way of attempts to refine the mapping of the locus with linkage analysis data gathered from individual families. The neural mechanism before HD direct neural pathway and indirect neural pathway is given in Fig. 2.3 and Fig. 2.4 respectively whereas during HD neural mechanism pathway is given in Fig. 2.5.

The polymorphic CAG triplet repeat in the gene is converted into a polyglutamine sequence of different lengths within the huntingtin protein [56]. Children of persons suffering from HD have a 50% chance of

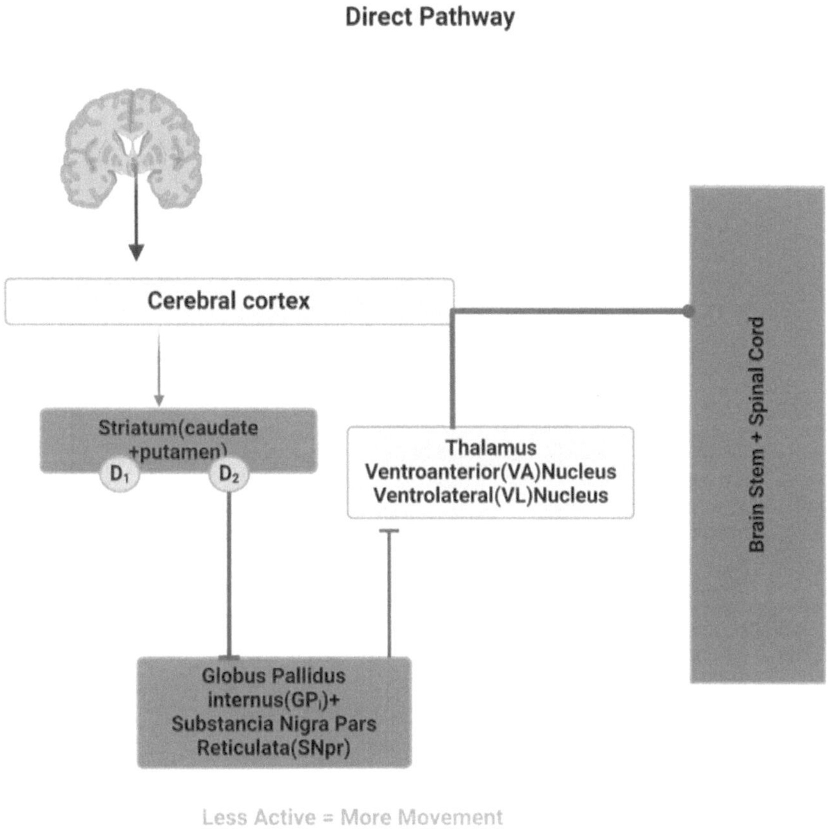

Figure 2.3 Neural Mechanism of the Direct Pathway Before Huntington's Disease.

inheriting the condition. Given that the typical onset of HD occurs after the age of 35, most patients have already had children before they begin to show symptoms of the disease. In 1987, the three countries of Canada, the UK, and the USA started up with trials for HD using RFLP i.e., Restriction Fragment Length Polymorphism analysis for both pre-symptomatic and prenatal diagnosis [57]. The HD mutation consists of a 200 kb long expanded trinucleotide CAG repeat found within the first 67 exons of the Huntingtin gene (HTT). Located on chromosome 4, this repeat leads to neurodegeneration, a toxic gain of function in the Huntingtin protein, and the symptoms characteristic of HD [58]. Recent personalized gene therapy approaches, such as "allele-specific" genetic treatment and "gene silencing" with antisense RNA molecules, show promise for treating inherited disorders, oligonucleotide design, manufacturing, and in vitro testing can

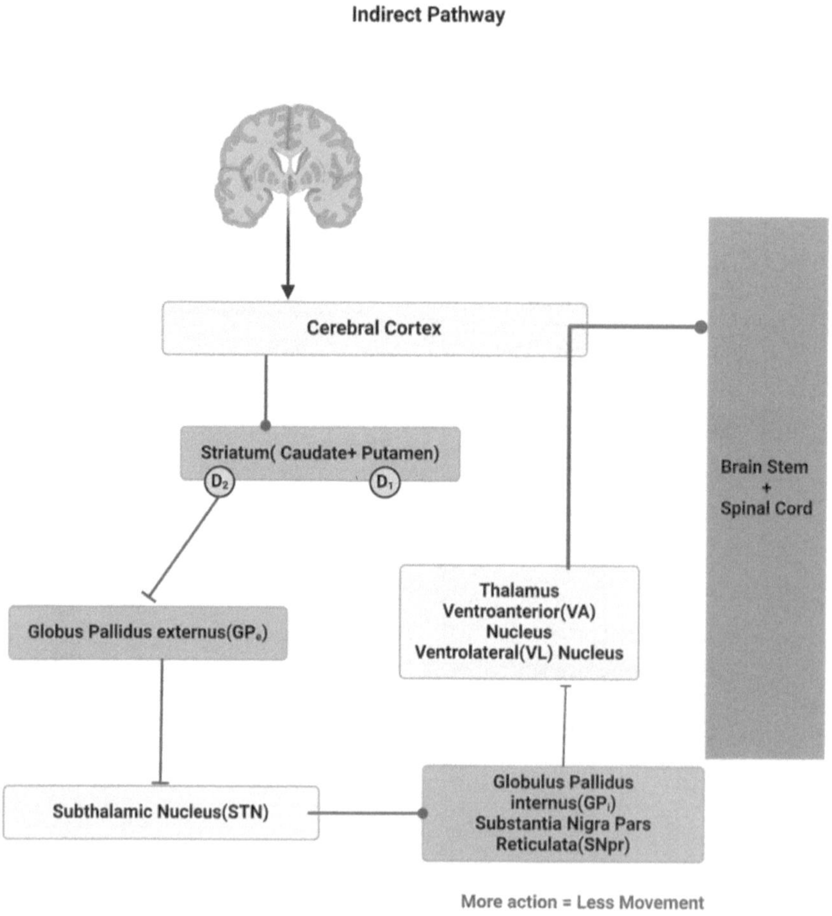

Figure 2.4 Neural Mechanism of the Indirect Pathway Before Huntington's Disease.

leverage allele-specific targeting of Huntingtin gene mRNA or specific areas (e.g., cag repeats, junction sites, or transcript polymorphisms) to reduce Huntingtin production [59].

2.5.2 Neurodevelopmental disorders

2.5.2.1 Autism-spectrum disorders (ASD)

Autism is a neurodegenerative disorder that significantly undermines an individual's interaction and social communication. This neurobehavioral syndrome is characterized by impaired communication skills, lack of social

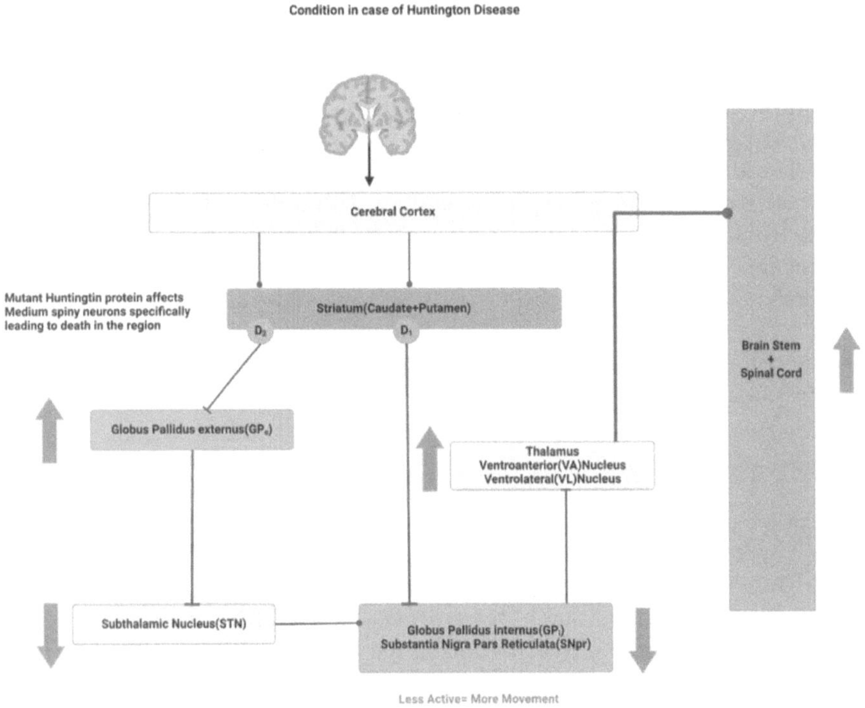

Figure 2.5 Neural Mechanism During Huntington's Disease Progression.

interaction, and language development skills. There are further behaviors repeated with a fixed frequency and intensity; ASD describes the whole series of symptoms characterizing this condition. While there has been no established reason behind the increasing incidence of autism, intervention at the very early stage plays a very important role in achieving long-term success. Again, with early support, a lot of help and care will still be required by an individual affected with autism for their entire lifetime [60]. The checking of children suffering from autism was primarily based on sensors and devices. There is an observation that the development of traditional tools for diagnosing children with autism is quickly being overtaken by the use of sensors and devices. IoT platforms have hastened the diagnosis of autism, which takes place among children between the ages of 2 to 3 years regardless of the significant state of the symptoms.

An autonomous health issue monitoring framework through wearable brain-reading sensors. The system sends data continuously to the caregivers of the autistic children. The authors are interested in tracing the brain waves detected by the sensors that can send a health report to the caregivers and doctors when the patients are in a distressed condition. This brain data provides more accurate predictions of diseases. With the help of an application "cloud computing", a patient's health status can be diagnosed based on retrieved parameters like heart rate, oxygen saturation, and body temperature. Data is collected from the mobile device and displayed on a PC or smartphone by using software that is equivalent to an MQTT lens. Amiri et al. [61] designed an IoT-based framework that uses a smartwatch to sense stereotypical behavior in children with autism. The accelerometer of the smartwatch tracks three stereotypical behaviors linked with autism. These are crying, hand flapping, and painting. The system developed by the authors gathers data from the involved sensors and transmits this information to the cloud for more in-depth analysis. As a result, the accuracy of the decision tree improves, benefiting not only parents but also healthcare professionals and caregivers.

2.5.2.2 Attention deficit-hyperactivity disorder (ADHD)

Attention deficit hyperactivity disorder (ADHD) is a neurodevelopmental illness identified in infancy that persists to adulthood. The symptoms of ADHD include inattention and hyperactivity/impulsivity, both of which affect executive functioning (ef). Children with ADHD sometimes struggle with sustained attention to tasks and activities. It affects approximately 6% to 8% of school-aged children worldwide. Roughly 75% of the children with ADHD (ages 5–2) maintain their criteria for the disorder during their teen years. Furthermore, 65% to 85% of that subset retains either full or partial criteria for ADHD into adulthood or has partial criteria and significant impairment because of the condition [62].

According to recent epidemiologic data, adults with ADHD have a prevalence of 4% to 5%, accounting for approximately 8 million individuals. Only a small percentage of these instances are diagnosed and treated. Other psychiatric and substance use problems also show a high incidence of ADHD [63]. Adult ADHD impairment can result from both core and accompanying symptoms, as well as long-term consequences. Adults seeking treatment may have had ADHD symptoms for up to 30 years and experience both direct and indirect effects of the illness. Academic problems and low self-esteem, which are very common presentations of ADHD in childhood, often have secondary consequences in adulthood. Adults with ADHD have a heightened vulnerability to injuries, smoking, and substance use disorders [64].

Follow-up examinations indicated that the pharmacological medications initial benefits were no longer as significant [65]. The findings indicate that commitment to behavioural therapy should be prioritized when treating persons with ADHD. Smartwatch technology holds promise for overcoming these limitations because it enables the development of software that can use

Cognitive Behavioural Therapy (CBT) via operant conditioning reinforcement techniques to increase desirable behaviours and decrease maladaptive behaviours in children with ADHD [66].

2.5.3 Traumatic and injury-related neural disorders

2.5.3.1 Traumatic brain injury (TBI)

Traumatic brain injury (TBI) is commonly called a "silent epidemic" [67] and ranks among the most important and regularly neglected public health issues because there is an estimated figure of 64 to 74 million people suffering from this annually [68, 69]. Most of the causes of TBI are motor vehicle accidents, falls, suicide by firearms, assaults, and participation in high-intensity sports [70]. Even though AI methods are quickly gaining increased acceptance in neurosurgery, their integration into clinical practice continues to be an evolving process [71]. Since most neuromonitoring data can be collected and the level of consciousness of patients keeps on fluctuating, the challenge of attaining speed and accuracy in clinical decision-making has become more challenging. Therefore, the CDSS is specifically designed to improve the delivery of health services by integrating targeted clinical knowledge, patient information, and other health data in forming medical decisions. AI performs several roles in clinical decision support systems, including real-time monitoring and analysis of health information regarding a patient and predicting any future medical events. This increases efficiency and effectiveness in the delivery of healthcare services. AI assists clinicians in swiftly recognizing circumstances and making appropriate medical judgments by evaluating massive volumes of data in a complex setting [72]. The very rapid advance in AI technology has allowed for the introduction of newer and sophisticated approaches: GMAI and DT technology, which can potentially revolutionize neurocritical care. These technologies are, as of now more theoretical, but still may add significantly to what could be accomplished with AI applications in this area [72].

2.5.3.2 Spinal cord injury (SCI)

Spinal cord injury (SCI) is an injury to the spinal cord caused by trauma from multiple factors. The most common causes of SCI include falls, gunshot injuries, motor vehicle accidents, and sports-related incidents. SCI has resulted in a range of complications, including neurogenic bladder, pressure ulcers, deep vein thrombosis, autonomic dysreflexia, and mental illness. SCI is synonymous with job loss and the emotional and financial consequences that accompany it. Rehabilitation from a spinal cord injury takes time and appears to require patience on the part of patients and families [73].

Rehabilitation for acute and subacute spinal cord injuries lasts six to twelve weeks, initiated at admission to the hospital with stabilization. Prevention of complications becomes a main focus during rehabilitation. Patients with complete injuries will need to be placed under intensive passive exercises with strict care to prevent the development of contractures, muscular atrophy, and pain during the acute phase [74]. The main aim of chronic rehabilitation in spinal cord injured patients is to be able to achieve independence in mobility. Ambulation can be done for exercise goals, social goals, or home goals and may be affected by the level of injury, age, weight, health condition, motivation, and spasticity. It's crucial to have walkers, crutches, and orthoses to enable chronic-stage ambulation.

2.5.4 Neuropsychiatric and mood disorders

2.5.4.1 Schizophrenia

Schizophrenia patients frequently exhibit distorted perceptions of causation, which can manifest as delusional ideation or references [75]. Deviant causal inferences in cognition can lead to skewed and impaired reasoning, as well as altered perceptions of others' mental states and social interactions [76]. Researchers are currently investigating in detail the brain mechanisms underlying cause-and-effect reasoning. Research using brain lesion and neuroimaging techniques has demonstrated a split between the automatic perception of causality and the more volitional process of cognitive inference that makes up the assessment of whether a causal relationship exists. These studies outline how different regions within the brain may correspondingly be more or less engaged in instinctive versus analytic thinking processes in carrying out the assessment of a causal relationship [77, 78].

A study involved the use of fMRI in normal subjects to investigate the activity of the brain in causal judgments for basic motion stimuli, both in physical and social contexts. It aimed to explore how the brain processes and interprets causality in different situations [79]. Causality judgments engaged a frontoparietal network more strongly than those regarding movement direction [80]. Recent imaging studies show that schizophrenia patients exhibit higher neural activity in inferior and middle frontal brain regions, indicating defective social judgments in visual events [81]. Schizophrenia often leads to social marginalization, in addition to its underlying causes [82]. Even when positive signs subside, most persons with schizophrenia continue to have a significant level of social impairment. There are fewer friends, lower marriage rates, and increased estrangement from family members outnumber the broader population [83].

2.5.4.2 Bipolar disorder (BD)

Bipolar disorder (BD) is a chronic illness that causes severe symptoms and can have a significant impact on sufferers and caretakers [84]. Bipolar disorder normally starts during adolescence or early adulthood, which after that has lasting hostile effects on the aspect of psychological and somatic health, educational achievements, professional possibilities, and interpersonal relationships. The consequences of BD can prevent the development of an individual and professional person and thereby affect all areas of life [85]. Many individuals with BD present to primary care doctors, but due to limited resources or experience, they may not obtain a thorough evaluation for a probable bipolar diagnosis. Early diagnosis can lead to effective therapy, improving both short-term and long-term outcomes [86].

Advanced technologies in healthcare have improved the treatment and follow-up of bipolar disorders and depression. Consultation and continuing care by telemedicine enhance accessibility while reducing the frequency of hospital re-admission [87]. Mobile health applications monitor trends in mood and adherence to medication, which provides feedback in real time for both patients and clinicians [88]. Physiological data on sleep and heart rate variability are monitored by wearable sensors that inform mood changes [89]. Additionally, AI-based systems process patients' data to predict mood swings and implement the treatment strategy. Individualized therapy would be taken through such methods that significantly improve the management of symptoms and overall results for mental health illnesses [90].

2.6 SOCIAL IMPACT OF NEURAL DISORDERS

2.6.1 Economic burden of neural disorders

Neural disorders are the second leading cause of death globally and the primary cause of disability. Death rates have doubled, increasing by 39% over three decades. The most significant rise in deaths and disability-adjusted life years (DALYs) occurred in low- and middle-income countries, despite a smaller overall increase in general DALYs [91]. Serious neurological illnesses in the USA are estimated to bear an annual cost of $800 billion in the United States, mainly dementias like Alzheimer's. This includes treatment, lost income from inability to work, and extra expenses for adaptive equipment, caregiving, etc., creating problems for patients, families, and healthcare systems.

2.6.2 Mental health and strategies to lessen stigma

There are five kinds of stigma: social stigma, self-stigma, association-based stigma, structural stigma, and stigma among health professionals. These definitions outline the aspects and means through which stigma affects different groups and individuals in society about the three levels of stigma: interpersonal, social, and individual. The social stigma hurts through asocial interactions with others. Self-stigma takes place because the attitudes of society are taken inside the mind. "Shame by association" is applied to family members of stigmatized persons. Structural stigma refers to problems of an institutional or systemic nature, which adversely limit rights and liberties for a particular group [92, 93]. Neurological illness characteristics that affect stigma were identified by Jones and colleagues as follows: visibility (hidden or visible), seriousness and progression, disruption of social and daily activities, aesthetic impact on others, fear and danger associated with the condition, and the perceived causes of the illness, which are aspects of psychological shame. It is recommended that clinicians ask about their patients' experiences of prejudice and stigma in the same way that they would about other social conditions. Addressing these difficulties, such as educating the family, should be integrated into the treatment plan.

2.6.3 Quality of life for patients and caregivers

2.6.3.1 Quality of life of caregivers

Carers experience stress and are possibly unable to lead an excellent QoL since caring for a patient requires a lot of time and energy. Many carers become jobless or part-time employees to ensure that they are capable of meeting their carer responsibilities. It must also be recalled that even when patients are well-controlled on medication and make few if any, physical demands, carers can still feel emotionally stressed out trying to give the care recipient the emotional support that they require. This makes it difficult to illustrate care, explain goals or activities that one enjoys, be thrust into caregiving against one's will, and lack an idea of what to expect or whether help is even available [94]. The functional dependency, cognitive limitation, disruptive behaviours of the care recipient, and lack of socialization are the reasons for the psychological stressors that the carers face. A range of sociodemographic factors, ways of coping, social support, relationship type, and financial status of both the caregiver and the care recipient contribute as additional stressors [95]. The sociodemographic characteristics of the care recipient and carer, including their age, gender, educational attainment, and financial situation, as well as their coping mechanisms, social support, and kind of relationship and background, are additional factors that contribute to stress on caregivers [96].

2.6.3.2 Quality of life of patients

Chronic conditions have a substantial negative influence on one's physical and mental health and necessitate lifelong medical care and lifestyle adjustments. They may result in discomfort, exhaustion, emotional difficulties, financial strain, and social isolation, all of which can lower patients' quality of life and interpersonal relationships [97]. Encouraging caregivers can negatively affect their health and performance. Supportive services reduce stress and improve patient outcomes through training, practical assistance, and financial aid [98]. All this results in disparities in education and training for this population, which affects their ability to obtain a job [99]. Extreme mental illnesses like depression mean that people have to be absent from work for longer periods; thus, even massive financial losses are incurred by the employees, companies, and indeed society. Average work absences of 5.6 hours a week are reported among those diagnosed with depression; others lose approximately 1.5 hours a week [100].

2.7. HEALTHCARE INNOVATIONS IN NEURAL DISORDER MANAGEMENT

2.7.1 AI and machine learning in diagnosis and treatment

Neurology, as an area of medicine, has recently experienced a great revolution with the incorporation of AI technologies. These have revolutionized the understanding of neurological disorders, the capacity to diagnose them, and the capacity to treat them. AI with its capacity to decipher complex patterns and analyze enormous volumes of data, is significantly advancing neurology in areas like early disease identification and customized treatment plans [101]. AI-powered BCIs help people who are suffering from severe NDs to connect and communicate in new ways. By interpreting brain impulses, these interfaces allow paralyzed people to regain some degree of autonomy over external devices. It enables people with severe neurological abnormalities to go beyond diagnosis and therapy, enabling a level of independence that was previously thought to be impossible [102].

2.7.1.1 Early detection and forecasting

It is tough to diagnose NDs on time with the ambiguity in symptoms. Large volumes of patient data, including genetic data and diagnostic results, can be analyzed by AI systems, so subtle clues that human specialists might omit may help doctors increase the accuracy of diagnosis. The Doppler effect is utilized in transcranial Doppler (TCD) ultrasonography, a non-invasive technique for diagnosing cerebrovascular diseases, to assess the hemodynamic and physiological characteristics of the main intracranial basilar arteries. When used in conjunction with other diagnostic imaging modalities for cerebrovascular illness, it can provide crucial hemodynamic information [103]. AI integration is significantly changing the complex network of neurological illnesses that impact the nervous system [104]. Algorithms powered by AI scan a range of patient data, such as genetic profiles, diagnostic results, and medical histories, so that they can identify subtle signs of neurological issues that people might miss [105]. AI can identify abnormalities in diseases like Parkinson's and Alzheimer's long before symptoms appear, allowing for more controllable therapies. A key component of diagnosis is neuroimaging. A variety of methods are included in neuroimaging, including PET, CT, MRI, SPECT, and AI is very good at analyzing this technique and the accuracy, effectiveness, and diagnostic potential of these techniques have been substantially enhanced by the use of AI technologies [106]. AI can also quantify brain structures, find anomalies, and monitor changes over time. These studies improve treatment planning by speeding up diagnosis and offering thorough insights [106]. AI systems, for example, can quickly analyze brain pictures to detect ischaemic regions in stroke diagnosis, leading to prompt therapies [107].

2.7.2 Advanced treatment of neural disorder

Neurology treatment approaches are being revolutionized by AI integration, which offers data-driven insights, tailored therapies, and enhanced clinical decision-making [108]. By examining thousands of patient data, ranging from genetic profiles to other analyses concerning treatment outcomes, AI indicates the best options for tailored therapy for patients who may face improvement through such approach and therapy. AI can forecast a disease's trajectory using patient data from the past. This makes it possible for neurologists to predict the development of a neurological illness, modify treatment strategies accordingly, and give patients and their families more accurate prognoses. Predictive analytics can also be useful in long-term care planning [109]. AI can help clinicians make well-informed medical decisions by analyzing drug interactions and forecasting possible side outcomes. Install AI-driven monitoring devices to track how well a patient is responding to treatment, including how well drugs are working and any side effects. Provide wearable technology or smartphone apps that let people log their symptoms in real time. AI can then analyze the data and give patients and healthcare professionals insights [110]. AI, by utilizing data-driven insights and personalizing care for each patient, can dramatically improve the efficacy and quality of treatment programs for neurological illnesses. To guarantee that AI complies with neurology's best practices and standards, medical experts should be included in the integration process [109].

2.7.3 Possible applications and uses of wearables in neurology

2.7.3.1 Identification of seizures

Several seizure-detecting devices have been developed. The Embrace wristwatch can identify atypical or involuntary muscle movements linked to convulsive or tonic-clonic seizures. It detects alterations in skin electric conductivity that are correlated with brain seizures [111].

With the use of electrodes affixed to the biceps, brain sentinel facilitates the identification of tonic-clonic seizures that originate in the motor cortex or propagate there. Similarly, another device called Seiz Alarm enables users experiencing small partial seizures to text, email, or call for assistance when it senses seizure-like motion. The user's location is shared via the phone or watch's Global Positioning System (GPS), and a diary feature records the start and end times of seizures. Lastly, the Inspyre wristwatch software notices a pattern of shaking, it will send out alerts via text and phone calls that include the event's duration, date, time, and GPS location.

2.7.3.2 Parkinson's disease (PD)

The signs and symptoms of PD measured by wearable technology include accelerometers and step counters. A 2-year study called mPower invites access to an app tracking change in dexterity, tremors, mobility, balance, gait, and memory through interactive exercises available to persons who are 18 years and older [112].

2.7.3.3 Sleep disorder

Numerous neurologic disorders impact a patient's ability to get enough quality sleep. Since they were available decades ago, wrist-worn actimetry sensors have been utilized and verified in sleep studies. One or more sensor types are included in sleep monitoring systems to measure physiologic tracking. Different new gadgets are available that use more direct interventions to enhance the quality of your sleep. The 2breathe device teaches users how to breathe in a way that promotes sleep by combining an app with a thoracic belt. Devices that distribute scents and those that use sound technologies are also used to encourage and/or induce sleep [113].

2.7.3.4 Suicide prevention devices

Some neurological disorders have enhanced their risk for suicidality. Research has been conducted to see if vocal frequencies and some language metrics can group people who suffer from depression, suicidal ideation, or intent. A depressed person may talk louder but has a decreased range of speech frequency while real-time monitoring of facial expressions will catch a slight inclination to commit suicide. When someone is contemplating suicide, small changes in their face may be picked up by real-time facial motion tracking. Assessing additional metrics (such as skin conductance and heart rate) may aid in identifying additional physiological alterations in those experiencing suicidal thoughts. Despite the encouraging nature of this research, scientists still need to assess the commercially accessible suicide prevention tools critically because they might not be clinically or empirically validated.

2.7.3.5 Assessment of neuropsychiatric relapse

Mind Lamp is a neuropsychiatric research tool that calculates the risk of any recurring mental conditions. A digital phenotype is developed by using time stamps, geolocation, cognitive tests, and questionnaires about the physical activity and symptoms of a person to monitor changes over time [114]. For instance, up to 40% of people with schizophrenia who are released from hospital-based care relapse. Relapse can be due to marital problems, job loss, increased self-harm, and a higher chance of cognitive deterioration [115]. To build a baseline profile or digital phenotype, the app utilizes passive data from timestamps, geolocation, and physical activity and active data from symptom surveys and cognitive tests. The app might track alterations over time to create relapse prediction models. The software can push users to execute interventions if an abnormality or relapse risk is detected in the hopes of lowering the relapse risk [116].

2.8 GLOBAL PERSPECTIVES OF NEUROLOGICAL DISORDERS

2.8.1 Neural disorder in the aging population

The Rotterdam study indicates that of two women and one man three will eventually suffer from dementia, stroke, or Parkinsonism in their lifetime. During the time frame of 1990–2016, the cases of neural disorders such as dementia, Parkinsonism, or stroke have increased by two or threefold [117]. Here we are taking cases of various neurological disorders like dementia, stroke, epilepsy, Parkinson's disease, and related disorders based on studies conducted all over the globe.

2.8.2 Alzheimer's disease (AD)

Alzheimer's disease is the most common form of dementia among older adults. This disease is characterized by the presence of neurofibrillary tangles and extracellular accumulations of beta-amyloid. Epidemiological studies show that the prevalence of AD increases with age, rising from 0.6% in individuals aged 65 to 69 to 22.2% in those aged 90 and older, approximately doubling every five years between the ages of 50 and 80 [16, 118]. Brain MRI is essential for the evaluation of the anatomy and physiology of the brain; differences in some volumes would also determine the diagnosis of Alzheimer's. Ridha et al. indicated that familial Alzheimer's patients had 5.5 years of hippocampal shrinkage and 3.5 years of whole-brain shrinkage before diagnosis. Cortical thickness is an essential marker for Alzheimer's disease. This parameter relates to a quicker progression of the disease and a faster decline in cognitive skills, especially at the temporoparietal junction. This feature can also be applied in the diagnosis of latent cases with the potential possibility of grading their severity, thereby enhancing early intervention techniques [119, 120].

2.8.3 Parkinson's disease (PD)

Parkinson's disease is the second leading neurological ailment after Alzheimer's, affecting around 1% of those over 60 and 5% of those over 85. In France, incidence rates are divided by age and are more frequently observed among older men and women in almost all age-related strata [121]. Advanced MRI techniques have unveiled a greater iron content in microsomes in the setting of pd because of the degeneration of dopaminergic neurons, which are markers of progressive diseases. A meta-analysis was conducted to determine that structural MRI distinguishes idiopathic PD from controls with 94% sensitivity and 90% specificity. Free water imaging by diffusion-weighted MRI (DWI) is also used to detect increased free water due to neuronal loss in the SNpc and thus to arrive at the diagnosis of PD [122].

2.8.4 Stroke

A stroke is a neurologic impairment caused by sudden vascular injury to the brain, that includes both cerebral infarction and subarachnoid hemorrhage. The lifetime stroke risk for middle-aged individuals is 20%, doubling every 10 years after 45, with 75% occurring in those over 65 [117]. Imaging studies provide critical information for the best stroke therapy. While radiologists have traditionally interpreted medical images intending to identify and track diseases, AI truly excels when working with imaging data to identify complex patterns and in creating quantitative grades of radiographic features that greatly improve diagnostic accuracy and efficiency [123].

2.9 CONCLUSION

Neural disorders range from neurodegenerative, and neurodevelopmental, to those caused by injury. Such neural disorders are part of the serious challenges to global healthcare systems. With millions affected worldwide by diseases such as AD, PD, and ASD, there is an imperative call for more accurate and effective diagnostic and treatment methods. This has revolutionized how neural health issues are approached through AI, IoT, and big data technologies to herald a new era in neural health care. Technological innovations, such as wearables and IoT, now enable real-time monitoring of symptoms, thus offering better care to patients afflicted with conditions like Parkinson's and epilepsy. Future trends also include gene therapy and neuro-regeneration, which may be the hope for HD. More importantly, case studies from low-income regions where resources are limited reveal how healthcare 6.0 technologies can help manage neural disorders. In a nutshell, the integration of AI, wearables, and more will present a new front in the management of neural disorders. Not only do the patient's needs to receive better care benefit from these advances but equally so, diagnoses, treatments, and monitoring for these conditions are hereby pushed forward to improve the quality of life of humankind on the global front.

2.10 FUTURE DIRECTIONS IN NEURAL HEALTH

Future neural health will be characterized by global collaboration, advanced healthcare technologies, and social policies. The development of big data, IoT, and AI has created novel opportunities for the diagnosis, treatment, and management of neurological illnesses. Early diagnosis and individualized treatment with AI-backed diagnostic tools for neurodegenerative disorders like Alzheimer's and Parkinson's will be developed. Major areas where innovations in wearable technology and continuous remote monitoring systems are expected to have a big role include conditions such as epilepsy and traumatic brain injuries. Probably of utmost significance is the collaboration across borders of research institutions, governments, and healthcare providers towards neural disorders. Data sharing and resource sharing would help hasten breakthroughs in neurodegeneration, gene therapy, and personalized medicine. Social policies that would bring equal opportunities to all despite the differences in the healthcare technologies of developed and low-income countries are also necessary to make these innovations applicable to every culture.

ACKNOWLEDGMENT

The authors are thankful to the Department of Pharmaceuticals, Ministry of Chemicals and Fertilizers, Government of India. All the figures are from www.biorender.com.

CREDIT AUTHORSHIP CONTRIBUTION STATEMENT

Sarasa Meenakshi, Krishna Murti, Ved Prakash: Conceptualization, **Mayank Mishra, Sushama Singh, Sarasa Meenakshi, Nitesh Kumar:** Writing – original draft preparation, visualization, **Sarasa Meenakshi, Ved Prakash, Nitesh Kumar, Nikhilesh Anand, Krishna Murti:** Supervision, writing – review and editing.

DECLARATION OF COMPETING INTEREST

The authors declare no competing or financial interests relevant to this article.

ABBREVIATIONS

AD	Alzheimer's disease
AI	Artificial intelligence
ALS	Amyotrophic lateral sclerosis
BD	Bipolar disorder
CAD	Computer aided diagnostic
CT	Computed tomography
EEG	Electroencephalography
fMRI	Functional magnetic resonance Imaging
fNIRS	Functional near infrared spectroscopy
IoT	Internet of Things
MEG	Magnetoencephalography
miRNA	micro-Ribonucleotide
ML	Machine learning
MPTP	Methyl phenyl tetrahydropyridine
MRI	Magnetic resonance imaging
ND	Neurological disease
NDDs	Neurodevelopmental disorders
PD	Parkinson's disease
PET	Positron emission tomography
SCI	Spinal cord injury
siRNA	Small interfering Ribonucleotide
SPECT	Single photon emission computed tomography
SZ	Schizophrenia
TBI	Traumatic brain injury

REFERENCES

[1] Gautam, R., and M. Sharma. "Prevalence and diagnosis of neurological disorders using different deep learning techniques: A meta-analysis." *J Med Syst* 44, no 2 (Jan 4 2020): 49. https://doi.org/10.1007/s10916-019-1519-7.

[2] Kennedy, D. P., and R. Adolphs. "The social brain in psychiatric and neurological disorders." *Trends Cogn Sci* 16, no 11 (Nov 2012): 559–72. https://doi.org/10.1016/j.tics.2012.09.006.

[3] Collaborators, GBDN. "2. N. Global, regional, and national burden of neurological disorders, 1990–2016: A systematic analysis for the Global

Burden of Disease Study 2016." *Lancet Neurol* 18, no 5 (2019): 459–80. https://doi.org/DOI: 10.1016/S1474-4422(18)30403-4.

[4] Feigin, Valery L., Emma Nichols, Tahiya Alam, Marlena S Bannick, Ettore Beghi, Natacha Blake, William J. Culpepper, *et al.* "Global, regional, and national burden of neurological disorders, 1990–2016: A systematic analysis for the Global Burden of Disease Study 2016." *The Lancet Neurology* 18, no 5 (2019): 459–80. https://doi.org/10.1016/S1474-4422(19)30411-9.

[5] Collaborators, GBDD. "GBD 2016 Dementia Collaborators Global, regional, and national burden of Alzheimer's disease and other dementias, 1990–2016: A systematic analysis for the Global Burden of Disease Study 2016." *Lancet Neurol* 18, no 1 (2019): 88–106. https://doi.org/10.1016/S1474-4422(18)30403-4.

[6] Dorsey, E. Ray, Alexis Elbaz, Emma Nichols, Nooshin Abbasi, Foad Abd-Allah, Ahmed Abdelalim, Jose C. Adsuar, *et al.* "Global, regional, and national burden of Parkinson's disease, 1990–2016: a systematic analysis for the Global Burden of Disease Study 2016." *Lancet Neurol* 17, no 11 (2018): 939–53. https://doi.org/10.1016/S1474-4422(18)30295-3.

[7] Chin, J. H., and N. Vora. "The global burden of neurologic diseases." *Neurology* 83, no 4 (Jul 22 2014): 349–51. https://doi.org/10.1212/WNL.0000000000000610.

[8] Lima, Aklima Akter, M. Firoz Mridha, Sujoy Chandra Das, Muhammad Mohsin Kabir, Md Rashedul Islam, and Yutaka Watanobe. "A comprehensive survey on the detection, classification, and challenges of neurological disorders." *Biology* 11, no 3 (2022): 469. https://doi.org/10.3390/biology11030469.

[9] Doi, Kunio. "Computer-aided diagnosis in medical imaging: Historical review, current status and future potential." *Computerized medical imaging and graphics* 31, no 4–5 (2007): 198–211. https://doi.org/10.1016/j.compmedimag.2007.02.002.

[10] McAfee, A., and E. Brynjolfsson. "Big data: The management revolution." *Harv Bus Rev* 90, no 10 (Oct 2012): 60–6, 68, 128. https://www.ncbi.nlm.nih.gov/pubmed/23074865.

[11] Kruse, C. S., R. Goswamy, Y. Raval, and S. Marawi. "Challenges and Opportunities of Big Data in Health Care: A Systematic Review." *JMIR Med Inform* 4, no 4 (Nov 21 2016): e38. https://doi.org/10.2196/medinform.5359.

[12] Onorati, F., G. Regalia, C. Caborni, M. Migliorini, D. Bender, M. Z. Poh, C. Frazier, *et al.* "Multicenter clinical assessment of improved wearable multimodal convulsive seizure detectors." *Epilepsia* 58, no 11 (Nov 2017): 1870–79. https://doi.org/10.1111/epi.13899.

[13] Okazaki, E. M., R. Yao, J. I. Sirven, A. Z. Crepeau, K. H. Noe, J. F. Drazkowski, M. T. Hoerth, *et al.* "Usage of EpiFinder clinical decision support in the assessment of epilepsy." *Epilepsy Behav* 82 (May 2018): 140–43. https://doi.org/10.1016/j.yebeh.2018.03.018.

[14] Sarica, A., A. Cerasa, and A. Quattrone. "Random forest algorithm for the classification of neuroimaging data in Alzheimer's Disease: A systematic review." *Front Aging Neurosci* 9 (2017): 329. https://doi.org/10.3389/fnagi.2017.00329.

[15] Salvatore, Christian, Antonio Cerasa, Isabella Castiglioni, F Gallivanone, A Augimeri, M Lopez, G Arabia, *et al.* "Machine learning on brain MRI data for differential diagnosis of Parkinson's disease and Progressive Supranuclear Palsy." *J Neurosci Methods* 222 (2014): 230–37. https://doi.org/10.1016/j.jneumh.2013.11.016.

[16] Lobo, A., L. J. Launer, L. Fratiglioni, K. Andersen, A. Di Carlo, M. M. Breteler, J. R. Copeland, *et al.* "Prevalence of dementia and major subtypes in Europe: A collaborative study of population-based cohorts. Neurologic Diseases in the Elderly Research Group." *Neurology* 54, no 11 Suppl 5 (2000): S4–9. www.ncbi.nlm.nih.gov/pubmed/10854354.

[17] Jack, C. R., Jr., T. M. Therneau, S. D. Weigand, H. J. Wiste, D. S. Knopman, P. Vemuri, V. J. Lowe, *et al.* "Prevalence of biologically vs clinically defined alzheimer spectrum entities using the national institute on aging-Alzheimer's Association Research Framework." *JAMA Neurol* 76, no 10 (Oct 1 2019): 1174–83. https://doi.org/10.1001/jamaneurol.2019.1971.

[18] Selkoe, D. J., Physicians American College of, and Society American Physiological. "Alzheimer disease: mechanistic understanding predicts novel therapies." *Ann Intern Med* 140, no 8 (Apr 20 2004): 627–38. https://doi.org/10.7326/0003-4819-140-8-200404200-00047.

[19] Querfurth, Henry W., and Frank M. LaFerla. "Alzheimer's disease." *N Engl J Med* 362, no 4 (2010): 329–44. https://doi.org/10.1056/NEJMra 0909142.

[20] Lopez, O. L., and L. H. Kuller. "Epidemiology of aging and associated cognitive disorders: Prevalence and incidence of Alzheimer's disease and other dementias." *Handb Clin Neurol* 167 (2019): 139–48. https://doi.org/10.1016/B978-0-12-804766-8.00009-1.

[21] Pardo-Moreno, T., A. Gonzalez-Acedo, A. Rivas-Dominguez, V. Garcia-Morales, F. J. Garcia-Cozar, J. J. Ramos-Rodriguez, and L. Melguizo-Rodriguez. "Therapeutic approach to Alzheimer's Disease: Current treatments and new perspectives." *Pharmaceutics* 14, no 6 (May 24 2022): 1117. https://doi.org/10.3390/pharmaceutics14061117.

[22] Martins, A. C., M. Y. Oshiro, F. Albericio, and B. G. de la Torre. "Food and Drug Administration (FDA) approvals of biological drugs in 2023." *Biomedicines* 12, no 9 (Sep 2 2024): 1992. https://doi.org/10.3390/biome dicines12091992.

[23] Wagstaff, A. J., and D. McTavish. "Tacrine. A review of its pharmacodynamic and pharmacokinetic properties, and therapeutic efficacy in Alzheimer's disease." *Drugs Aging* 4, no 6 (Jun 1994): 510–40. https://doi.org/10.2165/00002512-199404060-00006.

[24] Koul, B., U. Farooq, D. Yadav, and M. Song. "Phytochemicals: A promising alternative for the prevention of Alzheimer's disease." *Life (Basel)* 13, no 4 (Apr 12 2023): 999. https://doi.org/10.3390/life13040999.

[25] Jacobson, S. A., and M. N. Sabbagh. "Donepezil: Potential neuroprotective and disease-modifying effects." *Expert Opin Drug Metab Toxicol* 4, no 10 (Oct 2008): 1363–9. https://doi.org/10.1517/17425255.4.10.1363.

[26] Desai, A. K., and G. T. Grossberg. "Rivastigmine for Alzheimer's disease." *Expert Rev Neurother* 5, no 5 (Sep 2005): 563–80. https://doi.org/10.1586/14737175.5.5.563.

[27] Farlow, M. R. "Clinical pharmacokinetics of galantamine." *Clin Pharmacokinet* 42, no 15 (2003): 1383–92. https://doi.org/10.2165/00003088-200342150-00005.

[28] Olin, J., and L. Schneider. "Galantamine for Alzheimer's disease." *Cochrane Database Syst Rev* 3 (2002): CD001747. https://doi.org/10.1002/14651858.CD001747.

[29] Silva-Spinola, A., I. Baldeiras, J. P. Arrais, and I. Santana. "The road to personalized medicine in Alzheimer's disease: The use of artificial intelligence." *Biomedicines* 10, no 2 (Jan 29 2022): 315. https://doi.org/10.3390/biomedicines10020315.

[30] Yang, Jie, Xinyang Feng, Andrew F Laine, and Elsa D Angelini. "Characterizing Alzheimer's disease with image and genetic biomarkers using supervised topic models." *IEEE J Biomed Health Inf* 24, no 4 (2019): 1180–87. https://doi.org/10.1109/JBHI.2019.2928831.

[31] Wang, Xiaoqian, Jingwen Yan, Xiaohui Yao, Sungeun Kim, Kwangsik Nho, Shannon L Risacher, Andrew J Saykin, *et al.* "Longitudinal genotype–phenotype association study through temporal structure auto-learning predictive model." *J Comput Biol* 25, no 7 (2018): 809–24. https://doi.org/10.1089/cmb.2018.0008.

[32] Tam, A., C. Dansereau, Y. Iturria-Medina, S. Urchs, P. Orban, H. Sharmarke, J. Breitner, P. Bellec, and Initiative Alzheimer's Disease Neuroimaging. "A highly predictive signature of cognition and brain atrophy for progression to Alzheimer's dementia." *Gigascience* 8, no 5 (May 1 2019): giz055. https://doi.org/10.1093/gigascience/giz055.

[33] Zhou, T., K. H. Thung, X. Zhu, and D. Shen. "Effective feature learning and fusion of multimodality data using stage-wise deep neural network for dementia diagnosis." *Hum Brain Mapp* 40, no 3 (Feb 15 2019): 1001–16. https://doi.org/10.1002/hbm.24428.

[34] Ezzati, Ali, Danielle J. Harvey, Christian Habeck, Ashkan Golzar, Irfan A. Qureshi, Andrea R. Zammit, Jinshil Hyun, *et al.* "Predicting amyloid-β levels in amnestic mild cognitive impairment using machine learning techniques." *J Alzheimer's Dis* 73, no 3 (2020): 1211–19. https://doi.org/10.3233/JAD-191038.

[35] Lanka, P., D. Rangaprakash, M. N. Dretsch, J. S. Katz, T. S. Denney, Jr., and G. Deshpande. "Supervised machine learning for diagnostic classification from large-scale neuroimaging datasets." *Brain Imaging Behav* 14, no 6 (Dec 2020): 2378–416. https://doi.org/10.1007/s11682-019-00191-8.

[36] Nguyen, D. T., S. Ryu, M. N. I. Qureshi, M. Choi, K. H. Lee, and B. Lee. "Hybrid multivariate pattern analysis combined with extreme learning machine for Alzheimer's dementia diagnosis using multi-measure rs-fMRI spatial patterns." *PLoS One* 14, no 2 (2019): e0212582. https://doi.org/10.1371/journal.pone.0212582.

[37] Weiner, M. W., D. P. Veitch, P. S. Aisen, L. A. Beckett, N. J. Cairns, R. C. Green, D. Harvey, *et al.* "The Alzheimer's Disease Neuroimaging Initiative 3: Continued innovation for clinical trial improvement." *Alzheimers Dement* 13, no 5 (May 2017): 561–71. https://doi.org/10.1016/j.jalz.2016.10.006.

[38] Peng, Bo, Xiaohui Yao, Shannon L Risacher, Andrew J Saykin, Li Shen, Xia Ning, and ADNI. "Cognitive biomarker prioritization in Alzheimer's Disease using brain morphometric data." *BMC Med Inf Dec Mak* 20 (2020): 1–11. https://doi.org/10.1186/s12911-020-01339-z.
[39] Ezzati, Ali, Andrea R. Zammit, Danielle J. Harvey, Christian Habeck, Charles B. Hall, Richard B. Lipton, and Alzheimer's Disease Neuroimaging Initiative. "Optimizing machine learning methods to improve predictive models of Alzheimer's disease." *Journal of Alzheimer's Disease* 71, no 3 (2019): 1027–36. https://doi.org/10.3233/JAD-190262.
[40] Grassi, M., N. Rouleaux, D. Caldirola, D. Loewenstein, K. Schruers, G. Perna, and M. Dumontier. "Alzheimer's Disease Neuroimaging Initiative A novel ensemble-based machine learning algorithm to predict the conversion from mild cognitive impairment to Alzheimer's disease using socio-demographic characteristics, clinical information, and neuropsychological measures." *Front Neurol* 10 (2019): 756. https://doi.org/10.3389/fneur.2019.00756.
[41] Pusil, S., S. I. Dimitriadis, M. E. Lopez, E. Pereda, and F. Maestu. "Aberrant MEG multi-frequency phase temporal synchronization predicts conversion from mild cognitive impairment-to-Alzheimer's disease." *Neuroimage Clin* 24 (2019): 101972. https://doi.org/10.1016/j.nicl.2019.101972.
[42] Yan, Yu, Edward Somer, and Vicente Grau. "Classification of amyloid PET images using novel features for early diagnosis of Alzheimer's disease and mild cognitive impairment conversion." *Nucl Med Commun* 40, no 3 (2019): 242–48. https://doi.org/10.1097/MNM.0000000000000953.
[43] Geifman, Nophar, Richard E. Kennedy, Lon S. Schneider, Iain Buchan, and Roberta Diaz Brinton. "Data-driven identification of endophenotypes of Alzheimer's disease progression: implications for clinical trials and therapeutic interventions." *Alzheimer's Res Ther* 10 (2018): 1–7. https://doi.org/10.1186/s13195-017-0332-0.
[44] Wang, M., D. Zhang, D. Shen, and M. Liu. "Multi-task exclusive relationship learning for alzheimer's disease progression prediction with longitudinal data." *Med Image Anal* 53 (Apr 2019): 111–22. https://doi.org/10.1016/j.media.2019.01.007.
[45] Liu, X., J. Wang, F. Ren, and J. Kong. "Group guided fused Laplacian Sparse group Lasso for modeling Alzheimer's disease progression." *Comput Math Methods Med* 2020, no 1 (2020): 4036560. https://doi.org/10.1155/2020/4036560.
[46] Saif, Nabeel, Peter Yan, Kellyann Niotis, Olivia Scheyer, Aneela Rahman, Michael Berkowitz, Robert Krikorian, *et al.* "Feasibility of using a wearable biosensor device in patients at risk for Alzheimer's disease dementia." *J Prev Alzheimer's Dis* 7 (2020): 104–11. https://doi.org/10.14283/jpad.2019.39.
[47] Hunter, Matthew B., Natalie Jenkins, Clare Dolan, Hannah Pullen, Craig Ritchie, and Graciela Muniz-Terrera. "Reliability of telephone and videoconference methods of cognitive assessment in older adults with and without dementia." *J Alzheimer's Dis* 81, no 4 (2021): 1625–47. https://doi.org/10.3233/JAD-210088.

[48] Muurling, M., C. de Boer, R. Kozak, D. Religa, I. Koychev, H. Verheij, V. J. M. Nies, *et al.* "Remote monitoring technologies in Alzheimer's disease: Design of the RADAR-AD study." *Alzheimers Res Ther* 13, no 1 (Apr 23 2021): 89. https://doi.org/10.1186/s13195-021-00825-4.

[49] Cacabelos, R. "Parkinson's disease: From pathogenesis to pharmacogenomics." *Int J Mol Sci* 18, no 3 (Mar 4 2017): 551. https://doi.org/10.3390/ijms18030551.

[50] Braak, H., E. Ghebremedhin, U. Rub, H. Bratzke, and K. Del Tredici. "Stages in the development of Parkinson's disease-related pathology." *Cell Tissue Res* 318, no 1 (Oct 2004): 121–34. https://doi.org/10.1007/s00441-004-0956-9.

[51] Braak, H., and E. Braak. "Pathoanatomy of Parkinson's disease." *J Neurol* 247, no Suppl 2 (Apr 2000): II3–10. https://doi.org/10.1007/PL00007758.

[52] Chung, K. K., Y. Zhang, K. L. Lim, Y. Tanaka, H. Huang, J. Gao, C. A. Ross, V. L. Dawson, and T. M. Dawson. "Parkin ubiquitinates the alpha-synuclein-interacting protein, synphilin-1: implications for Lewy-body formation in Parkinson disease." *Nat Med* 7, no 10 (Oct 2001): 1144–50. https://doi.org/10.1038/nm1001-1144.

[53] Hughes, A. J., S. E. Daniel, S. Blankson, and A. J. Lees. "A clinicopathologic study of 100 cases of Parkinson's disease." *Arch Neurol* 50, no 2 (Feb 1993): 140–8. https://doi.org/10.1001/archneur.1993.00540020018011.

[54] O'Sullivan, Sean S., David R. Williams, David A. Gallagher, Luke A. Massey, Laura Silveira-Moriyama, and Andrew J. Lees. "Nonmotor symptoms as presenting complaints in Parkinson's disease: a clinicopathological study." *Movement disorders* 23, no 1 (2008): 101–06. https://doi.org/10.1002/mds.21813.

[55] Durbach, N., and M. R. Hayden. "George Huntington: The man behind the eponym." *J Med Genet* 30, no 5 (May 1993): 406–9. https://doi.org/10.1136/jmg.30.5.406.

[56] Ross, C. A., E. H. Aylward, E. J. Wild, D. R. Langbehn, J. D. Long, J. H. Warner, R. I. Scahill, *et al.* "Huntington disease: Natural history, biomarkers and prospects for therapeutics." *Nat Rev Neurol* 10, no 4 (Apr 2014): 204–16. https://doi.org/10.1038/nrneurol.2014.24.

[57] Farrer, L. A., R. H. Myers, L. A. Cupples, and P. M. Conneally. "Considerations in using linkage analysis as a presymptomatic test for Huntington's disease." *J Med Genetics* 25, no 9 (1988): 577–88. https://doi.org/10.1136/jmg.25.9.577.

[58] Harper, P. S. "*Huntington's disease*, 2nd edn, vol. 31." London: WB Saunders Co, 1996.

[59] Sah, D. W., and N. Aronin. "Oligonucleotide therapeutic approaches for Huntington disease." *J Clin Invest* 121, no 2 (Feb 2011): 500–7. https://doi.org/10.1172/JCI45130.

[60] Case-Smith, Jane, Lindy L. Weaver, and Mary A. Fristad. "A systematic review of sensory processing interventions for children with autism spectrum disorders." *Autism* 19, no 2 (2015): 133–48. https://doi.org/10.1177/1362361313517762.

[61] Amiri, Amir Mohammad, Nicholas Peltier, Cody Goldberg, Yan Sun, Anoo Nathan, Shivayogi V. Hiremath, and Kunal Mankodiya. "WearSense: Detecting autism stereotypic behaviors through smartwatches." *Healthcare* 5, no 1 (2017): 11. https://doi.org/10.3390/healthcare5010011.

[62] Biederman, J., M. C. Monuteaux, E. Mick, T. Spencer, T. E. Wilens, J. M. Silva, L. E. Snyder, and S. V. Faraone. "Young adult outcome of attention deficit hyperactivity disorder: A controlled 10-year follow-up study." *Psychol Med* 36, no 2 (Feb 2006): 167–79. https://doi.org/10.1017/S0033291705006410.

[63] Kessler, Ronald C., Lenard Adler, Russell Barkley, Joseph Biederman, C Keith Conners, Olga Demler, Stephen V. Faraone, *et al.* "The prevalence and correlates of adult ADHD in the United States: results from the National Comorbidity Survey Replication." *American Journal of psychiatry* 163, no 4 (2006): 716–23. https://doi.org/10.1176/ajp.2006.163.4.716.

[64] Wilens, T. E. "ADHD: prevalence, diagnosis, and issues of comorbidity." *CNS Spectr* 12, no 4 Suppl 6 (Apr 2007): 1–5. https://doi.org/10.1017/s1092852900025992.

[65] Wang, Christine H., Heather Mazursky-Horowitz, and Andrea Chronis-Tuscano. "Delivering evidence-based treatments for child attention-deficit/hyperactivity disorder (ADHD) in the context of parental ADHD." *Curr Psychiatry Rep* 16 (2014): 1–8. https://doi.org/10.1007/s11920-014-0474-8.

[66] Catala-Lopez, F., B. Hutton, A. Nunez-Beltran, M. J. Page, M. Ridao, D. Macias Saint-Gerons, M. A. Catala, R. Tabares-Seisdedos, and D. Moher. "The pharmacological and non-pharmacological treatment of attention deficit hyperactivity disorder in children and adolescents: A systematic review with network meta-analyses of randomised trials." *PLoS One* 12, no 7 (2017): e0180355. https://doi.org/10.1371/journal.pone.0180355.

[67] Vaishnavi, S., V. Rao, and J. R. Fann. "Neuropsychiatric problems after traumatic brain injury: unraveling the silent epidemic." *Psychosomatics* 50, no 3 (May-Jun 2009): 198–205. https://doi.org/10.1176/appi.psy.50.3.198.

[68] Dewan, Michael C., Abbas Rattani, Saksham Gupta, Ronnie E Baticulon, Ya-Ching Hung, Maria Punchak, Amit Agrawal, *et al.* "Estimating the global incidence of traumatic brain injury." *J Neurosurg* 130, no 4 (2018): 1080–97. https://doi.org/10.3171/2017.10.JNS17352.

[69] "The burden of dementia due to down syndrome, Parkinson's disease, stroke, and traumatic brain injury: A systematic analysis for the Global Burden of Disease Study 2019." [En eng]. *Neuroepidemiology* 55, no 4 (2021): 286–96. https://doi.org/10.1159/000515393.

[70] Miller, Gabrielle F., Scott R. Kegler, and Deborah M. Stone. "Traumatic brain injury–related deaths from firearm suicide: United States, 2008–2017." *Am J Public Health* 110, no 6 (2020): 897–99. https://doi.org/10.2105/AJPH.2020.305622.

[71] Reddy Kishor Kumar, Vijaya Sindhoori Kaza, P. R. Anisha, Mousa Mohammed Khurbani, Mohammed Shauib, and Sadaf Alam. "Optimizing barrier placement for intrusion detection and prevention in WSNs." *PLOS ONE*, February 2024. https://doi.org/10.1371/journal.pone.0299334

[72] Anisha, P. R., C. Kishor Kumar Reddy, Marlia Mohd Hanafiah, B. V. Ramana Murthy, R. Madana Mohana, and Y. V. S. S. Pragathi. "An intelligent deep feature based feature based metabolism syndrome prediction system for sleep disorder diseases." In *Multimedia Tools and Applications*, Springer, November 2023, https://doi.org/10.1007/s11042-023-17296-4

[73] Reddy, Kishor Kumar, P. R. Anisha, Marlia Mohd Hanafiah, Y. V. S. S. Pragathi, B. V. Ramana Murthy, and R. Madana Mohana. "An intelligent optimized cyclone intensity prediction framework using satellite images." *Springer Earth Science Informatics*, March 2023, https://doi.org/10.1007/s12145-023-00983-z

[74] Reddy, C. Kishor Kumar, P. R. Anisha, Tirupathi Reddy, B. Srinivasulu, D. Rambabu. "Light-weight real time weather forecasting simulation over Bangladesh using deep learning." *INT-JECSE* (2022): 449–465.

[75] Rizvi, A., S. R. Safwi, and M. A. Usmani. "Schizophrenia: Disability, clinical insights, and management. In: G. Bennett, E. Goodall (eds) *The Palgrave Encyclopedia of Disability*. Palgrave Macmillan, Cham, 2024, https://doi.org/10.1007/978-3-031-40858-8_119-1

[76] Herrington, J. D., C. Nymberg, and R. T. Schultz. "Biological motion task performance predicts superior temporal sulcus activity." *Brain Cogn* 77, no 3 (Dec 2011): 372–81. https://doi.org/10.1016/j.bandc.2011.09.001.

[77] Fonlupt, Pierre. "Perception and judgement of physical causality involve different brain structures." *Cognitive Brain Research* 17, no 2 (2003): 248–54. https://doi.org/10.1016/s0926-6410(03)00112-5.

[78] Fugelsang, Jonathan A., Matthew E. Roser, Paul M. Corballis, Michael S. Gazzaniga, and Kevin N. Dunbar. "Brain mechanisms underlying perceptual causality." *Cogn Brain Res* 24, no 1 (2005): 41–47. https://doi.org/10.1016/j.cogbrainres.2004.12.001.

[79] Blos, Johannes, Anjan Chatterjee, Tilo Kircher, and Benjamin Straube. "Neural correlates of causality judgment in physical and social context—the reversed effects of space and time." *Neuroimage* 63, no 2 (2012): 882–93. https://doi.org/10.1016/j.neuroimage.2012.07.028.

[80] Wende, K. C., A. Nagels, J. Blos, M. Stratmann, A. Chatterjee, T. Kircher, and B. Straube. "Differences and commonalities in the judgment of causality in physical and social contexts: an fMRI study." *Neuropsychologia* 51, no 13 (Nov 2013): 2572–80. https://doi.org/10.1016/j.neuropsychologia.2013.07.027.

[81] Pedersen, Anya, Katja Koelkebeck, Matthias Brandt, Melissa Wee, Kerstin Annika Kueppers, Harald Kugel, Waldemar Kohl, Jochen Bauer, and Patricia Ohrmann. "Theory of mind in patients with schizophrenia: is mentalizing delayed?" *Schizophr Res* 137, no 1–3 (2012): 224–29. https://doi.org/10.1016/j.schres.2012.02.022.

[82] Oliveira, Sandra E. H., Francisco Esteves, and Helena Carvalho. "Clinical profiles of stigma experiences, self-esteem and social relationships among people with schizophrenia, depressive, and bipolar disorders." *Psychiatry Res* 229, no 1–2 (2015): 167–73. https://doi.org/10.1016/j.psychres.2015.07.047.

[83] Rahman, A., A. Nag, and A. K. Bairagi. "A Hybrid Model for Recognizing Human Activity Using Extreme Learning." *2023 26th International Conference on Computer and Information Technology (ICCIT)*, Cox's Bazar, Bangladesh, 2023, pp. 1–6, doi: 10.1109/ICCIT60459.2023.10441574.

[84] Gaudiano, B. A., and I. W. Miller. "Patients' expectancies, the alliance in pharmacotherapy, and treatment outcomes in bipolar disorder." *J Consult Clin Psychol* 74, no 4 (Aug 2006): 671–6. https://doi.org/10.1037/0022-006X.74.4.671.

[85] Valente, S. M., and B. L. Kennedy. "End the bipolar tug-of-war." *Nurse Pract* 35, no 2 (Feb 2010): 36–45. https://doi.org/10.1097/01.NPR.0000367933.64526.3e.

[86] Manning, J. S. "Tools to improve differential diagnosis of bipolar disorder in primary care." *Prim Care Companion J Clin Psychiatry* 12, no Suppl 1 (2010): 17–22. https://doi.org/10.4088/PCC.9064su1c.03.

[87] Hilty, D. M., D. C. Ferrer, M. B. Parish, B. Johnston, E. J. Callahan, and P. M. Yellowlees. "The effectiveness of telemental health: A 2013 review." *Telemed J E Health* 19, no 6 (Jun 2013): 444–54. https://doi.org/10.1089/tmj.2013.0075.

[88] Bakker, D., N. Kazantzis, D. Rickwood, and N. Rickard. "Mental health smartphone apps: Review and evidence-based recommendations for future developments." *JMIR Ment Health* 3, no 1 (Mar 1 2016): e7. https://doi.org/10.2196/mental.4984.

[89] Lin, H-Y., S-L. Hwang-Gu, and SS-F. Gau. "Intra-individual reaction time variability based on ex-Gaussian distribution as a potential endophenotype for attention-deficit/hyperactivity disorder." *Acta Psychiatrica Scandinavica* 132, no 1 (2015): 39–50. https://doi.org/10.1111/acps.12393.

[90] Nag, A., *et al.* "TumorGANet: A transfer learning and generative adversarial network- based data augmentation model for brain tumor classification." *IEEE Access* 12 (2024): 103060–103081. doi: 10.1109/ACCESS.2024.3429633.

[91] Feigin, Valery L., Theo Vos, Emma Nichols, Mayowa O. Owolabi, William M. Carroll, Martin Dichgans, Günther Deuschl, *et al.* "The global burden of neurological disorders: Translating evidence into policy." *Lancet Neurol* 19, no 3 (2020): 255–65. https://doi.org/10.1016/S1474-4422(19)30411-9.

[92] Corrigan, Patrick. "How stigma interferes with mental health care." *Am Psychol* 59, no 7 (2004): 614. https://doi.org/10.1037/0003-066X.59.7.614.

[93] Corrigan, Patrick W., Jonathon E. Larson, and Nicolas Ruesch. "Self-stigma and the 'why try' effect: Impact on life goals and evidence-based practices." *World Psychiatry* 8, no 2 (2009): 75. https://doi.org/10.1002/j.2051-5545.2009.tb00218.x.

[94] O'Reilly, F., F. Finnan, S. Allwright, G. D. Smith, and Y. Ben-Shlomo. "The effects of caring for a spouse with Parkinson's disease on social, psychological and physical well-being." *Br J Gen Pract* 46, no 410 (Sep 1996): 507–12. www.ncbi.nlm.nih.gov/pubmed/8917868.

[95] Deimling, Gary T., and David M. Bass. "Symptoms of mental impairment among elderly adults and their effects on family caregivers." *J Gerontol* 41, no 6 (1986): 778–84. https://doi.org/10.1093/geronj/41.6.778.

[96] Haley, W. E., E. G. Levine, S. L. Brown, J. W. Berry, and G. H. Hughes. "Psychological, social, and health consequences of caring for a relative with senile dementia." *J Am Geriatr Soc* 35, no 5 (May 1987): 405–11. https://doi.org/10.1111/j.1532-5415.1987.tb04661.x.

[97] Ninou, A., E. Guthrie, V. Paika, E. Ntountoulaki, B. Tomenson, A. Tatsioni, E. Karagiannopoulou, *et al.* "Illness perceptions of people with long-term conditions are associated with frequent use of the emergency department independent of mental illness and somatic symptom burden." *J Psychosom Res* 81 (Feb 2016): 38–45. https://doi.org/10.1016/j.jpsychores.2016.01.001.

[98] Higgins, J. P., D. G. Altman, P. C. Gotzsche, P. Juni, D. Moher, A. D. Oxman, J. Savovic, *et al.* "The Cochrane Collaboration's tool for assessing risk of bias in randomised trials." *BMJ* 343 (Oct 18 2011): d5928. https://doi.org/10.1136/bmj.d5928.

[99] Kessler, R. C., P. Berglund, O. Demler, R. Jin, K. R. Merikangas, and E. E. Walters. "Lifetime prevalence and age-of-onset distributions of DSM-IV disorders in the National Comorbidity Survey Replication." *Arch Gen Psychiatry* 62, no 6 (Jun 2005): 593–602. https://doi.org/10.1001/archpsyc.62.6.593.

[100] Stewart, Walter F., Judith A. Ricci, Elsbeth Chee, David Morganstein, and Richard Lipton. "Lost productive time and cost due to common pain conditions in the US workforce." *JAMA* 290, no 18 (2003): 2443–54. https://doi.org/10.1001/jama.290.18.2443.

[101] Ahuja, Abhimanyu S. "The impact of artificial intelligence in medicine on the future role of the physician." *PeerJ* 7 (2019): e7702. https://doi.org/10.7717/peerj.7702.

[102] Yao, Z., H. Wang, W. Yan, Z. Wang, W. Zhang, Z. Wang, and G. Zhang. "Artificial intelligence-based diagnosis of Alzheimer's disease with brain MRI images." *Eur J Radiol* 165 (Aug 2023): 110934. https://doi.org/10.1016/j.ejrad.2023.110934.

[103] Gan, L., X. Yin, J. Huang, and B. Jia. "Transcranial Doppler analysis based on computer and artificial intelligence for acute cerebrovascular disease." *Math Biosci Eng* 20, no 2 (Jan 2023): 1695–715. https://doi.org/10.3934/mbe.2023077.

[104] Kumar, Y., A. Koul, R. Singla, and M. F. Ijaz. "Artificial intelligence in disease diagnosis: A systematic literature review, synthesizing framework and future research agenda." *J Ambient Intell Humaniz Comput* 14, no 7 (2023): 8459–86. https://doi.org/10.1007/s12652-021-03612-z.

[105] Surianarayanan, C., J. J. Lawrence, P. R. Chelliah, E. Prakash, and C. Hewage. "Convergence of artificial intelligence and neuroscience towards the diagnosis of neurological disorders-A scoping review." *Sensors (Basel)* 23, no 6 (Mar 13 2023): 3062. https://doi.org/10.3390/s23063062.

[106] Hosny, A., C. Parmar, J. Quackenbush, L. H. Schwartz, and Hjwl Aerts. "Artificial intelligence in radiology." *Nat Rev Cancer* 18, no 8 (Aug 2018): 500–10. https://doi.org/10.1038/s41568-018-0016-5.

[107] Monsour, R., M. Dutta, A. Z. Mohamed, A. Borkowski, and N. A. Viswanadhan. "Neuroimaging in the era of artificial intelligence: Current applications." *Fed Pract* 39, no Suppl 1 (Apr 2022): S14–S20. https://doi.org/10.12788/fp.0231.

[108] Segato, Alice, Aldo Marzullo, Francesco Calimeri, and Elena De Momi. "Artificial intelligence for brain diseases: A systematic review." *APL Bioeng* 4, no 4 (2020). https://doi.org/10.1063/5.0011697.

[109] Johnson, Kevin B., Wei-Qi Wei, Dilhan Weeraratne, Mark E. Frisse, Karl Misulis, Kyu Rhee, Juan Zhao, and Jane L. Snowdon. "Precision medicine, AI, and the future of personalized health care." *Clin Transl Sci* 14, no 1 (2021): 86–93. https://doi.org/10.1111/cts.12884.

[110] Jadczyk, Tomasz, Wojciech Wojakowski, Michal Tendera, Timothy D. Henry, Gregory Egnaczyk, and Satya Shreenivas. "Artificial intelligence can improve patient management at the time of a pandemic: the role of voice technology." *J Med Internet Res* 23, no 5 (2021): e22959. https://doi.org/10.2196/22959.

[111] Minen, Mia T., and Eric J. Stieglitz. "Wearables for neurologic conditions: Considerations for our patients and research limitations." *Neurol Clin Pract* 11, no 4 (2021): e537–e43. https://doi.org/10.1212/CPJ.0000000000000971.

[112] van Uem, J. M., T. Isaacs, A. Lewin, E. Bresolin, D. Salkovic, A. J. Espay, H. Matthews, and W. Maetzler. "A viewpoint on wearable technology-enabled measurement of wellbeing and health-related quality of life in Parkinson's disease." *J Parkinsons Dis* 6, no 2 (Mar 10 2016): 279–87. https://doi.org/10.3233/JPD-150740.

[113] Bianchi, M. T. "Sleep devices: wearables and nearables, informational and interventional, consumer and clinical." *Metabolism* 84 (Jul 2018): 99–108. https://doi.org/10.1016/j.mabol.2017.10.008.

[114] Torous, John, Jorge Rodriguez, and Adam Powell. "The new digital divide for digital biomarkers." *Digital Biomarkers* 1, no 1 (2017): 87–91. https://doi.org/10.1159/000477382.

[115] Emsley, Robin, Bonginkosi Chiliza, Laila Asmal, and Brian H. Harvey. "The nature of relapse in schizophrenia." *BMC Psychiatry* 13 (2013): 1–8. https://doi.org/10.1186/1471-244X-13-50.

[116] Barnett, Ian, John Torous, Patrick Staples, Luis Sandoval, Matcheri Keshavan, and Jukka-Pekka Onnela. "Relapse prediction in schizophrenia through digital phenotyping: a pilot study." *Neuropsychopharmacology* 43, no 8 (2018): 1660–66. https://doi.org/10.1038/s41386-018-0030-z

[117] Dumurgier, J., and C. Tzourio. "Epidemiology of neurological diseases in older adults." *Rev Neurol (Paris)* 176, no 9 (Nov 2020): 642–48. https://doi.org/10.1016/j.neurol.2020.01.356.

[118] Beghi, Ettore, Giorgia Giussani, Emma Nichols, Foad Abd-Allah, Jemal Abdela, Ahmed Abdelalim, Haftom Niguse Abraha, *et al.* "Global, regional, and national burden of epilepsy, 1990–2016: a systematic analysis for the Global Burden of Disease Study 2016." *Lancet Neurol* 18, no 4 (2019): 357–75. https://doi.org/10.1016/s1474-4422(18)30454-x.

[119] Dominguez-Fernandez, C., J. Egiguren-Ortiz, J. Razquin, M. Gomez-Galan, L. De Las Heras-Garcia, E. Paredes-Rodriguez, E. Astigarraga, C. Miguelez, and G. Barreda-Gomez. "Review of technological challenges in personalised medicine and early diagnosis of neurodegenerative disorders." *Int J Mol Sci* 24, no 4 (Feb 7 2023): 3321. https://doi.org/10.3390/ijms24043321.

[120] Dickerson, Bradford C., Akram Bakkour, David H. Salat, Eric Feczko, Jenni Pacheco, Douglas N. Greve, Fran Grodstein, *et al.* "The cortical signature of Alzheimer's disease: regionally specific cortical thinning relates

to symptom severity in very mild to mild AD dementia and is detectable in asymptomatic amyloid-positive individuals." *Cerebral Cortex* 19, no 3 (2009): 497–510. https://doi.org/10.1093/cercor/bhn113.

[121] Blin, P., C. Dureau-Pournin, A. Foubert-Samier, A. Grolleau, E. Corbillon, J. Jové, R. Lassalle, *et al.* "Parkinson's disease incidence and prevalence assessment in F rance using the national healthcare insurance database." *Eur J Neurol* 22, no 3 (2015): 464–71. https://doi.org/10.1111/ene.12592.

[122] Pavese, N., and Y. F. Tai. "Nigrosome imaging and neuromelanin sensitive MRI in diagnostic evaluation of Parkinsonism." *Mov Disord Clin Pract* 5, no 2 (Mar-Apr 2018): 131–40. https://doi.org/10.1002/mdc3.12590.

[123] Zeleňák, Kamil, Antonín Krajina, Lukas Meyer, Jens Fiehler, ESMINT Artificial Intelligence, Robotics Ad hoc Committee, Daniel Behme, *et al.* "How to improve the management of acute ischemic stroke by modern technologies, artificial intelligence, and new treatment methods." *Life* 11, no 6 (2021): 488. https://doi.org/10.3390/life11060488.

Chapter 3

Advancing explainable AI in healthcare methods, applications, and ethical implications

Swagata Ashwani

3.1 INTRODUCTION

Healthcare is significantly transformed by AI positively impacting patient care, diagnostics, and treatment methods with the potential to enhance the precision and efficiency of medical practices significantly. The need for Explainable AI (XAI) has emerged as a growing concern with the emergence of AI systems becoming ubiquitous [1]. The AI decision-making process needs to be transparent and interpretable in all fields and more so in healthcare as the implications and ramifications in healthcare are profound [2]. Transparent and Explainable AI decision-making is critical for enabling trust in the medical system and enabling healthcare professionals to feel confident about patient outcomes. AI algorithms tend to be complex, especially those based on deep learning as they tend to be opaque, making it challenging to comprehend the process of decision making. Given the challenges of understanding the decision-making progress, healthcare professionals as well as patients are wary of adopting AI technologies [3].

Therefore, developing XAI methods that are user-friendly and tailored to the expertise of healthcare practitioners is paramount. Such methods should facilitate actionable insights, enabling clinicians to comprehend AI recommendations and integrate them effectively in decision-making.

The ethical implications of deploying XAI in any field, more so in healthcare cannot be undermined. While deploying XAI, one must consider addressing the most critical issues such as relating to fairness, transparency, and accountability, as that is the only way to ensure usage of AI systems responsibly and equitably [4]. We must foster an ecosystem and an environment where humans and AI capabilities are collaborating and complementing each other and not competing against each other. This will ensure the explainability of AI systems can be further enhanced and we can navigate the ethical landscape more effectively. This collaboration is crucial for being assured that AI-assisted decisions align well with the values and needs of patients, thus reinforcing the human-centric nature of healthcare [5]. As we explore the advancements in XAI methods and their

DOI: 10.1201/9781003591085-3

applications in healthcare, this chapter will emphasize the importance of the integration of various ethical considerations into designing, developing and implementing AI technologies. By focusing on patient-centered outcomes and the collaborative potential of AI and human expertise, we can envisage a future where XAI becomes an indispensable tool in healthcare resulting in improved patient care and outcomes.

We are witnessing the development of precision algorithms with the advancements of AI in healthcare. These algorithms are adept at analyzing massive amounts of data that include electronic medical records, patient data, and medical images. These systems have demonstrated enhanced capabilities in the field of healthcare related to the diagnosis of disease, prediction of risks, and treatment planning. However, with the increasing complexity of the AI systems, it is getting harder for the inventor of these systems to comprehend how decisions are reached making the AI systems a black box. This lack of transparency poses significant challenges in healthcare, where there is no room for error and the aftermath of any such incorrect decisions could be life-threatening. Clinicians need to understand the rationale behind AI recommendations to validate them against their medical knowledge and experience. Patients, too, have a right to understand the factors influencing their diagnosis and treatment plans. XAI addresses these challenges by providing methods to interpret and explain AI decisions in a manner that is comprehensible to both healthcare professionals and patients.

The implementation of XAI in healthcare extends beyond mere technical solutions. It encompasses a broader approach to AI development and deployment that prioritizes interpretability from the outset. This approach involves designing AI systems with built-in explainability features, developing user interfaces that effectively communicate AI insights, and establishing protocols for integrating XAI into clinical workflows. XAI plays a critical role in addressing ethical concerns surrounding AI in healthcare. By providing transparency, XAI can help in the identification and mitigation of biases in AI systems, assuring fair delivery and fair care across diverse patient populations. It also supports the principle of informed consent by enabling patients to understand how AI influences their treatment planning and care by making informed decisions.

As we dig deeper into the world of XAI in healthcare, this chapter will explore the various methods and techniques used to enhance AI explainability, their applications across different medical domains, and the challenges and opportunities they present. We will examine case studies that present the practical implementation of XAI in healthcare settings, highlighting both successes and areas for improvement. Readers will gain a fair understanding of the current state of XAI in healthcare as they finish reading this chapter and also understand the potential of XAI to revolutionize patient care, and the critical considerations for its responsible and effective implementation [6]. As we continue to advance in this field, the goal remains clear: exploit AI for improvement in healthcare results while maintaining the trust, transparency, and ethical standards that are fundamental to the practice of medicine.

3.1.1 Key contribution

This chapter brings forth several important aspects with respect to the discussion around Explainable Artificial Intelligence (XAI) in the setting of healthcare. It also notes how XAI's role is particularly significant in garnering trust and transparency, which is central to the engagement of both clinicians and patients in AI-powered decision systems. In this way, the chapter illustrates how XAI can be an effective means of enhancing comprehension and acceptance of AI in the healthcare environment.

Apart from this, the chapter also discusses the most popular XAI methods, including LIME, SHAP, Integrated Gradients, and Concept Activation Vectors among others. Each of these approaches is presented in detail because they are believed to be useful in multiple surroundings in healthcare. The chapter discusses how these methods could be applied to the interpretation of complex AI models in order to give healthcare practitioners a better understanding of how AI systems make decisions.

The chapter also discusses the social challenges relating to the application of XAI in healthcare settings including issues dealing with fairness, responsibility, and patient rights. It stresses the necessity for diverse perspectives to identify and reduce the biases for the efficient use of AI in clinical settings. Such a concern with ethics gives rise to the necessity of AI systems that are transparent with respect to the rights and autonomy of the patient while also ensuring responsibility.

The chapter uses such real-life cases to prove the practicality of the integration of XAI into the clinical workflow as well as the complexities involved in the process. Instances from radiology, personalized medicine, and emergency care all demonstrate the diversity of XAI applications in various areas of healthcare. Such case studies show not only how XAI was implemented by practitioners but also the problems that were encountered in the process and the best ways to use XAI in clinical practice.

In addition, the chapter also presents some contemporary issues that warrant further research and how such issues have been addressed in the existing literature. It identifies the need for more contextualized and rigorous feasible XAI measures and issues of trade-offs between the interpretability of the model and its prediction ability. These research gaps narrow down the scope of various future studies to various possibilities that can help in uplifting XAI in health sector research.

The chapter has been presented in a sequential manner with clear transitions from one idea to another. The introduction brings out the relevance of XAI in the area of health seeking to explain the functionality of

XAI in enhancing trust, transparency, and AI ethics. After this, a comprehensive overview of various XAI methods such as LIME, SHAP, Integrated Gradients and Concept Activation Vectors is given, while highlighting their particular use cases and constraints within healthcare environments. The chapter then delves into the use of XAI patterns in disease diagnosis, recommending treatments, predicting risk, and analyzing medical images with appealing examples and case studies on these issues.

Ethics such as bias, accountability, lack of autonomy, and patient rights come last but are some of the most critical aspects regarding the application of XAI in the healthcare context. Use cases of XAI in clinical settings include radiology, precision medicine, and emergency medicine where some of the achievements, problems and lessons learnt in XAI adoption are discussed. To complete this, the chapter outlines the most significant and allowing research gaps for further development, including cross-discipline integration, policy issues and areas of future development in the XAI domain.

As a last note, the chapter restates its conclusions with special emphasis on the significance of XAI in the overall improvement of clinical AI solutions, highlighting their compliance, governance, and ethical aspects in the scope of healthcare. It provides a roadmap for future research and highlights the need for continued exploration of XAI techniques, ethical concerns, and practical applications in clinical settings.

3.2 EXPLAINABLE AI METHODS IN HEALTHCARE

Accountability in AI-driven decision-making processes is emerging as critical in healthcare for enhancing trust and understanding, and thus the need for integrating Explainable AI. This section explores several prominent XAI methods, including LIME, SHAP, Integrated Gradients, and Concept Activation Vectors, and compares their effectiveness and applicability in healthcare contexts. Figure 3.1 provides an overview of the landscape of model explainability within the healthcare domain. It categorizes different Explainable AI (XAI) methods based on their interpretability, transparency, and applicability to various healthcare applications. The diagram illustrates how methods such as LIME, SHAP, Integrated Gradients, and Concept Activation Vectors are positioned in relation to model complexity and the level of interpretability they provide, highlighting the trade-offs between model complexity and explainability.

3.2.1 How well humans can understand AI decisions

It is extremely important to understand the degree to which humans can understand decisions made by AI before we dive deep into the different Explainable AI methods.

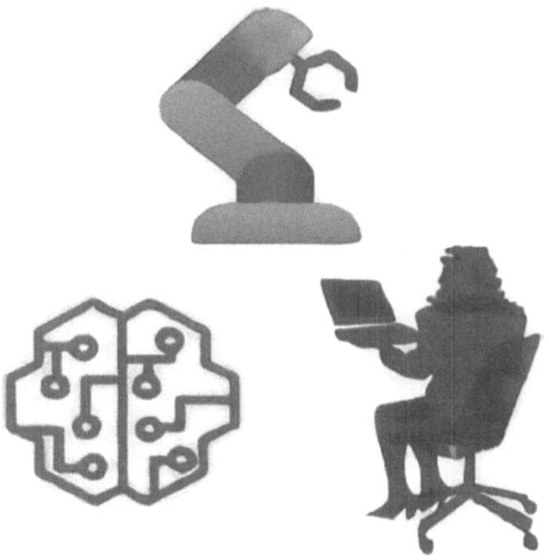

Figure 3.1 Model Explainability Landscape.

Understanding AI decisions is important for nurturing trust, enabling collaboration, and ensuring accountability as illustrated in Figure 3.1. However, AI systems—specifically complex machine learning models like neural networks—operate opaque to humans with little knowledge of the decision-making progress. The level of understanding varies based on several factors:

- **Complexity of the Model:** Simpler models like decision trees or linear regression offer straightforward interpretations, while more advanced models like deep learning networks, ensemble methods, and reinforcement learning systems can be difficult to interpret.
- **Domain Expertise:** Even if AI outputs are made explainable, users still need domain knowledge to understand the context of the decisions.
- **Cognitive Load:** Complex explanations can overwhelm users, reducing the usability of the insights AI offers. The goal is to balance interpretability with accuracy to make AI decisions understandable but also meaningful in practice.

3.2.2 How to foster trust and transparency in AI

In the healthcare domain where room for error is near zero, the cornerstones of AI adoption are transparency in the AI process of decision-making and trust in the systems incorporating AI. AI systems are increasingly making critical decisions, so it's essential that users—whether they are data scientists, policymakers, or end-users—trust the decisions the AI makes.

- **Trust:** For users to trust AI, they need to believe that its decisions are **accurate, fair, and unbiased.** Trust also depends on AI's ability to explain how it arrived at certain conclusions, providing insights into its decision-making process. Trust extends beyond accuracy and includes understanding if the AI behaves ethically and in line with societal norms.
- **Transparency:** Transparency involves making the workings of the AI system visible and explainable to the relevant stakeholders. This includes both technical and non-technical users. Transparency can be achieved through explainability (discussed in Section 3.2.3), auditability (allowing third parties to review AI processes), and clearly explaining the limitations and risks of AI systems.

  Transparency ensures that AI decisions are not only explainable but also accountable. Stakeholders should be able to trace decisions back to their source—whether it's an algorithm or data input—so that biases, errors, or faults can be identified and corrected.

3.2.3 Intrinsic vs. post-hoc explainability

Explainability is central to trust and transparency, as it allows humans a deep understanding of the process of decisions motivated by AI-composed systems. There are two kinds of explainability—intrinsic and post-hoc categories:

3.2.3.1 *Intrinsic explainability*

Models that are easy to interpret due to their design are classified as intrinsic. These models are transparent by nature meaning the decision-making process can be interpreted directly. Examples of intrinsically explainable models include:

- Linear Regression: The weights of the variables can be directly understood as the contribution made by each feature to the prediction-making process.
- Decision Trees: The process of making decisions is structured into a tree-like model where the reasoning behind decisions can be easily visualized. This can be seen in Figure 3.2.
- Rule-based Systems: Predefined set of rules that humans can follow and interpret the decision made by the AI-based system.

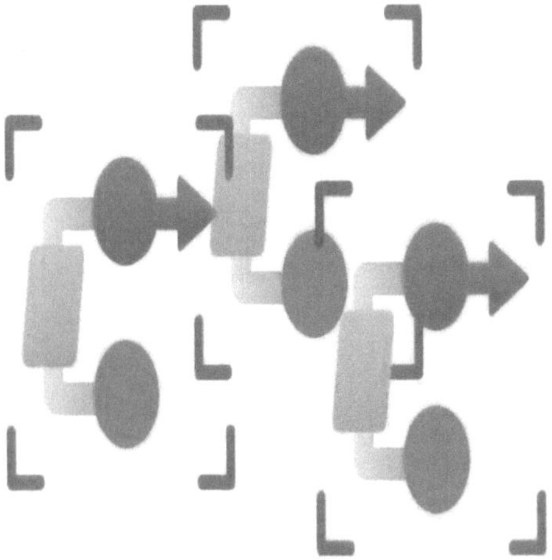

Figure 3.2 Decision Trees – Intrinsic Explainability Model.

3.2.4 LIME (Local Interpretable Model-agnostic Explanations)

LIME is a technique that explains the predictions made by any of the models in a local, interpretable manner. It is designed to work by using an interpretable model to approximate the complicated model that is simple and in the vicinity of the prediction being explained. This method is particularly useful in healthcare, where understanding the rationale behind AI predictions can significantly influence clinical decisions [7].

Key steps in LIME are depicted with an example in Figure 3.3.

- Selection of Data Point to explain.
  Perturbation.
- Model Prediction using the original model.
- Weight Assignment based on proximity.
- Local Model Training for new data points.
- Explanation Extraction from the simpler model.

Key Features of LIME:

- Model-agnostic: LIME can be applied to any machine learning model and does not require any modifications to the model.
- Local Interpretability: It focuses on explaining individual predictions and does not focus on explaining the overall model behavior thus making it suitable for case-specific insights.

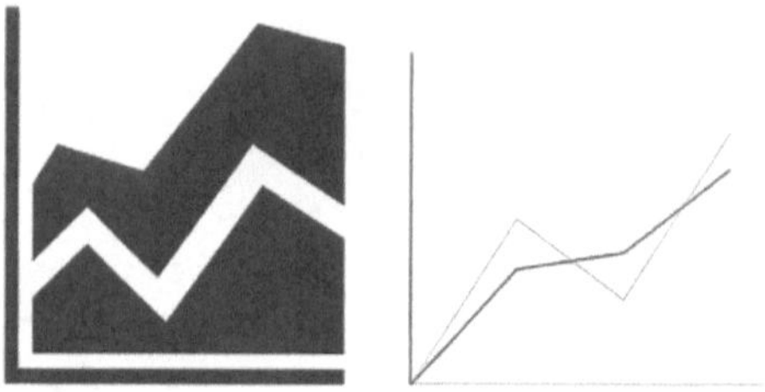

Figure 3.3 LIME Example.

Simplicity: By approximating complex models with simpler interpretable models (like linear models), LIME provides insights that are easier for healthcare professionals to understand [8].

Application in Healthcare:
LIME has been successfully applied in several healthcare scenarios, such as in predicting patient outcomes and isolating relevant features in medical imaging. For instance, it can help explain why a particular patient was classified as high risk for a disease, allowing clinicians to validate the model's reasoning against their medical knowledge.

3.2.5 SHAP (SHapley Additive exPlanations)

The SHAP technique is often used to interpret cooperative game theory-based model predictions. To provide a thorough understanding of the various ways in which distinct features affect the model's output, it gives each feature an important value for a specific prediction [9].

The key flow of SHAP is depicted with an example in Figure 3.4(a) and an example of SHAP value visualization is shown in Figure 3.4(b).

For a given instance, all possible subsets of features will be considered.

For each subset, the model's prediction will be compared with and without a particular feature.

Average these differences across all subsets to compute the SHAPLEY values for that feature.

Key Features of SHAP:

- Theoretical Foundation: SHAP is derived from Shapley values in cooperative game theory, ensuring fair and consistent feature attribution.
- Global and Local Interpretability: SHAP can provide insights at both the individual prediction level and the overall model level [10].

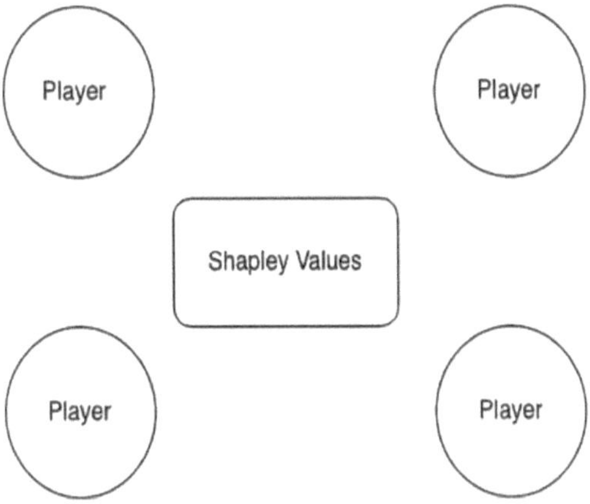

Figure 3.4(a) SHAP Example.

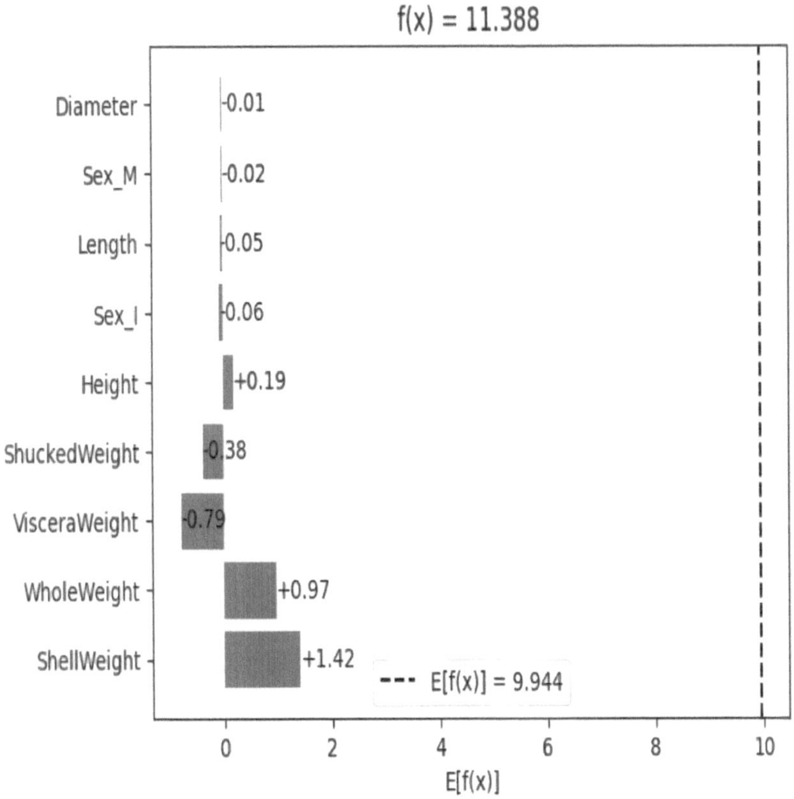

Figure 3.4(b) Example of SHAP Value Visualization.

3.2.6 Integrated gradients

Integrated Gradients attribute the output of a model to its input features to provide an explanation for deep learning models [11]. In order to integrate these gradients along a straight line from a baseline input to the actual input, the output gradients are computed in relation to the input features [12].
Key Features of Integrated Gradients:

- Deep Learning Focus: Specifically designed for deep learning models, making it suitable for complex healthcare applications like medical image analysis.
- Sensitivity: It considers the model output sensitivity to changes in input features, and thus provides insights into features that significantly impact predictions.
- Baseline Reference: The choice of a baseline input allows flexibility in understanding model behavior under different scenarios.

Integrated Gradients have been effectively used in medical imaging tasks, such as identifying regions of interest in radiological images. By highlighting which parts of an image contributed most to a diagnosis, this method enhances the interpretability of deep learning models in clinical practice.

3.2.7 Concept Activation Vectors (CAVs)

Concept Activation Vectors (CAVs) are a method for interpreting neural networks by associating specific concepts with their activations in the network. This technique allows for the examination of how certain high-level concepts influence model predictions [13].
Key Features of CAVs:

- Conceptual Understanding: CAVs provide insights into the model's understanding of specific concepts, such as "tumor" or "healthy tissue" in medical images.
- Layer-wise Interpretability: By analyzing activations at different layers of the network,

CAVs can reveal how concepts are represented throughout the model.

- Interactive Exploration: CAVs enable users to explore and visualize how different concepts affect predictions, facilitating a deeper understanding of model behavior.

3.2.8 Comparison of XAI methods in healthcare contexts

The selection of the XAI method depends on factors including specific healthcare applications, model complexity, and the need for interpretability.

Table 3.1 Summary of Key Characteristics and Applications of XAI Methods

XAI Method	*Key Features*	*Healthcare Applications*	*Strengths*	*Limitations*
LIME	Local interpretability, model-agnostic	Risk prediction, patient outcome analysis	Simple explanations, flexible	May not capture global model behavior
SHAP	Fair feature attribution, global/local insights	Disease progression, treatment response prediction	Comprehensive insights, strong theoretical foundation	Computationally intensive for large datasets
Integrated Gradients	Gradient-based, deep learning focus	Medical image analysis, pathology	Effective for deep learning models	Requires careful selection of baseline input
Concept Activation Vectors	Conceptual understanding, layer-wise analysis	Pathology, radiology	Reveals model's conceptual reasoning	May require extensive training data

Table 3.1 summarizes the key characteristics and applications of the discussed methods.

3.3 XAI APPLICATION IN HEALTHCARE

Explainable AI (XAI) has the wherewithal to transform healthcare by making improvements in various aspects such as improving the diagnosis of a disease and recommending the right treatment and predicting risks. This section explores the applications of XAI in these critical areas, highlighting how it can enhance trust and transparency in clinical care which are the cornerstone of any AI system.

3.3.1 Disease diagnosis

Accurate and timely disease diagnosis is essential for effective patient care. XAI methods can play a key role in assisting clinicians by furnishing insights into the reasoning behind AI-driven diagnoses. By understanding the factors that contribute to diagnosis, healthcare professionals can validate the decision-making process of the AI system by comparing it against their own medical expertise, fostering trust and collaboration between human and machine intelligence [14].

LIME can be particularly useful in disease diagnosis by providing local explanations for individual predictions. For example, in diagnosing heart disease, LIME can highlight the specific features (e.g., age, cholesterol levels, blood pressure) that contributed most to the AI's prediction for a particular patient. The specific information can help clinicians assess the validity of the diagnosis and identify areas where further investigation may be necessary. SHAP (Shapley Additive explanations) can aid in differential diagnosis by providing a comprehensive view of how various factors contribute to the likelihood of different diseases. By ranking the importance of symptoms, test results, and other relevant features, SHAP can help narrow down the list of potential diagnoses and guide clinicians toward the most likely condition. This can be particularly useful in complex cases where multiple diseases present similar symptoms.

3.3.2 Treatment recommendation

Selecting the most appropriate treatment plan is crucial for improving patient outcomes. XAI methods can assist clinicians in understanding the factors that influence treatment recommendations, enabling them to tailor therapies to individual patient needs and preferences [15].

3.3.2.1 Integrated Gradients for personalized treatment

Applying Integrated Gradients to deep learning models can identify the most influential factors in treatment recommendations. For instance, in oncology, Integrated Gradients can help explain which genetic markers or tumor characteristics are most predictive of a patient's response to a particular chemotherapy regimen. Clinicians can make well-informed decisions and facilitate shared decision-making by involving patients in the process by comprehending the rationale behind the AI's treatment recommendations.

3.3.2.2 CAVs for treatment adherence

Concept Activation Vectors (CAVs) can be used to explore how high-level concepts, such as treatment adherence or side effects, influence treatment recommendations. By analyzing the activations of these concepts in the AI model, clinicians can gain insights into the potential barriers to treatment success and develop a game plan to address them. For example, CAVs may reveal that a particular treatment is less likely to be recommended for patients with a history of non-adherence, prompting clinicians to implement interventions to improve adherence and optimize treatment outcomes.

3.3.3 Risk prediction

Predicting the risk of adverse health outcomes is crucial for preventive care and resource allocation. XAI methods can enhance the trust and transparency of risk prediction models, enabling clinicians to identify high-risk patients and implement targeted interventions. LIME can be used to describe the predictions of risk stratification models, helping clinicians understand what are the factors that contribute to a patient's risk profile. For instance, in predicting the risk of hospital readmission, LIME can highlight the specific factors (e.g., comorbidities, length of stay, social determinants of health) that increase a patient's likelihood of being readmitted. This information can guide clinicians in developing personalized discharge plans and post-discharge interventions to mitigate the risk of readmission. SHAP can be employed in chronic disease management to identify the key factors influencing disease progression and risk of complications [16]. By analyzing the SHAP values of various clinical and lifestyle factors, clinicians can prioritize interventions and tailor treatment plans to address the most significant contributors to a patient's risk. For example, in managing type 2 diabetes, SHAP can reveal the relative importance of factors such as diet, physical activity, medication adherence, and comorbidities in predicting the risk of diabetic retinopathy or cardiovascular complications [17].

3.3.4 Medical imaging analysis

AI has shown great promise in analyzing medical images for disease detection, classification, and monitoring. The interpretability of AI systems can be enhanced substantially by XAI methods enabling clinicians to validate their decisions and integrate them into their diagnostic and treatment workflows. Integrated Gradients when applied to DL models can be used for lesion detection in medical images, such as MRI or CT scans [18]. The regions that most contributed to AI's prediction can be highlighted and thus Integrated Gradients can help clinicians verify the accuracy of the lesion detection and assess the model's performance. This method is very useful to detect false positives or false negatives as they can have significant consequences such as in lung cancer screening or brain tumor detection. Concept Activation Vectors can be employed in medical imaging analysis to explore how the AI model's understanding of specific concepts, such as tumor grade or stage, influences its predictions. By analyzing the activations of these concepts in the model, clinicians can gain insights into the reasoning behind the AI's tumor grading or staging decisions. This information can help validate the AI's performance against established clinical guidelines and support clinicians in making informed treatment decisions based on the tumor's characteristics.

Figure 3.5 illustrates how LIME can be used to explain an AI's prediction in disease diagnosis. It can include a sample patient case, the AI's prediction, and a LIME explanation highlighting the most influential features contributing to the diagnosis.

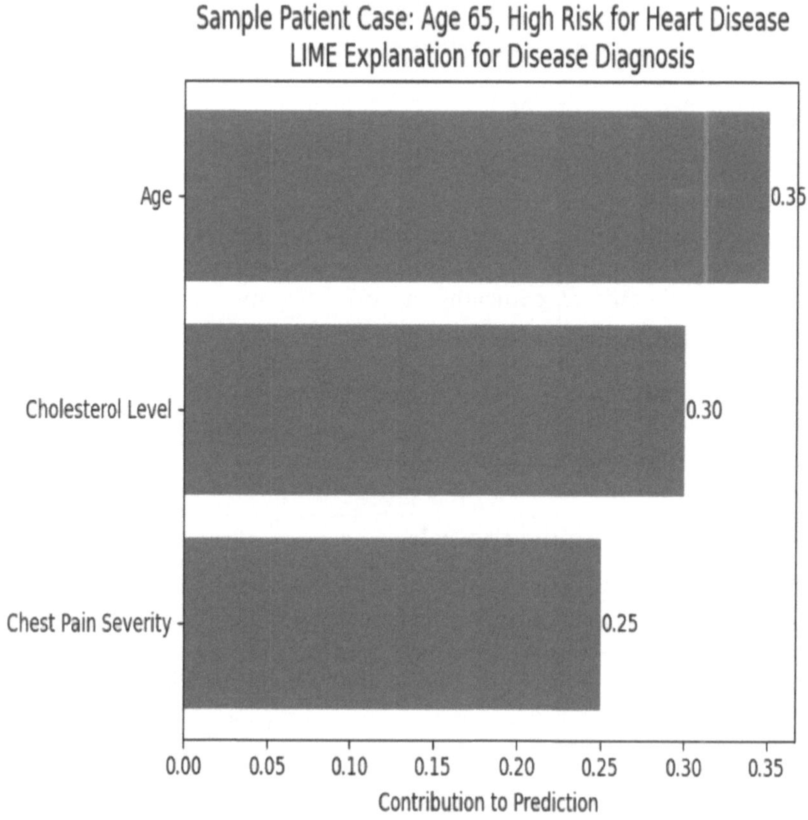

Figure 3.5 Example of LIME Explanation for Disease Diagnosis.

3.3.5 Advanced XAI techniques in healthcare

While the previously discussed methods provide valuable insights, more advanced XAI techniques can offer even deeper understanding of AI models in healthcare. This section explores some of these advanced methods and their specific applications in medical contexts.

3.3.5.1 Shapley Additive Explanations (SHAP) for multi-modal healthcare data

SHAP values are based on cooperative game theory. In healthcare, where data often comes from multiple sources (e.g., electronic health records, imaging, genomics), SHAP can be particularly useful.

Let's consider a model f(x) that predicts heart disease risk based on various factors. The SHAP value for a feature i is calculated as:

$$\varphi_i = \Sigma\left(S \subseteq N \setminus \{i\}\right)\left[|S|!\left(|N| - |S| - 1\right)! / |N|!\right]\left[f\left(S \cup \{i\}\right) - f(S)\right] \quad (3.1)$$

This equation describes the computation of the SHAP (SHapley Additive exPlanations) value for feature iii in a model f(x)f(x)f(x), which predicts the risk of heart disease based on various features (such as age, cholesterol level, blood pressure, etc.). SHAP values are a method to explain the contribution of each feature to the model's prediction for a specific instance by using principles from cooperative game theory, specifically Shapley values.

The Equation 3.1 above is defined where:

- *N* is the set of all features
- *S* is a subset of features
- *f(S)* is the prediction for feature subset *S*

For example, if we have features like age, blood pressure, and cholesterol levels, SHAP values would calculate the contribution of every feature into the final prediction, accounting for feature interactions.
Implementation:

1. Calculate SHAP values for each feature across a population of patients.
2. Identify the most significant contributors to heart disease risk.
3. Create personalized risk profiles and intervention strategies based on individual SHAP values.

3.3.5.2 Integrated Gradients for medical imaging analysis

Integrated Gradients (IG) is a gradient-based attribution method that can be particularly useful in medical imaging analysis. It satisfies the sensitivity and implementation invariance axioms, making it a reliable choice for explaining deep learning models in radiology.

The Equation 3.2 integrated gradient for the i-th feature is defined as:

$$IG_i(x) = \left(x_i - x_i'\right) \times \int\left(\alpha = 0 to 1\right)\left[\partial F\left(x' + \alpha\left(x - x'\right)\right) / \partial x_i\right] d\alpha \quad (3.2)$$

The Integrated Gradients (IG) method is a gradient-based technique designed to attribute the contribution of each feature (such as pixels in an image) to the output of a deep learning model. It is widely used in medical imaging analysis, particularly in fields like radiology, where understanding the model's decisions can be critical for diagnosis and treatment.

Where:

- x is the input image
- x' is the baseline image (usually a black image)
- F is the model's output
- α is the interpolation factor

In practice, this integral is approximated using a summation: $IG_i(x)$ is given by the Equation 3.3 ≈

$$\left(x_i - x_i'\right) \times \Sigma\left(k = 1\,to\,m\right)\left[\frac{\partial F\left(x' + \frac{k}{m} \times \left(x - x'\right)\right)}{\partial x_i}\right] \times \frac{1}{m} \tag{3.3}$$

The Integrated Gradients (IG) method is a powerful tool in medical imaging, particularly for interpreting deep learning models used in tasks like detecting pneumonia from chest X-rays. IG works by attributing the difference in the model's output between the actual input and a baseline (e.g., a black image) to each feature (e.g., pixels in an image). This attribution is achieved by calculating the integral of the gradients along the path from the baseline to the input image.

Implementation in medical imaging:

1. Apply IG to a CNN trained on chest X-rays for pneumonia detection.
2. Generate attribution maps highlighting regions most influential to the model's decision.
3. Overlay these maps on original images to guide radiologists' attention.

3.3.5.3 Concept Activation Vectors (CAVs) for interpretable genomics

CAVs allow us to interpret neural networks using human-friendly concepts. This can be particularly useful in genomics, where understanding the relationship between genetic patterns and high-level biological concepts is crucial.

To compute a CAV for a concept C:

1. Gather positive and negative examples of C.
2. Train a linear classifier to distinguish between these examples in the activation space of a chosen layer.

3. The vector normal to the decision boundary of this classifier is the CAV for C.

The conceptual sensitivity score *S(C,k,l)* for a concept *C*, class *k*, and layer *l* is defined by Equation 3.4 below:

$$S(C,k,l) = \left|\partial h\_k(l) / \partial l\right| \cdot v\_C \tag{3.4}$$

The Conceptual Sensitivity Score S(C,k,l)S(C,k,l)S(C,k,l) provides a way to measure the influence of a specific concept CCC on a model's prediction for a particular class kkk at a particular layer lll in the model. This score quantifies the sensitivity of the model's prediction with respect to the presence or absence of a concept, such as gene expression patterns in genomics. It is a useful tool for understanding how high-level concepts impact the predictions of deep learning models, especially in domains like genomics where concepts such as gene expression can be critical for predicting disease risk or drug response.

Where:

- *h_k(l)* is the logit for class *k*
- *v_C* is the CAV for concept *C*

Implementation in genomics:

1. Define concepts like "gene expression patterns associated with cancer."
2. Compute CAVs for these concepts using a dataset of gene expression profiles.
3. Calculate conceptual sensitivity scores to understand how model's predictions of cancer risk or drug response are influenced by these concepts.

3.3.5.4 Counterfactual explanations for treatment recommendations

Counterfactual explanations provide insights into how a model's output is affected by the changes in the input features. This can be particularly valuable in treatment recommendation systems.

To generate a counterfactual explanation:

1. Start with the original input *x* and desired output *y'*
2. Find *x'* that minimizes:

$$L(x,x')+\lambda \cdot l(f(x'),y') \tag{3.5}$$

Counterfactual explanations help in understanding how a model's output could change if certain input features were altered. In the context of treatment recommendation systems, counterfactuals can show how modifying certain patient characteristics (e.g., changing a medication dosage or symptom severity) might lead to a different treatment recommendation.

The above is the definition of Equation 3.5 where L is a distance metric, l is a loss function, and λ is a hyperparameter.

Implementation in treatment recommendation:

1. For a patient not recommended for a specific treatment, generate counterfactuals showing what changes would lead to a positive recommendation.
2. Provide clinicians with actionable insights, e.g., "If the patient's HbA1c level was 1% lower, the model would recommend treatment X."

3.3.5.5 *Anchors for robust clinical decision support*

Anchors provide high-precision rules that "anchor" a model's prediction. This is particularly useful in clinical decision support systems where clear, reliable rules are necessary.

An anchor *A(x)* is a rule that satisfies and is defined by Equation 3.6:

$$E[P(f(z)=f(x)) \mid A(x)=A(z)] \geq \tau \tag{3.6}$$

Anchors are an interpretable method used to provide high-precision rules that explain a model's prediction. These rules are particularly useful in fields like clinical decision support systems, where reliability and transparency are critical for decision-making. Anchors act as if-then rules that "anchor" the prediction of the model, meaning that when certain conditions (features) are satisfied, the model's prediction remains stable and unchanged, even when other aspects of the input data are perturbed.

Where:

- x is the instance being explained
- z is a perturbed version of x
- τ is a user-defined threshold (e.g., 0.95)

Implementation in clinical decision support:

1. Generate anchors for critical care decisions, e.g., "IF blood_pressure < 90 AND heart_rate > 120 THEN recommend_immediate_intervention."
2. Validate these rules with clinicians to ensure they align with medical knowledge and protocols.
3. Use anchors as a first-line explanation, backed up by more detailed methods like SHAP or LIME when necessary.

By implementing these advanced XAI techniques, healthcare AI systems can provide more nuanced, reliable, and actionable explanations, fostering greater trust and effectiveness in clinical settings.

3.4 ETHICAL IMPLICATIONS OF XAI IN HEALTHCARE

As AI continues to permeate healthcare, the ethical implications of its deployment become increasingly critical. Explainable AI (XAI) offers a pathway to address some of these ethical challenges by enhancing transparency, accountability, and trust. This section explores the ethical implications of XAI in healthcare, thereby shifting its focus on fairness and bias mitigation, accountability and transparency, trust between clinicians and AI systems, and informed consent and patient autonomy [19].

3.4.1 Fairness and bias mitigation

Fairness here refers to the principle that AI systems should operate without any sort of discrimination based on various attributes such as nationality, age or economic status. The discrimination should not be against any individual or group on any sensitive attribute. In healthcare, where decisions can significantly impact patient outcomes, ensuring fairness is paramount. Discriminatory practices can lead to unequal access to care, misdiagnosis, and inaccurate treatment recommendations [20].

Bias in AI can be due to many sources, including:

- Data Bias: If the data used for training the model is skewed and is not a fair representation of the sample, the AI model will be trained on data that is biased. For example, if a model has been trained on data from a specific section of age, race, ethnicity, or demographic group, it may perform poorly for underrepresented groups.
- Algorithmic Bias: If the algorithms are designed without consideration for fairness, the algorithms can introduce bias. For example, a risk prediction model may inadvertently prioritize certain features that correlate with specific demographic attributes.

- Human Bias: Bias can also stem from human decisions made during data collection, feature selection, and model training. If healthcare professionals unconsciously favor certain populations, this bias can be reflected in the AI system.

3.4.1.1 *Mitigating bias with XAI*

XAI can play a key role in the identification and mitigation of bias in healthcare AI systems. By providing interpretable insights into the decision-making process of the AI models, XAI allows stakeholders to scrutinize the factors thereby influencing predictions. This transparency can help identify biased patterns and facilitate corrective measures.

- Feature Importance Analysis: SHAP and LIME are techniques that can reveal which features are driving predictions. If certain features are found to disproportionately influence outcomes for specific demographic groups, stakeholders can take steps to adjust the model or the data used for training.
- Fairness Audits: Regular audits of AI systems can help ensure that they operate fairly across different populations. XAI methods can assist in evaluating model performance across demographic groups, enabling healthcare organizations to identify and address disparities.

3.4.2 Accountability and transparency

In healthcare, accountability is critical to ensure responsible and ethical usage of AI systems. AI systems are designed to make decisions that affect patient care and hence it is critical for the AI system to establish clear accountability for the decisions made. This accountability extends to architects, designers, data scientists, and developers of the AI system, healthcare organizations, and clinicians who utilize the AI systems [21].

Transparency is the ease with which users comprehend the decision made by the AI system. In healthcare, transparency is key for several reasons:

- Informed Decision-Making: Clinicians must understand how AI systems arrive at a decision and use it to make correct decisions about patient care. If an AI system suggests a treatment plan, clinicians should be able to assess the rationale behind that recommendation.
- Regulatory Compliance: Regulatory bodies require transparency in AI systems to meet ethical and legal standards. This includes understanding the data used for training, the algorithms employed, and the potential biases present in the system.

XAI enhances accountability by providing interpretable explanations for AI predictions. This transparency allows stakeholders to trace the reasoning behind decisions, facilitating accountability at multiple levels:

- Clinician Accountability: Clinicians can better understand the AI's recommendations and justify their decisions to patients and regulatory bodies. This accountability is crucial in maintaining trust in the healthcare system.
- Organizational Accountability: Healthcare organizations can be held accountable for the AI systems they deploy. By using XAI methods to audit and evaluate their AI systems, organizations can ensure that they are operating ethically and effectively.

3.4.3 Trust between clinicians and AI systems

Trust is a critical component of the clinician-patient relationship as well as in the interaction involving clinicians and AI systems. For AI to be effectively integrated into healthcare, clinicians must trust the technology and its recommendations. Several factors influence trust in AI systems:

- Accuracy and Reliability: Clinicians majorly trust AI systems that demonstrate high accuracy and reliability in their predictions. Continuous validation and performance monitoring are essential to maintain this trust [22].
- Explainability: Speaks of AI systems' capacity to give clear justifications for the choices they make. XAI methods that offer interpretable insights can help clinicians feel more confident in the AI's recommendations.
- User Experience: User-centric design of AI systems plays a key role in building trust. Intuitive interfaces and seamless integration into clinical workflows can enhance clinicians' willingness to rely on AI.

3.4.3.1 Fostering trust with XAI

XAI can foster trust between clinicians and AI systems by:

- Providing Clear Explanations: XAI methods can generate explanations that clinicians can easily understand, enabling them to assess the validity of AI recommendations.
- Encouraging Collaboration: By framing AI as a collaborative tool rather than a replacement for human expertise, XAI can help clinicians view AI systems as partners in patient care.

- Facilitating Continuous Learning: XAI can support a culture of continuous learning by allowing clinicians to provide fruitful feedback on AI recommendations, thereby significantly improving the system over time.

3.4.4 Informed consent and patient autonomy

Sharing information and seeking consent from patients is a fundamental principle in healthcare that ensures patients understand the risks, benefits, and alternatives of medical procedures and treatments. As AI becomes more integrated into healthcare decision-making, the concept of informed consent must evolve to encompass AI-driven recommendations. Several challenges arise when incorporating AI into the informed consent process:

- Complexity of AI Systems: Complex AI algorithms and AI systems sometimes make it difficult for patients to comprehend the interpretation of their data and how AI influences their care. This complexity can hinder patients' ability to provide informed consent [23].
- Data Privacy Concerns: Patients may have concerns about how their data is captured, collected, stored, and used by AI systems. Ensuring data privacy and security is essential for maintaining patient trust.
- Autonomy in Decision-Making: The utilization of AI in decision-making can raise questions about patient autonomy. Patients may feel that AI recommendations undermine their ability to make informed choices about their care.

XAI can enhance the informed consent process by:

- Simplifying Explanations: XAI methods can provide simplified explanations of how AI systems work and how they impact patient care. Patients can make informed decisions with the help of XAI.
- Empowering Patients: By providing patients with insights into the reasoning behind AI's decision-making, XAI can empower patients to engage in discussions about their care and make choices that align with their values and preferences.
- Addressing Privacy Concerns: XAI can help clarify how patient data is used in AI systems, addressing privacy concerns and fostering trust in the technology.

3.5 CASE STUDIES: IMPLEMENTING XAI IN CLINICAL SETTINGS

As Explainable AI (XAI) continues to make rapid advancements, it is essential to examine its practical implementation in clinical settings. This section presents two case studies to illustrate the application of XAI in radiology and personalized medicine, highlighting the benefits, challenges, and best practices associated with deploying XAI in real-world healthcare scenarios.

3.5.1 Case study 1: XAI in radiology

Radiology is a field where AI has demonstrated tremendous promise in assisting clinicians with tasks such as image interpretation, lesion detection, and diagnosis of disease. However, the opaque nature of many AI models which makes it challenging to understand the reasoning behind decision making has raised concerns about their interpretability and trustworthiness. XAI can address these concerns by providing insights into the reasoning behind AI-driven diagnoses and recommendations. In this case study, we explore the implementation of XAI in the radiology department of a large hospital. The hospital has deployed an AI system for the detection and classification of lung nodules in chest CT scans. The AI system is developed on a deep learning model that has achieved high accuracy in clinical trials. However, before fully integrating the system into clinical practice, the hospital aims to enhance its interpretability and transparency using XAI methods.

The hospital employs two XAI techniques to interpret the deep learning model:

1. Integrated Gradients: This method is used to identify the sections of the CT scan that significantly contribute to the AI's prediction of lung nodule presence and characteristics. By highlighting the most influential areas, clinicians can verify the AI's reasoning and assess its accuracy [24].
2. Concept Activation Vectors (CAVs): CAVs are used to explore how the AI model's understanding of specific concepts, such as nodule size, shape, and density, influences its predictions. By analyzing the activations of these concepts in the model, by understanding how the AI system makes decisions, doctors can make sure that it is consistent with their own clinical experience.

3.5.1.1 Benefits and challenges

The implementation of XAI in radiology has yielded several benefits:

- Enhanced Trust: By providing explanations for AI predictions that are easily interpretable, XAI has helped clinicians feel more confident in the AI system's recommendations, thereby leading to increased adoption and integration into clinical workflows.

- Improved Accuracy: The use of XAI has enabled clinicians to improve the AI system by identifying and correcting errors, leading to improved performance over time.
- Reduced Bias: XAI has helped the hospital identify and mitigate potential biases in the

AI system, ensuring that it operates fairly across different patient populations.

However, the hospital has also faced several challenges in implementing XAI:

- Data Availability: High-quality, annotated data is required for training the XAI model and the process of obtaining the data has been time-consuming and resource-intensive.
- Computational Complexity: The computational resources required for some XAI techniques, such as Integrated Gradients, when dealing with large datasets or complex models can be significantly high.
- Clinician Education: Continuous clinician training and education are needed to ensure clinicians can effectively interpret and utilize the explanations provided by XAI methods.

3.5.1.2 Best practices

Based on their experience, the hospital has identified several best practices for implementing XAI in radiology:

1. Involve Clinicians Early: Engage clinicians in the development and implementation process from the beginning to ensure that XAI methods address their needs and concerns.
2. Prioritize Interpretability: When selecting AI models for deployment, prioritize those that offer inherent interpretability or are compatible with XAI techniques.
3. Continuously Monitor and Evaluate: Regularly monitor the performance and accuracy of the AI system, and use XAI to identify areas for improvement.
4. Provide Clinician Training: Offer ongoing training and support to help clinicians understand and effectively utilize the explanations provided by XAI methods.

3.5.2 Case study 2: XAI in personalized medicine

The aim of personalized medicine is to curate the treatment plan to individual patients based on characteristics such as genetics, lifestyle, and environmental factors. AI has the potential to revolutionize personalized medicine by identifying complex patterns in patient data and making individualized treatment recommendations. However, the non-transparent nature of many AI models that makes it challenging to interpret decision-making processes can make it difficult for clinicians to understand and trust recommendations of the AI system. XAI can help bridge this gap by providing insights that are interpretable and explain the factors influencing treatment decisions. In this case study, we examine the implementation of XAI in a personalized medicine clinic that specializes in oncology. The clinic has developed an AI system that analyzes patient genomic data, clinical history, and lifestyle factors to predict treatment response and guide personalized therapy selection for cancer patients.

The clinic employs two XAI techniques to interpret the AI system's recommendations:

1. SHAP is used to identify the most influential factors contributing to the AI's treatment recommendations for each patient. By ranking the importance of various genomic markers, clinical features, and lifestyle factors, SHAP helps clinicians understand AI's decision-making process and assess their validity.
2. LIME is used to provide local explanations for individual treatment recommendations. By approximating the intricate AI model near a particular recommendation with a more straightforward and comprehensible model, LIME assists healthcare professionals in comprehending how patient-specific variables impact the AI's decision-making process.

3.5.2.1 Benefits and challenges

The implementation of XAI in personalized medicine has yielded several benefits:

- Improved Treatment Selection: By providing explanations that are easily interpretable for treatment recommendations, XAI has helped clinicians make informed decisions about personalized therapy selection, leading to better patient outcomes.
- Enhanced Patient Engagement: XAI has enabled clinicians to engage patients more effectively in shared decision-making by explaining the factors influencing treatment recommendations in a clear and understandable manner.
- Accelerated Research: The insights provided by XAI have helped researchers identify novel biomarkers and therapeutic targets, accelerating the development of new personalized medicine approaches.

However, the clinic has also faced several challenges in implementing XAI:

- Data Privacy Concerns: Patients may have concerns about how their sensitive genomic and personal data is being used by the AI system, which can hinder data sharing and collaboration.
- Regulatory Compliance: Ensuring AI systems and XAI methods comply with regulations and guidelines, such as data protection laws and clinical practice standards, can be complex and time-consuming.
- Clinician Resistance: Some clinicians may be hesitant to adopt XAI methods due to concerns about their reliability or a lack of understanding of how they work, which can slow down the integration of AI into clinical practice.

3.5.2.2 Best practices

Based on their experience, the clinic has identified several best practices for implementing XAI in personalized medicine:

1. Involving Patients in the Process: Involving patients in the development and implementation of XAI methods to address their concerns and ensure that the explanations provided are meaningful and useful.
2. Collaborate with Regulatory Bodies: Work closely with regulatory bodies to ensure that the AI system and XAI methods meet relevant standards and guidelines, and contribute to the development of new regulations that support the sound use of AI in healthcare.
3. Provide Comprehensive Clinician Training: Offer comprehensive training to clinicians on how to interpret and utilize the explanations provided by XAI methods, including hands-on workshops and case-based learning.
4. Continuously Evaluate and Refine: Regularly evaluate the performance and accuracy of the AI system and XAI methods, and use feedback from clinicians and patients to continuously refine and improve the system over time.

3.5.3 Case study 3: XAI in emergency department triage

This case study examines the implementation of an XAI-enhanced triage system in a busy urban emergency department (ED). The ED faced challenges with long wait times and inconsistent triage decisions. To address these issues, they implemented an AI-powered triage system that predicts patient acuity and recommends triage categories. However, the initial implementation faced resistance from staff due to its lack of transparency. The hospital integrated LIME (Local Interpretable Model-agnostic Explanations) into the triage system to provide interpretable explanations for each recommendation.

Key Features:

1. Real-time Explanations: For each patient, the system displays the top factors influencing the triage recommendation.
2. Visual Interface: A user-friendly dashboard shows the importance of different symptoms and vital signs.
3. Customizable Thresholds: Allows triage nurses to adjust sensitivity levels based on current ED capacity.

Outcomes:

1. Improved Consistency: Triage decisions became more consistent across different nurses and shifts.
2. Increased Efficiency: Average triage time decreased by 22%.
3. Enhanced Trust: Staff reported higher confidence in the AI system's recommendations.
4. Better Resource Allocation: More accurate triage led to improved patient flow and resource utilization.

Challenges Faced:

1. Initial Learning Curve: Staff required training to interpret and effectively use the XAI outputs.
2. System Updates: Keeping the XAI component aligned with updates to the underlying AI model proved challenging.
3. Edge Cases: Some complex cases still require override by experienced staff.

Lessons Learned:

1. Continuous Feedback Loop: Regular meetings with triage staff to gather feedback on the XAI system led to iterative improvements.
2. Flexible Implementation: Allowing staff to adjust the system's sensitivity helped balance AI assistance with human expertise.
3. Ongoing Education: Regular training sessions on interpreting XAI outputs were crucial for maintaining staff confidence and system effectiveness.

3.5.4 Comparative analysis of XAI implementations

To provide a broader perspective, let's compare key aspects of the three case studies, as depicted in Table 3.2:

Table 3.2 Comparative Analysis of XAI methods

Aspect	*Radiology (Case 1)*	*Personalized Medicine (Case 2)*	*ED Triage (Case 3)*
Primary XAI Technique	Integrated Gradients, CAVs	SHAP, LIME	LIME
Main Benefit	Enhanced trust in AI diagnoses	Improved treatment selection	Increased triage consistency
Key Challenge	Data availability	Regulatory compliance	Staff learning curve
Implementation Time	18 months	24 months	12 months
Staff Satisfaction	High	Moderate	Initially low, then high
Patient Impact	Faster, more accurate diagnoses	More personalized treatments	Reduced wait times

3.5.5 Best practices derived from case studies

Based on the experiences across these diverse implementations, we can extract some common best practices for XAI in healthcare:

1. Stakeholder Involvement: Engage clinicians, patients, and administrators early and throughout the implementation process.
2. Tailored Explanations: Customize XAI outputs to the specific needs and expertise levels of different user groups.
3. Phased Implementation: Start with a pilot program and gradually expand, allowing for adjustments based on feedback.
4. Continuous Monitoring: Regular assessment of the impact of XAI on clinical decisions, patient outcomes, and workflow efficiency.
5. Ethical Considerations: Establish clear guidelines for data privacy, algorithmic bias mitigation, and human oversight.
6. Integration with Workflow: Ensure that XAI tools seamlessly integrate into existing clinical workflows to maximize adoption.
7. Flexibility and Adaptability: Design systems that can evolve with changing healthcare needs and advancing AI technologies.

3.6 FUTURE DIRECTIONS AND RECOMMENDATIONS

As Explainable AI (XAI) in healthcare continues to evolve, it is necessary to identify future directions and make recommendations that can enhance the effectiveness, trustworthiness, and ethical deployment of AI systems. This section outlines key areas for future research, the need for balancing performance and interpretability, regulatory considerations, and the importance of interdisciplinary collaboration.

3.6.1 Research gaps and opportunities

Despite the significant advancements in XAI, several research gaps remain that present opportunities for further exploration:

1. Understanding Human-AI Interaction Research is needed to get a better understanding of how clinicians and patients interact with AI systems. This includes studying how explanations provided by XAI methods influence decision-making, trust, and acceptance of AI recommendations. Investigating the cognitive processes involved in interpreting AI outputs can help refine XAI techniques to enhance usability and effectiveness [25].
2. Developing Robust Evaluation Metrics – There is a need to identify robust metrics that are standardized to evaluate the effectiveness of XAI methods in healthcare. Current evaluation frameworks often focus on model performance (e.g., accuracy, precision) without adequately assessing the interpretability and usability of explanations. Developing robust metrics that are standardized and capture the quality and impact of XAI explanations on clinical decision-making is essential.
3. Addressing Domain-Specific Challenges – Different healthcare domains may require tailored XAI approaches. For instance, the interpretability needs in radiology may differ from those in personalized medicine or genomics. Research should focus on developing domain-specific XAI methods that address the unique challenges and requirements of various healthcare specialties.
4. Mitigating Bias and Ensuring Fairness – While XAI can certainly help identify and eradicate bias in AI systems to a large extent, more research is needed to develop effective strategies for ensuring fairness in healthcare AI. This includes exploring how XAI can be used to audit AI systems for bias, as well as developing techniques to create fairer training datasets and algorithms.

3.6.2 Balancing performance and interpretability

A key challenge in deploying AI [26] systems in healthcare is balancing the model performance with interpretability. High-performing models, particularly deep learning algorithms, often operate as opaque with no inference into decision making which makes it challenging for clinicians to understand the reasoning for a decision. Conversely, a model may be easily interpretable but may not provide high accuracy. The following techniques are suggested to balance performance [25] and interpretability in models:

1. Hybrid Approaches – Research should explore a hybrid approach that combines the power and strength of complex models with the ease of interpretable methods. For instance, using ensemble methods that integrate both black-box models and interpretable models can provide clinicians with accurate predictions while maintaining a level of interpretability.
2. Interpretable Deep Learning Models – There is a lot of interest in developing deep learning models that are inherently interpretable. Research efforts should focus on creating architectures that provide built-in interpretability without compromising performance. Techniques such as attention mechanisms, which highlight important features in the input data, can enhance interpretability while maintaining model accuracy.
3. User-Centric Design – The design of XAI systems should prioritize user needs and preferences. Engaging clinicians in the design process can help ensure that explanations are easy to comprehend, relevant, and actionable. User studies and user research can provide deep insights into how clinicians interpret AI outputs and what types of explanations are most helpful in clinical practice.

3.6.3 Regulatory considerations

Regulatory frameworks must evolve to address the unique challenges posed by XAI as AI technologies become more integrated into healthcare. Recommendations for implementing regulatory considerations:

1. Establishing Standards for XAI – Regulatory bodies should establish clear standards and guidelines for the deployment of XAI in healthcare. These standards should address issues related to transparency, accountability, and ethical considerations, ensuring that AI systems are used responsibly and effectively.
2. Ensuring Data Privacy and Security – Data security and privacy must be given top priority in legal frameworks due to the growing usage of patient data in AI systems. This involves making sure that regionally specific legislative frameworks, including the Health Insurance Portability and Accountability Act (HIPAA) in the US and the General Data Protection Regulation (GDPR) in Europe, are followed. XAI techniques ought to be created with patient privacy in mind and offer insightful data.
3. Facilitating Collaboration Between Regulators and Developers – Collaboration between regulatory bodies and AI developers is mandatory to create a supportive environment suitable for innovation while ensuring patient safety. Regular dialogue can help identify emerging

challenges and opportunities, leading to more effective regulatory frameworks that keep pace with technological advancements.

3.6.4 Interdisciplinary collaboration

Successful implementation of XAI in healthcare requires multi-disciplinary collaboration:
Recommendations for implementing interdisciplinary collaboration:

1. Collaboration Between Clinicians and Data Scientists – Interdisciplinary collaboration between clinicians and data scientists is crucial for developing AI systems that meet the needs of healthcare professionals. Clinicians can provide deep and valuable insights into clinical workflows, patient care, and the explanations that are most relevant and useful, while data scientists can apply their expertise in AI and machine learning to create effective models.
2. Engaging Ethicists [27] and Social Scientists – Incorporating perspectives from ethicists and social scientists can help ensure that XAI systems are deployed in an ethical and socially responsible way. Engaging these experts can provide insights into the societal implications of AI technologies, including issues related to privacy, bias, fairness, and the impact on patient autonomy.
3. Fostering Collaboration Across Institutions – Collaboration between healthcare institutions, academic researchers, and industry partners can facilitate knowledge sharing and innovation in XAI. Collaborative initiatives, such as research consortia and public-private partnerships, can help advance the field by pooling resources, expertise, and data.

3.6.5 Emerging XAI techniques for healthcare

As the field of XAI evolves, new techniques are being developed that show promise for healthcare applications: Emerging XAI techniques specific to healthcare are listed below:

1. Concept-based Explanations – Concept-based explanations aim to fill in the gap between high-level and low-level features that are more intuitive for clinicians. For instance, in medical imaging, instead of highlighting individual pixels, these methods can identify and explain in terms of anatomical structures or pathological patterns.
2. Causal XAI – Causal XAI methods focus on understanding the causal relationships between inputs and outputs, rather than just correlations. This approach can be particularly valuable in healthcare,

where understanding the underlying mechanisms of diseases and treatments is crucial.

3. Interactive XAI – Interactive XAI systems allow users to explore and interrogate AI models in real time. This can be especially useful in clinical settings where clinicians may need to investigate specific aspects of a model's decision-making process [28].
4. Temporal XAI – Many healthcare applications involve time-series data, such as continuous monitoring of patient vital signs or disease progression over time. Temporal XAI methods are needed to explain predictions based on these complex temporal patterns.

3.6.6 Integration of XAI into clinical workflows

XAI needs to be seamlessly integrated into existing critical workflows for it to be effective in healthcare. Recommendations for integrating XAI [29] into clinical workflows are listed below:

1. Real-time Explanations – Develop XAI systems that can provide explanations in real-time, enabling clinicians to incorporate AI insights and make informed decisions without causing delays.
2. Contextual Explanations – Create XAI systems that can adapt their explanations based on the specific clinical context, the role of the user, and the stage of the decision-making process.
3. Multi-modal Explanations – Healthcare often involves diverse data types, including imaging, text, and numerical data. XAI systems should be able to provide coherent explanations that integrate insights from these different modalities.
4. Integration with Clinical Decision Support Systems – Incorporate XAI into existing Clinical Decision Support Systems (CDSS) to enhance their effectiveness and trustworthiness.

3.6.7 Education and training for XAI in healthcare

As XAI becomes more prevalent in healthcare [30], there's a growing need for education and training:

Suggestions for education and training for XAI in healthcare are provided below.

1. Curriculum Development – Develop curricula for medical schools and continuing education programs that include training on AI and XAI in healthcare.
2. Interdisciplinary Training – Create training programs that bring together clinicians, data scientists, and ethicists to foster a shared

understanding of the challenges and opportunities in XAI for healthcare.

3. Patient Education – Develop resources to educate patients about the use of AI systems in healthcare and how XAI can be used to help them understand and engage with AI-driven decisions affecting their care.

3.7 CONCLUSION

Adoption of XAI is crucial for making artificial intelligence systems explainable in the healthcare decision-making processes. With AI systems deployed across virtually every aspect of patient management, diagnosis, treatment, and risk assessment, XAI becomes a valuable tool that helps bridge the existing gap between patients and these intelligent systems. This chapter has discussed different XAI techniques like LIME, SHAP, Integrated Gradients, and CAV, and has compared their effectiveness and drawbacks in the healthcare domain. Furthermore, further topics of ethical concern, specific to XAI including fairness, accountability, and mitigation of bias have been mentioned, underlining the significance of the ethical utilization of AI in clinical practice.

The application of XAI in radiology and personalized medicine has revealed that XAI can enhance clinician trust and patient benefits, in practice. Specific governance approaches to XAI, data protection, and cross-disciplinary coordination and cooperation of clinicians, data scientists and ethicists will be essential in the promotion of safe and effective application of AI in medicine. XAI, as a method aimed at the interpretability of AI's results, as well as promotion of its ethical implications and collaboration with human professionals, may gas AI's further integration into the sphere as a tool that enriches professionals' work and enhances patient care.

REFERENCES

1. Xu, X., He, P., Wu, W., & Zhang, J. (2018). Industry 4.0–enabled smart manufacturing in the context of lean manufacturing: A conceptual framework. *International Journal of Production Research, 56*(8), 2788–2800. DOI: 10.1080/00207543.2018.1443227
2. Tao, F., Zhang, H., Liu, A., & Nee, A. Y. C. (2019). Digital twin in industry: State-of-the-art. *IEEE Transactions on Industrial Informatics, 15*(4), 2405–2415. DOI: 10.1109/TII.2018.2873186
3. Rezaei, J., Ortt, R., & Scholten, V. (2018). Industry 4.0 and lean manufacturing: A systematic literature review and future research directions. *Journal of Manufacturing Technology Management, 29*(6), 909–936. DOI: 10.1108/JMTM-12-2017-0508
4. Schwab, K. (2016). The Fourth Industrial Revolution: What it means and how to respond. *Foreign Affairs*. DOI: 10.1007/978-3-319-62479-9

5. Xu, L . D., He, W., & Li, S. (2014). Internet of Things in industries: A survey. *IEEE Transactions on Industrial Informatics, 10*(4), 2233–2243. DOI: 10.1109/TII.2014.2300753
6. Kumar, A., & Sharma, M. (2022). Industry 5.0: Vision and implications for manufacturing. *Journal of Cleaner Production, 319*, 128746. DOI: 10.1016/j.jclepro.2021.128746
7. Wang, G., Gunasekaran, A., & Ngai, E. W. T. (2016). Big data analytics in logistics and supply chain management: Certain investigations for research and applications. *International Journal of Production Economics, 176*, 98–110. DOI: 10.1016/j.ijpe.2016.03.014
8. Holzinger, A., Biemann, C., Pattichis, C. S., & Kell, D. B. (2017). What do we need to build explainable AI systems for the medical domain? arXiv preprint arXiv:1712.09923. DOI: 10.48550/arXiv.1712.09923
9. Gerke, S., Minssen, T., & Cohen, G. (2020). Ethical and legal challenges of artificial intelligence-driven healthcare. In Adam Bohr and Kaveh Memarzadeh (eds.) *Artificial Intelligence in Healthcare* (pp. 295–336). Academic Press. DOI: 10.1016/B978-0-12-818438-7.00012-5
10. Cabitza, F., Rasoini, R., & Gensini, G. F. (2017). Unintended consequences of machine learning in medicine. *JAMA*, 318(6), 517–518. DOI: 10.1001/jama.2017.7797
11. Ribeiro, M. T., Singh, S., & Guestrin, C. (2016). Why should I trust you?: Explaining the predictions of any classifier. In *Proceedings of the 22nd ACM SIGKDD International Conference on Knowledge Discovery and Data Mining* (pp. 1135–1144). DOI: 10.1145/2939672.2939778
12. Lundberg, S. M., & Lee, S. I. (2017). A unified approach to interpreting model predictions. In *Proceedings of the 31st International Conference on Neural Information Processing Systems* (pp. 4768–4777).DOI: 10.48550/arXiv.1705.07874
13. Sundararajan, M., & Oscherwitz, T. (2019). Axiomatic attribution for deep networks. In *Proceedings of the 36th International Conference on Machine Learning* (pp. 1–10). DOI: 10.48550/arXiv.1703.01365
14. Caruana, R., Lou, Y., Gehrke, J., Koch, P., Sturm, M., & Elhadad, N. (2015). Intelligible models for healthcare: Predicting pneumonia risk and hospital 30-day readmission. In *Proceedings of the 21st ACM SIGKDD International Conference on Knowledge Discovery and Data Mining* (pp. 1721–1730). DOI: 10.1145/2783258.2788613
15. Rajkomar, A., Oren, E., Chen, K., Dai, A. M., Hajaj, N., Hardt, M., ... & Dean, J. (2018). Scalable and accurate deep learning with electronic health records. *NPJ Digital Medicine*, 1(1), 1–10. DOI: 10.1038/s41746-018-0029-1
16. Holzinger, A., Langs, G., Denk, H., Zatloukal, K., & Müller, H. (2019). Causability and explainability of artificial intelligence in medicine. *Wiley Interdisciplinary Reviews: Data Mining and Knowledge Discovery*, 9(4), e1312. DOI: 10.1002/widm.1312
17. Holzinger, A., Malle, B., Kieseberg, P., Roth, P. M., Müller, H., Reihs, R., & Zatloukal, K. (2017). Towards the augmented pathologist: Challenges

of explainable AI in digital pathology. arXiv preprint arXiv:1712.06657. DOI: 10.48550/arXiv.1712.06657

18. Mehrabi, N., Morstatter, F., Saxena, N., Lerman, K., & Galstyan, A. (2021). A survey on bias and fairness in machine learning. *ACM Computing Surveys (CSUR)*, 54(6), 1–35. DOI: 10.1145/3457607
19. Doshi-Velez, F., & Kim, P. (2017). Towards a rigorous science of interpretable machine learning. In *Proceedings of the 34th International Conference on Machine Learning*. DOI: 10.48550/arXiv.1702.08608
20. Lipton, Z. C. (2018). The mythos of model interpretability. *Communications of the ACM*, 61(10), 36–43. DOI: 10.1145/3233231
21. Mittelstadt, B. D. (2019). Principles alone cannot guarantee ethical AI. *Nature Machine Intelligence*, 1(11), 501–507. DOI: 10.1038/s42256-019-0103-5
22. Wachter, S., Mittelstadt, B., & Floridi, L. (2017). Why a right to explanation of automated decision-making does not exist in the General Data Protection Regulation. *International Data Privacy Law*, 7(2), 76–99. DOI: 10.1093/idpl/ipx005
23. Holzinger, A., Carrington, A., & Müller, H. (2020). Measuring the quality of explanations: The evaluation of explainable AI. *Journal of Artificial Intelligence Research*, 69, 125–150. DOI: 10.1613/jair.1.12192
24. Gunning, D., & Aha, D. (2019). DARPA's Explainable Artificial Intelligence (XAI) Program. *AI Magazine*, 40(2), 44–58. DOI: 10.1609/aimag.v40i2.2850
25. Tonekaboni, S., Joshi, S., McCradden, M. D., & Goldenberg, A. (2019). What clinicians want: Contextualizing explainable machine learning for clinical end use. *Proceedings of Machine Learning Research*, 106, 359–380. DOI: 10.1002/widm.1379
26. Reddy, K. K., Kaza, V. S., Anisha, P. R., Khurbani, M. M., Shauib, M., & Alam, S. (2024). Optimizing barrier placement for intrusion detection and prevention in WSNs. *PLOS ONE*. https://doi.org/10.1371/journal.pone.0299334
27. Anisha, P. R., Kishor Kumar Reddy, C., Hanafiah, M. M., Murthy, B. R., Mohana, R. M., & Pragathi, Y. V. S. S. (2023). An intelligent deep feature based feature based metabolism syndrome prediction system for sleep disorder diseases. In *Multimedia Tools and Applications*, Springer. https://doi.org/10.1007/s11042-023-17296-4
28. Reddy, C. K. K., Anisha, P. R., Hanafiah, M. M., Pragathi, Y. V. S. S., Murthy, B. R., & Mohana, R. M. (2023). An intelligent optimized cyclone intensity prediction framework using satellite images. *Springer Earth Science Informatics*. https://doi.org/10.1007/s12145-023-00983-z
29. Reddy, C. K. K., Anisha, P. R., Reddy, T., Srinivasulu, B., & Rambabu, D. (2022). Light-weight real time weather forecasting simulation over Bangladesh using deep learning. *INT-JECSE*. 4616–4633.DOI: 10.9756/INT-JECSE/V14I3.602

Chapter 4

From neurons to algorithms

Enhancing machine learning with neuroscientific insights

Areesha Fatima, Kishor Kumar Reddy C, Srinath Doss, and Herat Joshi

4.1 INTRODUCTION

The interaction between neuroscience and AI has become of great interest, at least in these times when we try to capture the intricate functionalities of the human brain into computational systems. The nucleus of this interaction is neurons: the fundamental units of the brain and its framework for communication – action potentials and synaptic transmission. These biological processes underpin cognition and learning and inspire the design of artificial neural networks (ANNs), which power many applications of modern AI. Machine learning (ML), one of the areas in AI, uses such neural-inspired architectures to enable systems to learn from data and to improve their performance over time. Drawing insights from neuroscience involves researching what ought to give AI models their efficiency and capabilities to perform such complex tasks under the thresholds of human cognition, which requires some level of reasoning and adaptability. This paper explores the nature of biological neurons, and their comparison with artificial counterparts in machine learning and abstracting neural functionality in ANNs, to illustrate how the insight into neural processes informs and improves AI technology. We venture into this combined perspective from neuroscience and computation, where exciting breakthroughs may unfold in new directions in creating smarter AI and more sophisticated systems for human communication and understanding.

The remaining chapter is arranged as follows: the subsections discuss the biological and artificial neurons. Section 4.2 covers the neuroscience-inspired learning mechanisms. Section 4.3 delves into the hierarchical structure of the brain and its similarity with deep learning. Section 4.4 focuses on the neuroscientific theories of learning and their impact on algorithms. Section 4.5 discusses neural computation and symbolic reasoning. Section 4.6 focuses on neural efficiency and resource optimization. Section 4.7 concludes this chapter.

DOI: 10.1201/9781003591085-4

4.1.1 Biological neurons

Biologically, neurons are basic components of the human brain nervous system, which capture and process information. They function in a liquid electrolyte and exchange information through gaps, or synapses, between the dendrite of postsynaptic neurons and the axon of presynaptic neurons [1]. Each neuron is divided into several parts: the cell body or soma, dendrites, an axon, and synapses. Within the cell, body are found the nucleus and other vital organelles that sustain the health and functioning of the neuron. Surrounding the cell body are dendrites, tree-like extensions that receive incoming signals from other neurons. These signals are often in the form of chemical messengers, called neurotransmitters, which bind to receptors on the dendrites to initiate electrical changes within the neuron.

A neuron generates an electrical impulse known as an action potential when it has received enough excitatory inputs. This impulse travels down the axon, a long, thin projection that acts as a conduit for transmitting the signal from the cell body to other neurons or target tissues. The axon is often insulated by a fatty layer called the myelin sheath, which speeds up signal transmission. Axon terminals, which form synapses with other neurons' dendrites or cell bodies, are at the axon's tip. A synapse is where the neurons talk to each other. It is made up of a presynaptic neuron, which transmits the signal, and a postsynaptic neuron, which receives it. Figure 4.1 illustrates the key components of a biological neuron, including the cell body, dendrites, axons, and synapses [1].

The action potential reaching the axon terminal causes the release of neurotransmitters stored inside the synaptic vesicles. These chemicals are released into the synaptic cleft-the minute gap between neurons, where they may bind to receptors on the postsynaptic neuron. The binding of chemicals

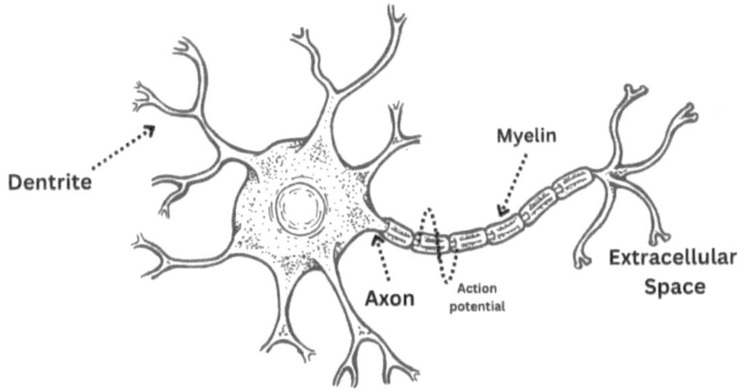

Figure 4.1 Structure of a Biological Neuron.

causes ion channels in the membrane of receiving neurons to open, leading to the inflow or outflow of ions, which can stimulate or inhibit a neuron. If these excitatory signals reach a threshold, then the postsynaptic neuron fires off its action potential and therefore continues the propagation of the flow of information.

Neurons are much more than passive conductors of signals; they can process all information that reaches them in terms of the complex play between excitatory and inhibitory inputs. Each neuron makes thousands of synaptic connections with other neurons, so there's a complex network underlying all brain functions: from sensory perception to higher-order cognition. This synaptic connection is continually modified as a function of experience in a process known as synaptic plasticity, which plays a crucial role in learning and memory. It is simply since neurons are capable of considerable communication between themselves in their speed, and flexibility, which makes it possible for the brain to perform its real-time complex spectrum of functions.

4.1.2 Artificial neural networks

Biological neurons and artificial neurons are conceptual representations that have vast differences in complexity and functionality. Biological neurons are complex cells present in the human brain, undertaking processing and communication of information through electrochemical impulses. Complex structure is made up of dendrites, the cell body, axons, and synapses. Biological neurons receive tens of thousands of synaptic inputs from other neurons and create electrical signals called action potentials in the axon that propagate to other neurons. These synaptic connections have changing strengths and plasticity with time, thereby enabling adaptation, learning, and the wide range of functions that are associated with brain functionality. This process is influenced by many factors, including types of neurotransmitters, timing of signals, and ongoing synaptic modifications, which render biological neurons highly dynamic and capable of sophisticated processing.

Artificial neurons that form the building blocks of models of machine learning, such as ANNs, are highly simplified representations of their biological counterparts. In ANN design, artificial neurons take on a set of numerical inputs, apply weights to them, sum the inputs, and feed through an activation function (like a sigmoid or ReLU function). What is passed along to other artificial neurons within the network is the output. While dealing with continuous signals and complex chemical interactions, biological neurons are in sharp contrast to artificial neurons. Artificial neurons deal with fixed numerical values which may make the process more mathematical and deterministic than necessary. Whereas biological neurons operate within an enormous highly interconnected network that is mutable, artificial neurons are usually organized in structured layers (input, hidden,

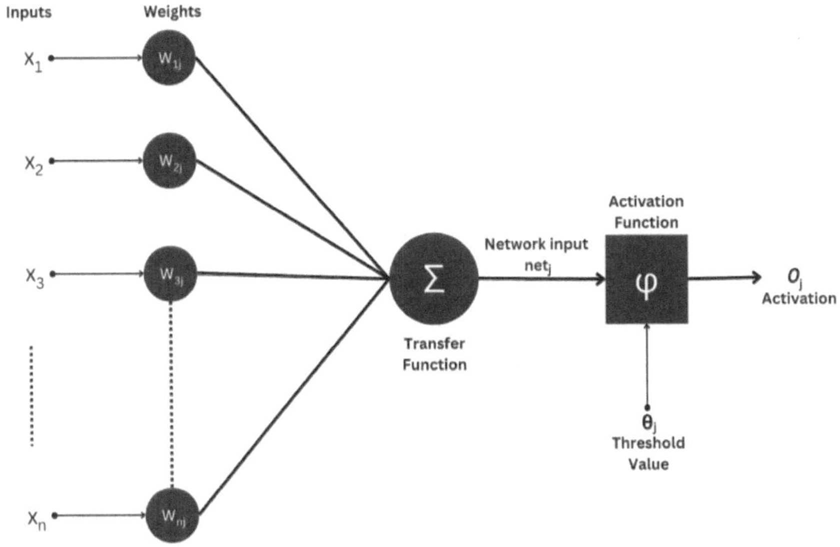

Figure 4.2 Structure of Artificial Neurons.

and output layers) but normally have static connections during inference. Figure 4.2 illustrates its inputs, weights, summation, activation function, and output. This diagram emphasizes how artificial neurons abstract the complexities of biological neurons for computational purposes.

Inspired by this basic concept of biological neurons to receive inputs, and generate outputs, the design abstracts much biological complexity from it. For example, artificial neurons do not capture signal timing or the kind of synaptic plasticity seen in the biological system. Instead, it uses gradient-based learning algorithms like backpropagation during the training cycle to update weights in an attempt to imitate the notion of learning in a far simpler and computationally practical manner. This oversimplification had allowed artificial neurons to be able to carry out tasks, such as image and natural language recognition, but lacked the full explanation of the biological fidelity of real neural systems.

Table 4.1 highlights the key differences and similarities between biological neurons and artificial neurons, providing insights into their respective structures, communication methods, learning mechanisms, energy efficiency, and temporal dynamics.

Artificial neurons mimic their natural counterparts but bear many performance and adaptability restrictions. Artificial neural networks have emerged as a potential model system for understanding neural circuits, as some huge-scale task-optimized ANNs have exceeded classical neuronal

Table 4.1 Comparison of Biological and Artificial Neurons

Feature	*Biological Neurons*	*Artificial Neurons*
Structure	Complex structure with dendrites, axons, and synapses	Simplified architecture with inputs, weights, and activation functions
Communication	Discrete spikes (action potentials)	Continuous values (activation outputs)
Learning Mechanism	Synaptic plasticity (e.g., STDP)	Gradient descent and backpropagation
Energy Efficiency	Highly energy-efficient	Often requires significant computational resources
Temporal Dynamics	Dependent on spike timing	Generally, static activation based on inputs

models in capturing brain activity. A common criticism of using ANNs to simulate brain circuits is that ANNs just create a new, similarly complex system to replace the original, sophisticated one [2]. The critical limitation in artificial neurons is based on level abstraction; biological neurons work under real conditions, where electrochemical signals occur continuously and depend on synaptic plasticity, neurotransmitter release, or even the timing of signal transmission events. On the other hand, artificial neurons render this process discrete at a mathematical level simply stated as follows: inputs are weighted, summed, and fed through an activation function. This simplification does not capture the nuanced, time-sensitive nature of biological processing, which may end up making artificial neurons less adaptive and flexible.

Another limitation lies in the rigidity of learning. Biological neurons continuously adapt based on feedback in real-time, implementing some mechanisms like Hebbian learning and synaptic plasticity; in this way, the brain can respond flexibly to new information. Artificial neurons, in contrast, are based on predefined learning algorithms. For example, there is gradient descent and backpropagation, where neuron weights are updated only during the training phase. This static learning process makes artificial neurons incapable of adapting themselves after completing training. Bio-neurons, on the other hand, never get rigid throughout life. Another significant difference lies in the energy efficiency of these two. With 86 billion neurons, the brain can function at maximum energy efficiency, at approximately 20 watts. On the other hand, artificial neural networks, especially deep networks, devour huge amounts of computational resources and energy, particularly when training phases are ongoing. This renders them unsuitable for low-power or real-time computing, which biological neurons accomplish with ease.

4.2 NEUROSCIENCE-INSPIRED LEARNING MECHANISMS

4.2.1 Hebbian learning

The neuroscience concept "cells that fire together, wire together" comes from Hebbian learning, a framework derived in 1949 by the Canadian psychologist Donald Hebb [3]. One of the cornerstones of this premise supposes that the more often two neurons are coactivated, the greater the connection between them becomes, so communication between them flows more easily into the future [4]. Or, put another way, if one neuron is continually used to activate another, the bond between them gets strengthened at the synapse. This biological process is central to how the brain learns, adapts, and stores information and determines everything from how memory is formed to how a particular skill is acquired. Hebbian learning typifies how experience and repeated stimulation modulate neural circuits, resulting in long-lasting alterations to behavior and cognitive functions.

This notion has motivated learning rules in artificial networks directly, especially in algorithms for unsupervised learning. In machine learning, Hebbian learning translates to the thought that artificial neurons adjust their weights based on the extent of correlation of their inputs with the neuron's activation. Put simply, if two connected artificial neurons tend to activate in concert often enough, the connection weight of the synapse is increased. Unlike standard backpropagation used in supervised learning featuring labeled data with explicit error correction, Hebbian learning-inspired models function by pattern and correlation detection within the data without external supervision [3]. These principles form the basis of many developed self-organizing maps, principal component analysis, and early associative memory networks. Although Hebb's idea is very biologically inspired, simplicity is somewhat lacking in his learning rule compared to the approach that is computationally more efficient for large-scale tasks and implements more complex learning mechanisms within deep learning. Still, it remains a seminal idea connecting neuroscience to machine learning.

4.2.2 Spike-timing-dependent plasticity

Spike-timing-dependent plasticity is a biological learning mechanism where the strength of any connection between two neurons is adjusted based on their detailed spike timing. Initially originating from classical training and Hebbian synaptic plasticity, the notion of sustained synaptic plasticity (STDP) surfaced in the 1990s upon the identification of the significance of time in the polarity of enduring synaptic alterations [5]. The STDP type of long-term synaptic change is brought on by the relative order of pre- and postsynaptic spiking activity. [5]. In STDP, if a presynaptic neuron fires just before a postsynaptic neuron, the synaptic connection between them becomes strengthened, called long-term potentiation. If, on the other hand, the postsynaptic neuron fires before the presynaptic neuron, the connection weakens; this is known as long-term depression (LTD) [6]. This timing-dependent plasticity lets neurons refine their synaptic strengths according to temporal patterns, making STDP an important mechanism for learning and memory formation in the brain. It allows neurons to learn causal relationships because one neuron's impact on another can progressively strengthen over many repetitions of their firing. At various synapses, there are many fundamental types of STDP with significant differences, which are likely due to both synapse specialization and diverse experimental settings [7].

STDP significantly influences the building of machine learning models, especially within the area of spiking neural networks (SNNs). Spiking neural networks try to model neural dynamics by incorporating the timing of spikes into learning algorithms. Unlike artificial neural networks, where inputs and outputs are continuous values, SNNs deal with discrete spikes over time, for potentially more biologically realistic and energy-efficient learning processes [8]. Future machine learning models may be dynamically more adaptive than current systems, and the systems may adapt to static patterns, but to temporal sequences and even to causal dependencies by mechanisms similar to STDP. This would make it particularly suitable for tasks like real-time decision-making, processing of sensory input, or all the applications requiring some form of temporal awareness, such as robotics or speech recognition. The emphasis of STDP on time further introduces one possible route to more power-efficient computation: spiking neurons would fire only when computationally useful, thereby avoiding the redundant operations that do occur in the traditional models.

4.2.3 Neural plasticity and adaptability

Neural plasticity is the brain's ability to adapt and be reorganized upon exposure to new information, experiences, or changes in the environment. The plasticity of the brain is known to be partially modified through synaptic connections, with the strengthening of frequently used pathways and the weakening or elimination of unused ones. The brain is constantly rearranging itself with synaptic plasticity and neurogenesis, improving efficiency and flexibility in the performance of new tasks or recovery from damage. It is exactly this flexibility that allows human beings to acquire new skills, modify behavior with changing environments, or continuously improve their performance without the need for explicit instructions or retraining. Although the study of plasticity has long been a focus of neuroscience, deep learning has just lately been interested in this field [9].

Incorporation of similar principles of neural plasticity into machine learning could greatly enhance the ability of models to adapt in real time to this evolution. Conventional models of machine learning, especially those based on deep learning, take an extensive retraining process when faced with new information or a changing environment, which takes a long time as well as high computational cost. But if they are designed to reflect the principles of neural plasticity, dynamic models could change internal parameters on the fly as new data comes in, hence a system that can be much more responsive and adaptive than it would be with retraining from scratch; it could learn on the fly and adapt to non-static environments such as financial markets or autonomous driving scenarios or personalized healthcare. Mechanisms that may potentially be embedded to allow models to fine-tune themselves incrementally, much like the strengthening and weakening of synaptic connections in the brain, may make machine learning systems more efficient by reducing this constant dependence on human supervision and therefore allowing them to operate in real-world, real-time contexts with greater autonomy and accuracy.

4.2.4 Spiking neural networks (SNNs)

Biological neurons communicate mainly in discrete spikes or action potentials: rapid changes in the electrical charge of a neuron's membrane. However, when a neuron receives enough input from its synaptic connections, it will generate an action potential, a brief, rapid depolarization followed by a return to the resting state. This spike is an all-or-nothing response; once initiated, it propagates along the axon and is transmitted to other neurons via synapses. The frequency and timing of such spikes encode information about the strength and nature of input signals. Thus, a stronger stimulus may result in a higher firing rate. Certain patterns of spikes may be used to convey distinct information about this aspect of biological neurons by the intricate ways in which they communicate.

Figure 4.3 shows the architecture of SNNs. The incoming signal is converted into spikes by passing it through filters that have characteristic

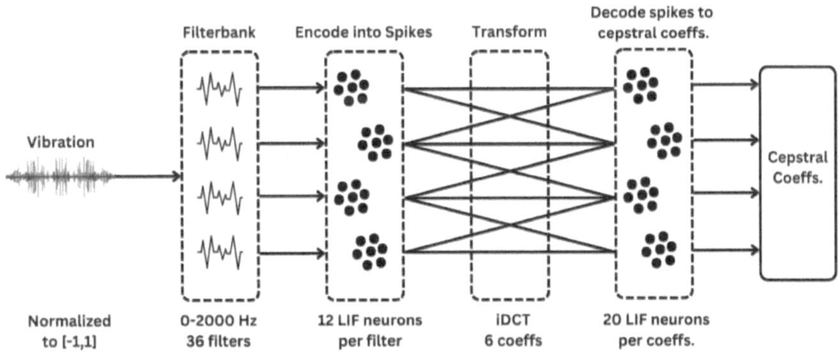

Figure 4.3 Schematic of the SNN Architecture.

frequencies that are logarithmically separated. Each filter has a set of spiking neurons assigned to it. After completing the first layer's output, the second layer receives the results of the inverse DCT transformation. The weights on the links between the layers carry out the change. Decoding from the second layer yields the cepstral coefficients. The L2-norm is used to determine how many extracted coefficients are needed to capture more than 99% of the energy in the input signal. Both the number of ensembles and cepstral coefficients are identical [10].

Artificial Intelligence has seen SNNs emerging as a model of computation that closely mimics the temporal dynamics of biological neurons. This fast rise in AI is sometimes attributed to the 2012 ImageNet competition, in which a team of academics from the University of Toronto submitted AlexNet, a deep Convolutional Neural Network (CNN) with a top-5 error of 10.8% lower than the second-best result [11]. Contrasting with traditional artificial neural networks that process information using real numbers and static activation functions, SNNs compute in discrete spikes, mimicking how biological neurons work. Neurons in SNNs communicate in terms of spikes generated based on their respective input signals, and the times of these spikes play a significant role in information processing. This temporal coding explains why SNNs can catch complex temporal patterns and dependencies within the data with high resolutions, making them very well adapted for applications involving high-resolution temporal processing, such as speech recognition and sensory processing [12].

Probably one of the significant advantages of SNNs is their potential for energy-efficient computing. Biological systems use a negligible amount of energy, and SNNs are engineered to realize these efficiency levels. SNNs function only when the spikes occur. In such an architecture, power is saved by orders of magnitude more than that of traditional ANNs that process all inputs in real time without a need for constant consumption of power. In the computation model with events, a lot of data can be processed in an SNN while having no long-term need to constantly consume power. As a result, they are especially promising in applications for edge computing and Internet of Things devices, where the efficiency of power consumption is emphasized.

The inclusion of temporal dynamics in SNNs also opens up new opportunities in the development of more biologically inspired learning algorithms. The native training methods of SNNs can be classified into supervised learning with gradient descent and spike backpropagation, and unsupervised learning with local learning rule at the synapse [13]. Techniques such as spike-timing-dependent plasticity, based on the difference in timing of spikes, can be adopted in facilitating learning in SNNs. This will enable the networks to learn adaptively based on the temporal relationships between the inputs and thus lead to more subtle approaches to learning that are therefore more similar to real biological mechanisms of learning. Advances in SNN research make their ability to combine energy efficiency, temporal processing, and biologically inspired learning rules an attractive alternative to traditional machine learning models that lead the way for more intelligent and adaptable systems operating closer to biological computation.

4.3 HIERARCHICAL STRUCTURE OF THE BRAIN AND DEEP LEARNING

4.3.1 Cortical hierarchies

The human brain hierarchically processes information; it analyses the sensory inputs at multiple levels of complexity, with each abstraction level pulling out higher-order features. One of the best and most clear examples of this is seen within the visual cortex, which is organized into several distinct layers and areas along an evolutionary hierarchy of increasing complexity, and each subset of layers and areas of the cortex serves a different purpose in visual processing. Visual features, such as edges, colors, and motion, are first discovered by primary visual neurons at these early stages [14]. As information continues to flow through layers of the cortex, progressively more complex features start to be identified, including shapes and patterns, and eventually, objects and even faces. This hierarchical processing allows the brain to integrate so much visual information in such an efficient way, converting raw sensory input to meaningful perceptions, step by step through these stages of abstraction.

It is this concept of hierarchical information processing that has underpinned much of the development of deep learning architectures, particularly in convolutional neural networks (CNNs). These mirror-layered designs in the visual cortex of the brain are just stacks of convolutional layers that filter higher-level features from raw image data. The initial layers notice simple patterns and the deeper layers combine to notice more complex structures of patterns, quite analogous to the visual cortex. Such a hierarchal design enables CNNs to obtain outstanding performance in the areas of image classification and object detection as they can learn to identify complex patterns in data through successive transformations. The beauty of these deep learning models is that they exploit the natural organization of the brain by drawing upon cortical hierarchies, which enhance features, give better generalization, and result in better efficiency in processing visual information to thereby bridge the gap between biological and artificial intelligence.

4.3.2 Convolutional neural networks (CNNs)

A CNN is designed to mirror the hierarchical structure of the human visual system by following how the brain processes visual information in layers.

The initial layers involved in extracting low-level features from raw input images are edges, textures, and basic shapes in a CNN. This is achieved through convolutional operations where small filters slide over the image, computing local patterns, and showing significant features. These low-level features then propagate through to the deeper layers of the network, which pool and refine them to produce more complex representations, similar to the visual cortex that receives simple elements and builds them up into objects and patterns.

Because information flows through this network, each successive layer might be capturing progressively more abstract features through layers, from basic lines and shapes early to more complex structures, such as parts of objects, textures, and eventually the whole objects or scenes in the deeper layers. This layered approach allows CNNs to create a rich feature hierarchy, which enables them to learn and recognize complex patterns effectively in images. Plus, pooling layers are typically alternated with convolutional layers, which subsample the feature maps, so that downsampling maintains the critical information; it is not unlike how the brain reduces input data to concentrate on the most salient features. It is this hierarchical feature extraction that makes CNNs especially well-suited to visual tasks, capable of achieving state-of-the-art performance in image classification, object detection, and many other applications, all drawing on principles originally derived from the natural organization of processing in the brain.

4.3.3 Attention mechanisms and cognitive focus

Attention in the brain is the basic cognitive process that helps us selectively focus on certain stimuli and exclude inappropriate information at a particular moment. Therefore, it is also crucial for negotiating a complex environment and the optimal use of cognitive resources. The mechanisms and brain regions that take part in the process of attention include, above all, the prefrontal cortex, responsible for controlling attentional control, to enable higher-level functions like decision-making, planning, and goal-oriented behavior. It interacts with the parietal lobes, which gather sensory information and serve to guide attentional resources to stimuli of interest. The thalamus also serves as a relay for sensory signals; it controls the flow of information into the cortex and is responsible for determining which sensory inputs are prioritized by attention.

The brain uses both bottom-up and top-down mechanisms of attention. Bottom-up attention refers to the stimulus-driven attention that makes the brain respond automatically to anything relatively new and salient in the environment, such as a loud, sudden noise or flash of light. Top-down attention involves control of attention through an individual's goals, expectations, and prior knowledge to focus on specific tasks or relevant information while blocking out specific distractions. This interplay between these mechanisms allows for the process of adaptive resource allocation in the brain, which escalates important stimuli for learning and memory. In addition, dynamic attention shifts in the brain play a significant role in daily activities since they allow the human system to respond to ever-changing situations and monitor information according to its needs or objectives at the time. Such an intricate orchestration of attentional processes underscores the brain's remarkable capacity to manage and optimize performance in a world where competing stimuli abound.

Thus, it makes the self-attention within transformers similar to biological attention mechanisms since this makes it possible for the models to focus on any given subset of inputs depending on the contextual value. The human brain works based on neural processes to assess stimulus relevance to make a person focus on what matters and filter out distractions. This is achieved through a dynamic interaction of cognitive resources whereby regions such as the prefrontal cortex and parietal lobes cooperatively dictate which information is processed at greater levels via their salience and relevance to an ongoing task. Likewise, self-attention in transformers works by calculating the connections between all elements of an input, whether this be words within a sentence or pixels in an image, and as such, allows a model to compute weighted representations of all inputs. This happens in mechanisms that give more attention scores to more relevant tokens, which means that models should pay more attention to the parts of the input that most significantly contribute to the overall context.

Biological and artificial attention mechanisms are particularly good at processing complex, structured data. In biological systems, the brain dynamically makes adjustments in what to pay attention to based on what's demanded by the situational setup, which makes it better fitted for interpreting and responding to the environment. Self-attention layers in transformers accomplish this by computing attention scores between each token concerning every other token in the input sequence. That is how it contextualizes dependencies and relationships, bringing it much closer to a richer understanding of data. This hierarchical representation enables Transformers to excel marvellously at applications such as language translation text summarization and image recognition. In much the same way that the brain adjusts its pattern of attention to maximize cognitive performance in reaction to environmental stimuli, self-attention in Transformers enables AI models to reallocate their processing resources in real time, thus making them better at understanding and generating complex data streams. This congruence between biological and artificial mechanisms of attention only underlines the impact that neuroscience can have on the development of complex AI architectures.

4.4 NEUROSCIENTIFIC THEORIES OF LEARNING AND THEIR IMPACT ON ALGORITHMS

4.4.1 Reinforcement learning and the dopamine system

The brain's reward system, particularly the role played by dopamine, plays a critical role in behavior shaping and learning in reinforcement learning. In both biological and artificial intelligence, dopamine is a neurotransmitter that transmits the signals of rewards, motives, or pleasures, thus making it an essential part of the brain's learning mechanism. When a stimulus leads to the occurrence of positive reinforcing outcomes or rewards, dopamine neurons in the ventral tegmental area (VTA) and the nucleus accumbent get excited by reinforcement between that action and the rewarding outcome. This natural feedback mechanism encourages the repetition of responses that lead toward favorable outcomes and discourages those that do not; it, therefore, facilitates adaptive learning in dynamic environments.

The principles from the brain's dopamine system have heavily influenced the reinforcement learning algorithms engineered to optimize decision-making in the intelligent artificial realm [15]. These algorithms maximize what is learned by living organisms by trying out methods and correcting strategies to suit rewarding interactions with their environment, all based on the cumulative reward signals utilized by the model to maximize the accumulation of rewards over time. The concept of the reward signal in these algorithms is similar to the way dopamine appears in the brain, the positive feedback strengthens associations of specific actions with their effects. Techniques such as Q-learning and policy gradients advance on this, updating values or policies based on received rewards from a computation similar to how the human mind learns through experience. Further, the thought process of temporal difference learning in reinforcement learning has sounded just like that, as any reward the brain can predict for its future from its current actions more promisingly gives it a more discerning understanding of long-term consequences. By taking principles from the reward mechanism of the brain, reinforcement learning algorithms have been proven to be more effective at solving complex tasks such as game playing, robotics, and resource management. This is an example of how neuroscience and artificial intelligence work together to enable adaptive learning systems.

4.4.2 Predictive coding in the brain

Predictive coding is the fundamental process within neuroscience whereby the brain makes predictions of incoming sensory information and adjusts them according to actual sensory feedback. Information fed into this organization is viewed as not being received passively but actively made predictions based on what it can expect to perceive in light of previous experiences, knowledge, and contextual clues. Whenever sensory input arrives the brain compares this to its prediction, and calculates the difference, or "prediction error". If there is a match between actual sensory inputs and the prediction reinforcement of the prediction takes place. If there is some difference between actual sensory inputs and predictions of the brain then it updates its predictions so that future errors are at a minimum, therefore, in a way, learning from a mismatch. This adaptive mechanism enhances the way information is processed in the brain, so that it focuses more on novel or unexpected stimuli, whereas responses to familiar patterns are streamlined. Many layers form a layered structure in the hierarchical generative models typically used in predictive coding [16].

This concept of predictive coding somewhat mirrors the way modern models in machine learning, most notably deep learning, work, where predictions and feedback upon incorrectness improve the models' performance. For example, in neural networks, a prediction is derived based on input data, and the output is compared with actual results. Then, through backpropagation, the parameters of the model are adjusted by relating the predicted output to the actual output, just as occurs in the error of the brain of the prediction. It allows a model to continually refine its understanding and precision over time, much like the brain fine-tunes its predictions based on experience. This predictive framework enables both biological and artificial intelligence systems to learn and adapt efficiently and hence perform better in complex tasks. It is this synergy between the concept of predictive coding in the brain and prediction-driven learning in AI that underscores the influence of neuroscientific principles in the development of advanced machine-learning algorithms [17].

Table 4.2 outlines key neuroscientific principles, describing their significance and corresponding applications in AI, showcasing how insights from the brain can enhance machine learning models.

Table 4.2 Key Neuroscientific Principles and Their Applications in AI

Neuroscientific Principle	*Description*	*AI Application*
Sparse Coding	Representing information using a small number of active neurons	Model pruning and feature selection
Spike-Timing-Dependent Plasticity (STDP)	Learning based on the timing of spikes	Temporal learning in Spiking Neural Networks (SNNs)
Predictive Coding	The brain predicts sensory input and adjusts based on errors	Adaptive learning algorithms
Hierarchical Processing	Information processed at multiple levels	Deep learning architectures
Energy Efficiency	Optimization of neural processes to minimize energy use	Energy-efficient AI models for resource-constrained devices

4.4.3 Cognitive neuroscience in human learning

Cognitive neuroscience sheds insight that could be used to significantly enhance the design and effectiveness of AI models, as in natural language learning systems, wherein the ultimate aim is communication with humans. Therefore, cognitive neuroscience explains how the brain processes information, learns, and remembers and hence elucidates very basic principles of human learning, memory, and language acquisition. These principles, when adopted into AI models by developers, can help create systems that better present cognitive processes similar to that of human beings: in short, hence more engaging for users and have better learning outcomes [18].

This way, for instance, language learning models could be informed by some of the knowledge ascertained on how people learn languages—such as the importance of context, repetition, or meaningful interactions in actual learning. Spaced repetition research from cognitive neuroscience shows that learners learn by re-exposure, and meaningful discussions provide context and relevance, again, methods that AI, in its models of language learning, can integrate into itself through adaptive learning techniques, in which content is adapted to a specific learner's progress and preferences.

This further means that the human cognition social and emotional aspect makes AI interactions more intuitive and human-like. Studies have proven that emotional engagement plays a huge part in motivation and retention of learning. Designing AI systems that can detect and respond to users' emotional states—through natural language processing in detecting sentiment or tone, among others—will surely create an environment of better support in learning, thereby promoting persistence and engagement.

Table 4.3 compares traditional AI language models with neuromyotonic AI models, emphasizing the benefits of integrating neuroscientific insights into language learning systems, particularly contextual understanding,

Table 4.3 Benefits of Integrating Neuroscience with AI in Language Learning

Aspect	*Traditional AI-Language Models*	*Neurosymbolic AI Models*
Contextual Understanding	Limited context processing	Enhanced context integration through symbolic reasoning
Personalization	Fixed learning pathways	Adaptive learning based on user interaction and feedback
Explainability	Often opaque decision-making	Clearer rationale through symbolic logic
Engagement	Basic interaction	Emotionally responsive interfaces that adapt to user states
Knowledge Transfer	Rigid transfer of learning	Flexible application of learned concepts across domains

personalization, explainability, engagement, and knowledge transfer. In addition, knowledge of how the human brain structures and retrieves information can be used as guidelines when structuring content within an AI system to match up with human thought patterns. For example, the way information is presented can be structured in such a manner to use pre-existing knowledge and mental models that thereby will help in achieving better comprehension and retention. The findings from cognitive neuroscience can thus be used to make AI models learn better but also interact in a way that's more impactful and human-centered than before, therefore making the user experience richer in applications such as language learning.

4.4.4 Brain-computer interfaces (BCI)

Here is an example of the intersection of neuroscience and AI in the continuous development of interfaces shown for BCIs, which are increasingly promising direct enhancements to machine learning systems. A brain-machine interface, or BCI, is a collaboration that permits direct electrical signal transmission from neurons to an external equipment or system, such as a computer or robotic arm [19]. Brain-computer interfaces allow one to have a direct connection between the brain and external devices for the collection of neural signals that are interpretable and translatable into actionable data. What it does is harness insights from neuroscience about how the brain processes information and produces motor commands, which create a very different kind of input stream that traditional sensors and interfaces can't provide. Thus, it can be integrated with machine learning algorithms to develop systems adaptive to users' neural patterns and will have applications more personalized and responsive to users' needs.

Indeed, in assistive technology, BCIs can be most compellingly applied, to allow disabled individuals to control prosthetic limbs or even computers purely by thought. Machine learning models used in the context of brain-computer interfaces can, in theory, adapt unique neural data from users, which may help progressively increase the accuracy and responsiveness of the interface. This adaptability not only enhances user experience but may allow the system to learn and evolve based on the neural patterns of a particular user, thus offering a much more fluid interaction.

Brain-computer interfaces are further expected to enhance human-machine interaction by elaborating states of cognitive, emotional, and decision-making processes. Real-time analysis of brain activity may provide smart systems with feedback to improve behavior per the mental condition of the user, which could help create a more intuitive and engaging form of interaction. To achieve interaction with the outside world and control the external environment, a brain-computer interface (BCI) system can directly transform the information given by the brain into commands that can operate external devices and substitute human limbs or phonation organs

[20]. An example of this would be how a BCI keeps track of a learner's levels of attention and engagement, thereby creating an adaptive learning environment that responds to their needs and optimizes educational outcomes.

It is most likely that the integration of neuroscience and AI in BCI technology shall be the source of innovative solutions across various domains-from healthcare and rehabilitation to gaming and virtual reality-and can open up avenues for improved machine learning systems, raising great questions regarding the future of human cognition, agency, and interaction with technology, deeper understanding of the brain, and simultaneously growing the capabilities of AI.

4.5 NEURAL COMPUTATION AND SYMBOLIC REASONING

4.5.1 Biological symbolic representation

The most interesting area of research is that which combines neural computation with symbolic reasoning. This is an interesting area because it points toward the intricate interplay between several cognitive processes. Neural computation is concerned more directly with the distributed networks of neurons in the brain, which receive sensory information and learn through patterns and relationships. Symbolic reasoning, however, deals with abstract concepts, rules, and relationships. Such duality suggests that the brain cannot rely purely on either end of the computational spectrum but is likely to utilize a balance of both to perform higher-order cognitive functions like language, problem-solving, and decision-making.

There is some evidence that regions within the brain may be uniquely specialized for symbolic processing. For instance, areas inside the left hemisphere, specifically the inferior frontal gyrus and angular gyrus, have been perceived as necessary elements for language processing and mathematical reasoning. Such areas may coactivate with other association networks within the cortex that perform some of the underlying neural computation for learning and memory. This allows the human mind to transform sensory feelings into representations, hence facilitating abstraction and rules used by logic. The concept is simply an example: for example, in solving a mathematical equation, the brain may be using neural networks so that the required quantities and their relationships are represented as part of that which is calculated while representing symbolic abilities through manipulating the equations with conclusions drawn out.

The integration of neural computation and symbolic reasoning may also play an important role in other cognitive processes, such as analogical or metaphorical thinking. These higher-order cognitive abilities make the brain bridge diverse concepts with common attributes to guarantee innovative problem-solving and creative thinking. In addition, the architecture of the brain is not only meant to retrieve information speedily but to use symbolic representations to enhance understanding and flow of ideas in communication. Even as cognitive neuroscience continues the in-depth exploration of brain mechanisms, a clearer vision of how these two processes work together can come to the fore, offering valuable insights into human cognition and eventually the development of artificial intelligence systems created to try to emulate these capabilities. This synergy between neural computation and symbolic reasoning brings out the highly remarkable capability of the brain to navigate complex environments and find problem solutions in multifaceted ways of information processing.

4.5.2 Neuromyotonic AI

Neuromyotonic AI is a new direction that seeks to integrate the best abilities of deep learning with symbolic logic. It is a disciplined endeavor to enhance the capability of artificial systems to do highly complex reasoning tasks. Traditional models of deep learning are great at recognizing patterns and learning from vast sets of data; however, they tend to falter at tasks requiring explicit reasoning, generalization, and manipulation of abstract concepts. Symbolic AI is in contrast extensively based on many years of rich tradition that enables advanced reasoning and problem-solving through formal logic and structured representations but often lacks fluidity and scalability in handling unstructured inputs like images and natural language [21].

As with many other things, deep learning has recently had a significant influence on neurosymbolic AI. While earlier neurosymbolic AI research frequently strayed from conventional artificial neural network topologies, this seems to express, on the other hand, an almost exclusive concentration on deep learning methodologies as the neural substrate [22]. Neuromyotonic approaches attempt to build systems in which artificial intelligence systems use the strengths of both neural and symbolic processing by combining both paradigms. This would thus integrate much more fine-grained understanding and reasoning capabilities, which would allow systems to not only identify patterns in data but also reason about the relationships, rules, and hierarchies implicit in that data. For instance, a neuromyotonic AI may search a visual scene with deep learning approaches that have identified objects while at the same time using symbolic reasoning to determine the relationships of those objects, such as knowing that the cat is on the mat or that the person is feeding the dog.

Another benefit that neuromyotonic AI may bring with it is better explanations and interpretability. The addition of symbolic logic to these systems makes it possible for them to elucidate further the reasoning behind their decisions through more transparent information about their logic processes. That is, it makes it more understandable to people how conclusions are reached. Neuromyotonic frameworks also facilitate cross-domain knowledge transfer, which permits AI systems to apply learned concepts to new scenarios, a problem whose neural counterparts suffer frequently from. Continued progress in this kind of research in neuromyotonic AI promises revolutionary applications, from natural language processing to robotics and the most complex decision-making and automated reasoning attempts, which might take it more toward intelligent, adaptive AI systems, designed to think and reason like human beings.

4.6 NEURAL EFFICIENCY AND RESOURCE OPTIMIZATION

4.6.1 Energy efficiency in the brain

The human brain is very economical in its energy usage. It works at a power of approximately 20 watts, which is equivalent to the amount of energy used by a dim light bulb. For that, even though it makes up only 2% of the total body weight, at rest, it uses about 20% of the total energy expenditure of the body. It is attributed to a few complex mechanisms that enhance the utilization of energy without affecting cognitive performance. Its activity levels directly determine its energy usage, but it has several methods with which it reduces energy dissipation. For example, it employs local processing strategies: neurons sensitive to specific stimuli increase their efficiency due to sparse coding that activates only a small number of neurons at any moment in time, thereby reducing energy consumption on average.

One fundamental aspect of brain development and function may be the efficiency of the brain's energy cost exchange for information processing or the partial derivative of information processing concerning energy cost [23]. Effective signalling techniques include the reliance on action potentials, also called spikes in biology. This method allows information to travel rapidly with low energy expenditure from one neuron to another. All of this can be accomplished through an all-or-nothing firing mechanism that provides speed in communication without the continuous expenditure of energy, dissimilar from the traditional computing systems reliant on constant power usage. In addition, the brain's structure, with its extremely well-connected network of neurons, allows for parallel processing, so many cognitive tasks can be handled simultaneously without a proportionate increase in the consumption of energy. These fuel efficiencies also underline the evolutionary adaptation [24] of the brain for survival as they inspire new avenues of improving energy-efficient artificial intelligence systems. Researchers attempt to create AI models that can carry out intricate tasks with a reduction in energy requirements tenfold thus answering one of the biggest challenges in advancing computational technologies. AI applications for optimizing energy efficiency are many and powerful, with great potential to cut costs, minimize environmental effects, and reduce energy usage [25].

Table 4.4 presents a comparison of energy consumption between the human brain and various AI models, highlighting the efficiency of the brain

Table 4.4 Energy Consumption of the Human Brain Compared to AI Models

Entity	*Power Consumption (Watts)*	*Functionality*
Human Brain	~20 watts	Complex cognitive tasks, real-time processing
Standard Deep Learning Model	300-500+ watts	Image recognition, natural language processing
Spiking Neural Network	Variable (potentially < 20 watts)	Temporal processing, energy-efficient computations
Mobile AI Model	5-20 watts	Lightweight tasks, adaptive to resource constraints

in performing complex tasks compared to traditional and emerging AI systems [26].

4.6.2 Optimizing AI models

The insights neuroscience developed about the energy efficiency of the brain can provide quite a large amount of information for optimization techniques in machine learning, more for device-constrained applications such as mobile phones, IoT devices, and embedded systems. When assessing, categorizing, or enhancing current systems or data, an optimization algorithm is a crucial tool for determining which option, out of all the potential alternatives, is optimal [27]. There is a cognitive ability of the brain to manage complex performance tasks with very minimal amounts of energy, which makes it an invaluable model for drawing AI algorithms that value efficiency without sacrificing any performance. One principle borrowed from neuroscience, though in application to quite a different field, is sparse coding. Here, only a subset of neurons should be active in the representation of information to minimize energy expenditure. In machine learning models, sparse representations can be developed where only a few parameters are active during computation; data can thus be processed efficiently while conserving energy [12].

Another critical component of the brain's efficiency is its dependency on parallel processing, so much can be processed simultaneously without a huge increase in power usage. This principle could inspire the development of distributed machine-learning techniques that take advantage of parallel processing between multiple cores or devices, optimizing resources and enhancing the speed of computation [7]. Other techniques include model pruning and quantization, which can simulate some of the functional mechanisms of the brain: removal of redundant weights or decreased precision of computation, respectively [28]. The former reduces the overall computational load, and the latter reduces the energy requirements.

Understanding the dynamic nature of synaptic connections and the adaptive use of resources based on current tasks by the brain may help in designing adaptive machine-learning systems [29]. These would vary in complexity and resource use according to what a specific task might require, much like the brain adjusts neural pathways to different stimuli or conditions. Finding integration within neuroscience-inspired approaches may make AI models more efficient to start with using under-resourced environments, leading to even more sustainable technologies that are even more efficient by the principles of biological intelligence. This amalgamation enhances the capabilities of machine learning but also generates more intelligent yet resource-aware AI applications well-suited for this new digital age [30].

4.7 CONCLUSION

Long-term integration of neuroscience with artificial intelligence may unlock tremendous potential by exploiting principles in brain functions to generate much smarter and more efficient AI. Biological neurons, for example, are noteworthy for more complex processes, such as synaptic plasticity, energy-efficient signaling, and temporal dynamics; these serve as templates for the optimization of machine learning models. Incorporating neuroscience insights, such as Hebbian learning and spike-timing-dependent plasticity, has been shown to considerably improve AI. An excellent example is that of spiking neural networks (SNNs) that resemble the spike-based communication of the brain, a route in which neuroscience has informed AI towards more biologically plausible systems, and also much more energy-efficient systems.

The hierarchical organization of cortical processing in the brain-inspired architecture in deep learning results, among other things, in breakthroughs in image and pattern recognition using convolutional neural networks. Neuromyotonic AI aspires to unify neural and symbolic reasoning to handle more complex tasks, which again shows how biologically inspired insights can elevate the abilities of AI. The interplay between the advancements of neuroscience and AI can make AI adaptive, energy efficient, and relevant to real-world challenges. This convergence not only lays a foundation for much more advanced AI systems but also opens new exciting paths in understanding the human brain and machine intelligence, ways for further investigation and innovation, and so forth.

REFERENCES

[1] Sarkar, T., Lieberth, K., Pavlou, A., et al., "An organic artificial spiking neuron for in situ neuromorphic sensing and biointerfacing",

Nature Electronics 5, 774–783, 2022, https://doi.org/10.1038/s41928-022-00859-y

[2] Chung, S., & Abbott, L. F., "Neural population geometry: An approach for understanding biological and artificial neural networks", *Current Opinion in Neurobiology*, 70, 137–144, 2021, https://doi.org/10.1016/j.conb.2021.10.010

[3] Ororbia, A., et al., "A review of neuroscience-inspired machine learning.", arXiv preprint arXiv:2403.18929, 2024, https://doi.org/10.48550/arXiv.2403.18929

[4] Ororbia, A. G., & Kelly, M. A., "A neuro-mimetic realization of the common model of cognition via Hebbian learning and free energy minimization.", *Proceedings of the AAAI Symposium Series*, 2(1), 2023, https://doi.org/10.1609/aaaiss.v2i1.27702

[5] Debanne, D., & Inglebert, Y., "Spike timing-dependent plasticity and memory", *Current Opinion in Neurobiology*, 80, 102707, 2023, https://doi.org/10.1016/j.conb.2023.102707

[6] Vogeti, S., Boetzel, C., & Herrmann, C. S., "Entrainment and spike-timing dependent plasticity – A review of proposed mechanisms of transcranial alternating current stimulation", *Frontiers in Systems Neuroscience*, 16, 2022, https://doi.org/10.3389/fnsys.2022.827353

[7] Zheng, H., Wu, Y., Deng, L., Hu, Y., & Li, G., "Going deeper with directly-trained larger spiking neural networks", *Proceedings of the AAAI Conference on Artificial Intelligence*, 35(12), 11062–11070, 2021, https://doi.org/10.1609/aaai.v35i12.17320

[8] Liu, F., Zhao, W., Chen, Y., Wang, Z., Yang, T., & Jiang, L., "SSTDP: Supervised Spike Timing Dependent Plasticity for efficient spiking neural network training", *Frontiers in Neuroscience*, 15, 2021, https://doi.org/10.3389/fnins.2021.756876

[9] Lyle, C., Zheng, Z., Nikishin, E., Avila Pires, B., Pascanu, R., & Dabney, W., "Understanding Plasticity in Neural Networks", In A. Krause, E. Brunskill, K. Cho, B. Engelhardt, S. Sabato, & J. Scarlett (Eds.), *Proceedings of the 40th International Conference on Machine Learning* (Vol. 202, pp. 23190–23211). PMLR, 2023, https://proceedings.mlr.press/v202/lyle23b.html

[10] Vathakkatil Joseph, G., & Pakrashi, V., "Spiking neural networks for structural health monitoring", *Sensors*, 22, 9245, 2022, https://doi.org/10.3390/s22239245

[11] Nunes, J. D., Carvalho, M., Carneiro, D., & Cardoso, J. S., "Spiking neural networks: A survey," *IEEE Access*, 10, 60738–60764, 2022, https://doi.org/10.1109/ACCESS.2022.3179968

[12] Nag, A., et al., "TumorGANet: A transfer learning and generative adversarial network- based data augmentation model for brain tumor classification," *IEEE Access*, 12, 103060–103081, 2024, doi: 10.1109/ACCESS.2024.3429633.

[13] Yamazaki, K., Vo-Ho, V-K., Bulsara, D., & Le, N., "Spiking neural networks and their applications: A review", *Brain Sciences*, 2022, https://doi.org/10.3390/brainsci12070863

[14] Piasini, E., Soltuzu, L., Muratore, P., et al., "Temporal stability of stimulus representation increases along rodent visual cortical hierarchies", *Nature Communications,* 12, 4448, 2021, https://doi.org/10.1038/s41467-021-24456-3

[15] Chakroun, K., Wiehler, A., Wagner, B., et al., "Dopamine regulates decision thresholds in human reinforcement learning in males", *Nature Communications,* 14, 5369, 2023, https://doi.org/10.1038/s41467-023-41130-y

[16] Millidge, B., Seth, A., & Buckley, C. L., "Predictive coding: A theoretical and experimental review", 2021, https://doi.org/10.48550/arXiv.2107.12979

[17] Smith, R., Badcock, P., & Friston, K. J., "Recent advances in the application of predictive coding and active inference models within clinical neuroscience", *Psychiatry and Clinical Neurosciences*, 75(1), 3–13, 2021, https://doi.org/10.1111/pcn.13138

[18] Nastase, S. A., Goldstein, A., & Hasson, U., "Keep it real: Rethinking the primacy of experimental control in cognitive neuroscience", *NeuroImage*, 222, 117254, 2020, https://doi.org/10.1016/j.neuroimage.2020.117254

[19] Mudgal, S. K., Sharma, S. K., Chaturvedi, J., & Sharma, A., "Brain computer interface advancement in neurosciences: Applications and issues", *Interdisciplinary Neurosurgery*, 20, 100694, 2020, https://doi.org/10.1016/j.inat.2020.100694

[20] Bonci A, Fiori S, Higashi H, Tanaka T, Verdini F., "An introductory tutorial on brain–computer interfaces and their applications", *Electronics*, 2021, https://doi.org/10.3390/electronics10050560

[21] Wan, Z., Liu, C.-K., Yang, H., Li, C., You, H., Fu, Y., Wan, C., Krishna, T., Lin, Y., & Raychowdhury, A., "Towards cognitive AI Systems: A survey and prospective on neuro-symbolic AI", 2024, https://doi.org/10.48550/arXiv.2401.01040

[22] Hitzler, P., Eberhart, A., Ebrahimi, M., Sarker, M. K., & Zhou, L., "Neuro-symbolic approaches in artificial intelligence", *National Science Review*, 9(6), 2022, https://doi.org/10.1093/nsr/nwac035

[23] Shao, F., & Shen, Z., "How can artificial neural networks approximate the brain?", *Frontiers in Psychology*, 13, 2023, https://doi.org/10.3389/fpsyg.2022.970214

[24] Reddy, V., Elango, N. M., & Kishor Kumar Reddy, C., "Diabetes Kaggle dataset adequacy scrutiny using factor exploration and correlation", *International Journal of Recent Technology and Engineering*, 8, 1S4, 2019.

[25] Olatunde, T. M., Okwandu, Akande, D. C., & Sikhakhane, Z. Q., "Reviewing the role of artificial intelligence in energy efficiency optimization", *Engineering Science & Technology Journal*, 5(4), 1243–1256, 2024, https://doi.org/10.51594/estj.v5i4.1015

[26] Reddy, V., Elango, N. M., & Kishor Kumar Reddy, C., "Internet of things based early detection of diabetes using machine learning algorithms: DPA", *International Journal of Innovative Technology and Exploring Engineering*, 8, 10, 2019.

[27] Abdolrasol, M. G. M., Hussain, S. M. S., Ustun, T. S., Sarker, M. R., Hannan, M. A., Mohamed, R., Ali, J. A., Mekhilef, S., Milad, A., "Artificial

neural networks based optimization techniques: A review", *Electronics*, 2021, https://doi.org/10.3390/electronics10212689
[28] Andrade-Talavera, Y., Fisahn, A., & Rodríguez-Moreno, A., "Timing to be precise? An overview of spike timing-dependent plasticity, brain rhythmicity, and glial cells interplay within neuronal circuits", *Molecular Psychiatry*, 28, 2177–2188, 2023, https://doi.org/10.1038/s41380-023-02027-w
[29] Rahman, A., Nag, A., & Bairagi, A. K., "A hybrid model for recognizing human activity using extreme learning," *2023 26th International Conference on Computer and Information Technology (ICCIT)*, Cox's Bazar, Bangladesh, 2023, 1–6, doi: 10.1109/ICCIT60459.2023.10441574.
[30] Nag, A., Das, B., Sil, R., Hameed, A. A., Bhushan, B., & Jamil, A., "A Survey on Image-Based Cardiac Diagnosis Prediction Using Machine Learning and Deep Learning Techniques", In F. P. García Márquez, A. Jamil, I. S. Ramirez, S. Eken, A. A. Hameed (Eds.), *Computing, Internet of Things and Data Analytics. ICCIDA 2023. Studies in Computational Intelligence* (Vol. 1145). Springer, Cham, 2024, https://doi.org/10.1007/978-3-031-53717-2_44

Chapter 5

Optimizing neural disorder treatment through federated learning and multi-institutional data collaboration

Monika Singh T, Kishor Kumar Reddy C, Jagadeshwari Puttanapura, and Srinath Doss

5.1 INTRODUCTION

Neural diseases, or neurological diseases, is a term that describes a group of diseases involving the nervous system, which comprises both the brain and the spinal cord; and peripheral nerves. These encompass diseases, including Alzheimer's disease, Parkinson's disease, epilepsy, and multiple sclerosis. They greatly impact the person's efforts toward leading an ordinary lifestyle, as they cause all forms of damage to the motor systems, memory, cognitive structures, or even sensory detection. As the world is ageing along with the population, there is an increase in neural disorder cases, which suggests that it poses a serious growing burden on healthcare systems worldwide. Despite the recent breakthroughs in neuroscience, many neural disorders are still not well understood [1]. The attention of researchers is primarily focused on disentangling the complex conditions involving genetics, molecules, and environmental situations that initiate the disease. Another challenge is the complexity of approaching treatments for such diseases due to the fragile nature of the brain, with such interference disrupting the fine balance of its functions. This complexity underlines the need to innovate diagnostics as well as therapeutic strategies.

Neurological conditions can take an assortment of forms and may only rarely be associated with minor loss of cognitive control to highly disabling physical impairments. Amyotrophic lateral sclerosis (ALS), Huntington's disease, as well as traumatic injury to the brain, are some of the disorders that result in a high decline in a patient's health leading to long-term use of medical treatment. Environmental exposures and infections, as well as autoimmune responses, are the most potent contributors to the condition of specific neurologic disorders. Neuroinflammatory processes have become central features in the pathogenesis of many diseases, providing new therapeutic possibilities [2]. However, one of the greatest challenges for these diseases relates to their early detection; the symptoms usually appear at a

DOI: 10.1201/9781003591085-5

time when crucial neural tissue damage has already been done. The families and caregivers also suffer significant emotional and financial costs. This explains the crucial requirement of enhanced preventive measures and early interventions along with support systems to deal with the rising challenges presented by neurological disorders.

Figure 5.1 shows different categories of neurological diseases. The diagram expands the cause of various conditions, such as being due to vascular and neuromuscular as well as neural developmental problems and trauma, among others, psychological disorders, dementia, autoimmune diseases, infections, and other neurological impairments. Each category herein has a distinct origin of neurological disease.

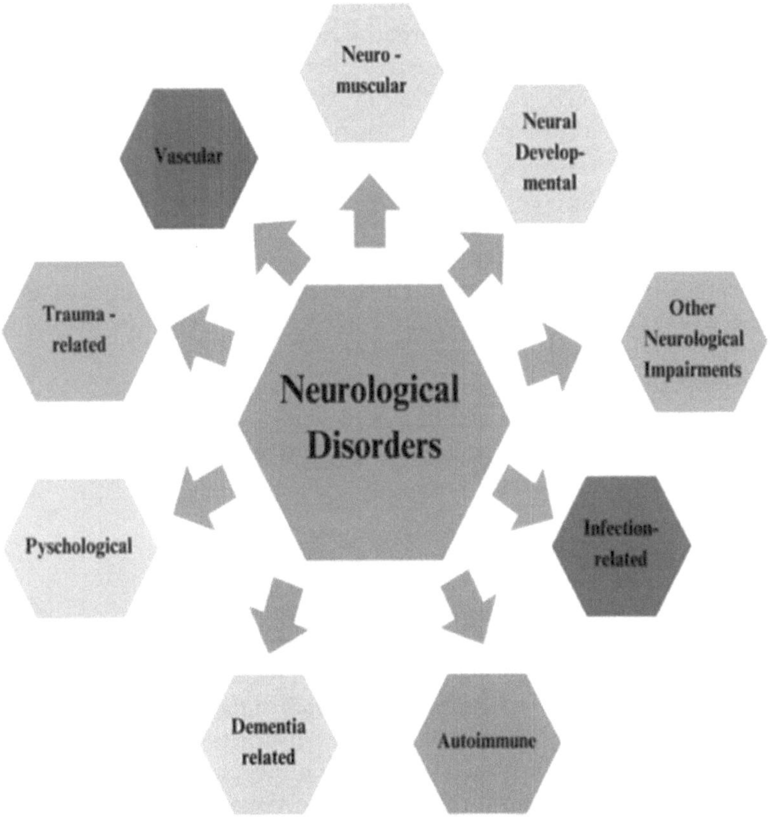

Figure 5.1 Types of Neurological Diseases.

5.1.1 Challenges

Neural disorders are not that easy to treat as the nervous system, involved with structures and functioning parts, is quite complex. Most neurological diseases progress imperceptibly: even when symptoms begin, they often appear only after prolonged silent progression of the disease process. The necessary treatment cannot be initiated early enough, for when the diagnosis is actually made, the damage is already irreversible. Most treatments of neurological disorders besides human immunodeficiency viruses (HIV) and dementia [3] are concerned with the alleviation of symptoms rather than slowing the progression of disease, thereby leaving patients with a chronic condition requiring long-term care. Another major challenge is the blood-brain barrier, a physiological defence that keeps many substances out of the brain from the bloodstream. While it protects it against toxins and infections, this barrier excludes many useful drugs from reaching the target, thus making it difficult for potentially effective treatments to reach their mark. Moreover, neural disorders are highly heterogeneous; that is, while effective for one patient, these treatments might not work for another [4]. This heterogeneity complicates the development of universal therapies, in turn, emphasizing the need for personalized medicine in treating neural diseases. The treatment of neurological disorders requires specialized care, including, and apart from, medical experience, advanced diagnostic instruments, and complex medications. However, most healthcare systems are challenged to offer enough support in such areas, which further complicates these disorders by giving rise to problems in accurate diagnosis and effective treatment [5]. The resulting misdiagnosis, with attendant delay, exacerbates symptoms and augments the burden on patients and caregivers alike. The points above require a more holistic approach – areas critical to this challenge include improved access to care, investment in research to increase diagnostic and therapeutic options, and public awareness regarding neurological conditions.

5.1.2 Necessity of data-centric methods

The last few years have witnessed a huge spike in the popularity of the data-driven approach that includes Artificial Intelligence (AI), Machine Learning (ML), and Big Data Analytics in the study of neural disorders. These technologies enable the analysis of massive amounts of data that include genetic information, neuroimaging, as well as patient histories among many others. These analyses can, in turn, be used to bring out previously undetectable patterns. These insights can then be turned to the advantage of clinicians, empowering them to make better-informed diagnoses, forecast the likely course of a disease, and even design personified treatment plans tailored to each patient's needs. Indeed, data-driven models can revolutionize drug discovery to predict what new compounds are likely to have an effect and where they might be toxic in much earlier terms than the traditional clinical trials. Therefore, from the faster identification of the potential candidate, saving time and cost would come from reducing years and millions of dollars needed to bring new medicines to market. Further development of research into neural disorders may result in the unlocking of completely new therapies for millions of sufferers around the world while introducing the application of data-driven techniques together with traditional approaches.

Table 5.1 shows how the data-driven approaches have such high advantages over traditional methods in the diagnosis, personalizing treatment, predicting the progression of disease, discovering drugs and integrating data from patients into promising advancements in the treatment of neural disorders.

The chapter's main contribution will be a very informative discussion regarding how Federated Learning (FL) could change the diagnosis and treatment of neural disorders under the setting of multi-institutional data collaborations. It portrays the critical elements of federated learning methodologies, the roles that FL assumes in improving health, and its applications to optimize treatment for diseases such as epilepsy, Alzheimer's, and Parkinson's. Challenges in data sharing for healthcare, ethical concerns

Table 5.1 Importance of Data-Driven Approaches

Aspect	*Traditional Approaches*	*Data-centric Methods*	*Benefits of Data-centric Methods*
Diagnosis	It is based on the clinical symptoms and physical examinations	Uses an AI to analyze neuroimaging, genetic, and clinical data	Improved accuracy and earlier detection
Treatment Personalization	One-size-fits-all treatments	Machine learning models suggest personalized treatment plans	Customized treatments based on individual profiles
Disease Progression Prediction	It is difficult to predict without long-term monitoring	Predictive models analyze patient data to forecast progression	Anticipates disease progression for proactive intervention
Drug Discovery	It is time-consuming and costly drug trials	AI predicts drug efficacy and potential side effects	Speeds up drug discovery and reduces trial costs
Data Integration	Fragmented patient records and limited data sources	Combines diverse datasets (e.g., genetics, imaging, symptoms)	Holistic view of patient health and comprehensive analysis

with privacy-preservation techniques, and how FL may unlock possibilities for breakthroughs in personalized medicine are among the areas that this paper will bring to attention. Case studies and practical insights from this work should help advance the understanding of the shape that FL may bring to the future landscape of healthcare delivery or spur cooperative institutional efforts.

The following is the order of the remaining sections of this chapter: Section 5.2 refers to the overview of federated learning and its methodologies; Section 5.3 is entitled with a focus on the importance of cross-institutional data sharing to develop research results; Section 5.4 contains findings concerning the application of federated learning in neurology; Section 5.5 presents the detailed procedure for the data collection and preprocessing; Section 5.6 discusses model design and training processes particularly with federated learning; Section 5.7 refers to issues and solutions when applying federated learning in healthcare; Section 5.8 outlines the applications of federated learning in neural disorder treatments; Section 5.9 discusses ethical, legal, and regulatory considerations; Section 5.10 focuses on future directions and research possibilities; and Section 5.11 is the conclusion that summarizes overall implications on the basis of findings. The last section provides a number of references through which all the sources are recognized in the course of research.

5.2 AN OVERVIEW OF FEDERATED LEARNING

Federated learning is essentially a decentralized approach to machine learning for training models distributed across multiple devices or servers that do not move local data to any centralized location. Here, the participating device or server trains a local model on its data and sends just model updates (e.g., gradients) to some central server that aggregates them in order to improve the global model. This is contrasted sharply with the traditional machine learning scenario, which often needs the central collection of data for training models, hence relating issues of privacy and scalability [6]. The three key principles underlying federated learning are decentralization, privacy preservation, and communication efficiency. Federated learning saves the data directly on devices, which means that gaining and maintaining privacy is immediate and not susceptible to breach. It also minimizes the need to transfer large datasets which can be expensive and time-consuming from a computation point of view. An important aspect of federated learning is that it is robust for environments in which devices may have intermittent connectivity or computational capabilities, so appropriate for the use cases in real-time smartphones, Internet of Things (IoT) devices, and Edge computing.

Figure 5.2 is the representation of a federated learning system's workflow. This begins at Step 1 where a global model is initiated and shared with

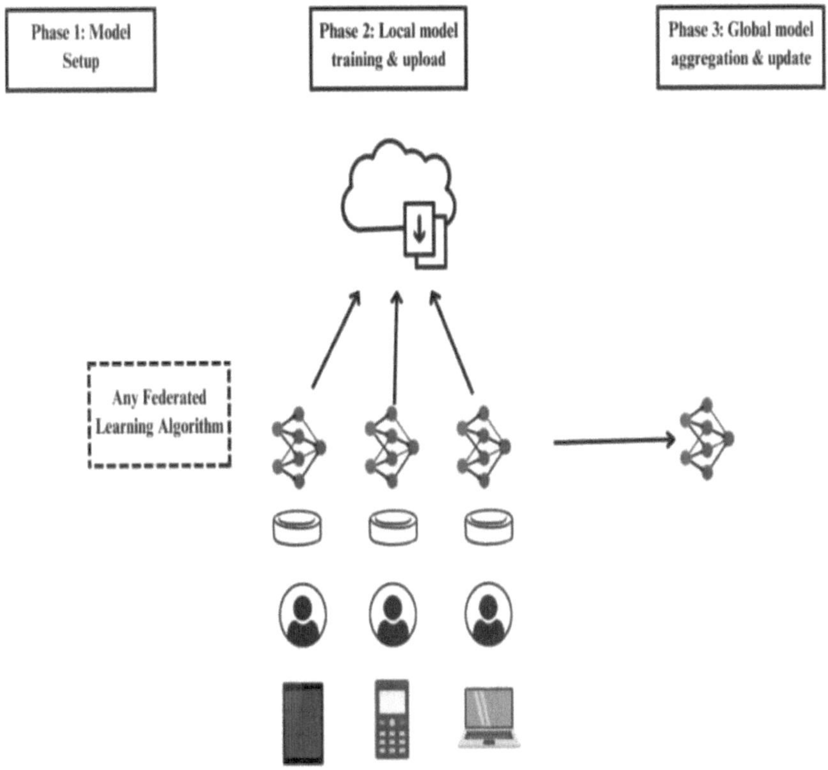

Figure 5.2 Federated Learning Flow: Distributed Model Training and Aggregation.

several devices, including smartphones, tablets, and laptops. Each of these devices has local data, and using that in Step 2, the devices continue to train local models based on their personal data and forward the locally learned models to a central server. In Step 3, the central server aggregates updates from all of the devices for cleaning and updating the global model. This application is controlled through a federated learning algorithm in which raw data resides on the local devices but contributes to the improvement of a global model.

A key advantage of federated learning is its focus on privacy-preserving machine learning. Classic centralization for machine learning typically involves the transfer of sensitive data to a central server. Thus, there is a huge risk of privacy violations and data breaches [7]. By contrast, federated learning minimizes such at-risk practices by averting the exit of raw data off local devices. It aligns perfectly with the data privacy regulations, including the General Data Protection Regulation (GDPR), which has highly emphasized the protection of personal information. It incorporates differential privacy and secure aggregation techniques to add more layers of security to data. Differential privacy adds controlled noise to the model updates in the aggregated result to prevent the recovery of individual data points. Secure aggregation makes sure that the individual updates are encrypted before they are transmitted to the central server so that even if an attacker intercepts the communication, he can't access raw updates [8]. Such privacy-preserving techniques become of prime importance in making machine learning possible in sensitive domains like healthcare and finance.

Applications in Healthcare

Healthcare is a sector where federated learning is quite relevant, considering general problems of privacy and silos of data. Patient information is poorly distributed and can hardly be shared within hospitals and institutions of research because of sensitive privacy. With these settings, probably institutions would have the chance to collaborate on training models collectively and information-sharing without revealing private details of certain patients [9]. A variety of predictive models based on model testing for disease diagnosis, personalized treatment, and medical image analysis can be developed in diversified datasets. Federated learning makes it possible to design AI-based solutions for healthcare, such as architectures of the Internet of Medical Things (IoMT), clinical trial optimization, and precision medicine [10]. All these solutions can become critical in the management and control of patient care and treatment strategies during a pandemic. For instance, hospitals can use federated learning to collectively train models on heart disease prediction or on cancer detection from medical images in such a way that patient data remains inside the safe confines of the hospital. That is to say, [11] the models would probably be closer to the truth using a decentralized approach, for it could be able to pool data variety from several institutions simultaneously with an ability to respect regulatory requirements and preserve patient records' confidentiality. Therefore, future fast medical research may critically depend upon more robust and privacy-preserving AI systems.

5.3 CROSS-INSTITUTIONAL DATA SHARING AND ITS IMPORTANCE

Institutional data sharing across institutions is important in scientific research, particularly in the health sector because access to diverse, high-scale datasets is important in producing robust and generalizable insights. Individual institutions may have limited or fragmented data that may be biased in some instances if used in isolation. Pooling data from various institutions provides researchers with broader and more varied datasets, thereby enhancing the quality and accuracy of the outcomes of the research [12]. This kind of collective approach helps researchers trace events that

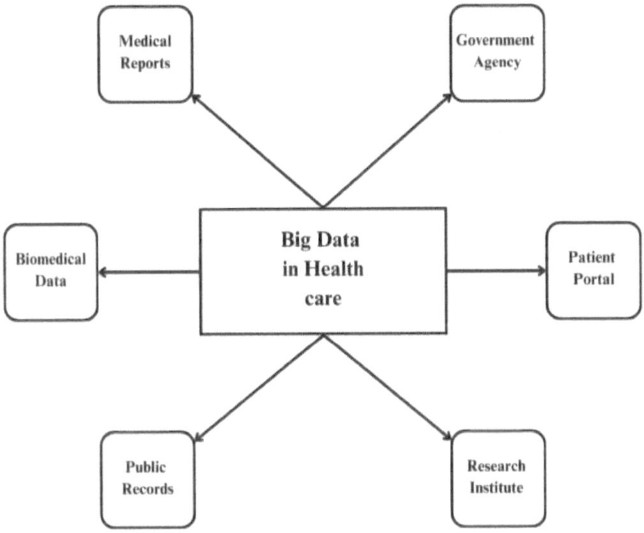

Figure 5.3 Sources of Big Data.

may not appear from research based solely on a single institution. Cross-institutional data sharing has delivered many groundbreaking achievements in healthcare, with examples being delivery in personalized medicine, population health management, and epidemiological research. Predictive models of diseases, such as cancer or cardiovascular conditions, require diverse data from varied populations and environments. Collaborative efforts in data work also hasten innovation because other researchers can work with earlier work from each other and discover quicker, more impactful medical interventions. Ultimately, the aggregate power of shared data drives evidence-based decisions in both clinical care and public health [13].

Figure 5.3 shows diverse sources of big data in healthcare. These sources encompass medical reports, clinical records, biomedical data, electronic health records, public records, and generic databases. In addition, data is pulled from governmental agencies, patient portals, and research institutes. These diverse sources together derive a more complete understanding of patient health and help in the process of research, treatment, and healthcare management.

5.3.1 Challenges of data sharing in healthcare

Whereas the benefits of data sharing are well apparent, it is not possible for healthcare to succeed in its attempt at effective cross-institutional collaboration. One of the significant challenges is healthcare data fragmentation [14]. Institutions usually store their data in different forms because standards and systems differ. This sets a virtually unsurmountable barrier for data sharing or integration, making large-scale collaboration very challenging. There is also this fear of sharing data with institutions, particularly in matters relating to competitive advantage and intellectual property, hence slowing down collaboration.

Table 5.2 explains the different hurdles experienced by healthcare centers while trying to communicate data between institutions. This can greatly impact the effectiveness of cross-institutional collaboration.

Table 5.2 Challenges of Data Sharing in Healthcare

Challenge	*Description*	*Impact*
Data Fragmentation	Healthcare data is often stored in different formats, systems, and standards across institutions.	Some disadvantages are lack of interconnectivity which makes integrating or analyzing data from different sources nearly impossible.
Lack of Standardization	Inconsistent data standards (e.g., coding, formats) across institutions stops interrupt hinder effective data exchange.	Leads to data silos, making cross-institutional collaboration and data integration complex and error-prone.
Privacy Concerns	Sharing patient data raises concerns about violating privacy regulations like HIPAA and GDPR.	Limits the extent to which sensitive data can be shared, hindering collaborative research and clinical insights.
Data Security Risks	Transferring data between institutions increases the risk of unauthorized access or breaches.	Compromises patient confidentiality and can result in legal and financial consequences for institutions.
Institutional Reluctance	Institutions may be unwilling to share data due to competitive concerns or fear of losing intellectual property.	Slows collaboration and restricts access to valuable data that could enhance healthcare research.
Ethical Considerations	Concerns over patient consent and the ethical use of shared healthcare data.	Limits the sharing of data, as patients may not agree to or be informed about cross-institutional data use.
Data Ownership Issues	Uncertainty about who owns the data, especially in collaborations between private and public institutions.	Can lead to disputes, delays, and challenges in sharing data for research or clinical purposes.
Technical Infrastructure	Inadequate or outdated IT infrastructure in some institutions impedes secure and efficient data sharing.	Creates bottlenecks in data transfer, affecting the quality and speed of collaborative efforts.

The other major issue is patient privacy. Healthcare data are very sensitive, and therefore need to be very confidential, as is proposed through the Health Insurance Portability and Accountability Act (HIPAA) in the United States and GDPR in Europe [15]. Such laws mandatorily require organizations with very strict requirements on how data may be shared, stored, and processed, which often complicates efforts in data sharing. Thus, the issues of ethics are involved, so that even with de-identified data, patients might not be ready to share their information across the institutions. The complexities of legal and ethical rules form big barriers to multi-institutional collaboration in the data in healthcare.

5.3.2 Dealing with data privacy and security concerns

Data privacy and security are always of significant concern for institutes, especially when operating in areas like medicine, which handle sensitive data concerning patients. Traditional methods of data sharing are very dangerous since a centralized storage configuration can provide significant security weaknesses and open up avenues for breaches in effective collaboration to mitigate these concerns [16]. One such approach is federated learning, which allows institutions to train on the same machine learning model without ever necessarily sharing data. A federated learning system doesn't move the data to a central location but lets all institutions train a local model and share only the model parameters and gradients, and then combine them into a global model. This way, raw data never leaves the local environment. Risks in terms of privacy were lowered highly by this approach.

In addition to federated learning, another very strong tool for enhancing the security of multi-institutional data collaboration is differential privacy. Differential privacy works by adding properly calibrated noise to the outputs of data; their contribution from any single data point is obfuscated. This technique is very effective and particularly useful in the types of sharing within institutions or when aggregations are to be released to the public [17]. Applying differential privacy will help defend against data reverse-engineering attacks that could expose individual data from the shared datasets by preventing attackers from determining which specific records exist in the shared dataset while allowing for the overall utility of the data to be preserved for analysis.

Homomorphic encryption raises the level of security through the computation of encrypted data. In this approach, the data is still encrypted during processing. So, the institution or entity that actually analyzes the data will never receive unencrypted data. Homomorphic encryption allows entities to share datasets in encrypted form for collaborative analysis without violating any secrecy. Although such technology is computationally intensive, recent advances in computational technology make it much more practical for large-scale collaborations, especially when it comes to healthcare areas and where maintaining patient anonymity becomes the paramount issue. Lastly, collaboration tools such as blockchain technology are also emerging to ensure the integrity and security of data in multi-institutional collaborations. Blockchain offers its distributed ledger system – a tamper-proof, transparent record of access and sharing data events so that all transactions are traceable and secure; with these features, institutions can ensure that trust is generated in the collaboration process, knowing that data has not been altered or accessed without authorization. This may be highly useful in clinical trials or in research networks, where the integrity and provenance of data are of utmost importance.

There are many multi-institutional collaborative models regarded as blueprints in cross-institutional health data sharing. Such a model includes the Global Alliance for Genomics and Health (GA4GH), which seeks to leverage international collaboration in genomics research by developing standards for equitable access, efficient management, and proper control of genomic and health-related data that respect participant and host sovereignty. GA4GH focuses on creating standard data-sharing practices across institutions and designing secure technologies for collaborative work in research on genomics. Another instance is the Observational Health Data Sciences and Informatics (OHDSI) initiative, which provides open-source tools and resources for standardized analytics across diverse health datasets. This would enable institutions to share and analyze real-world health data without compromising privacy, thereby using data harmonization and distributed analytics. The collaboration frameworks would be much more significant in dealing with common challenges facing healthcare, such as the development of new therapies, better decision-making at clinical levels, and an improved understanding of disease progression. Through these models, institutions pool resources and gain access to larger datasets, which work together with them to advance the broad field of healthcare research.

5.4 OPTIMIZING NEURAL DISORDER TREATMENT WITH FEDERATED LEARNING

Many advances have been made in personalized medicine and cooperative healthcare in optimizing treatments for neural disorders through federated learning. Neural disorders like epilepsy, Alzheimer's, Parkinson's, and mental health disorders are complex; hence, treatments have to be provided along pretty complex lines based on data rather than usual rules that can be applied to all patients. Federated learning allows these health institutions to work together in developing strong machine learning models by sharing insights obtained from decentralized data without sharing patient information. This approach enhances the diagnostics of models on predictability and personalizes treatment planning, thus enabling more accurate and effective interventions. Usage of diverse data across multiple institutions also opens a chance for innovative solutions in the diagnosis and management of neurology disorders, which is private and secure.

5.4.1 Current approaches to the diagnosis and treatment of neurological diseases

Clinical testing, neuroimaging, genetic testing and analysis of spinal biomarkers are diagnostic and therapeutic approaches for many neurological diseases such as Alzheimer's, Parkinson's and epilepsy. Magnetic Resonance Imaging (MRI), Computed Tomography (CT) scanning, Electroencephalography (EEG) and Positron Emission Tomography (PET) scanning are used to detect structural or functional abnormalities in the brain, while genetic testing assesses the genetic predisposition to certain diseases such as Huntington's and certain forms of infectious diseases [18]. However, these diagnostic tools are not always very precise and a common source of misdiagnosis – very often at the early stages, when many neurodegenerative diseases come. A large proportion of neural disorders also have an extremely high interindividual variability in their respective rates of progression, which complicates treatment plans. The treatments for neural disorders are symptomatic rather than curative. The levodopa and other medications, control, in a manner of speaking, the motor symptoms of Parkinson's disease continuously but arrest the disease process; the treatment of Alzheimer's disease consists of medications that temporarily make the short-term cognitive functions of the patient improve but do not halt neurodegenerative degeneration. Such an approach, combined with difficulties in early detection, suggests that even more precise techniques would be data-driven to offer personal insights to the patients for better overall outcomes. Despite all the recent breakthroughs in medical technology, the necessity of optimizing ways in the approach to diagnosis and treatment of neural disorders has arisen. Most methods that are currently in use remain dependent on small-scale, institution-specific data and are far from achieving a robust, generalized model that can be used for diagnosis and the treatment of diseases of this kind. It is precisely for these reasons that innovative techniques, such as federated learning, may become promising means of collaboration and precision medicine.

A federated learning approach could therefore revolutionize the diagnosis of neural disorders to a great extent, as it would enable collaboration between multiple institutions without revealing the identity of the patients. The current diagnostic models are, however, based on extremely limited datasets from individual hospitals or research centres, where even the richness and nuances of neural disorders may not be captured fully. It addresses the problem by enabling institutions to train local models on their datasets but share only model parameters rather than raw data.

This strategy utilizes the power of distributed data and helps in the creation of more comprehensive and accurate diagnostic tools. In the case of neural disorders, federated learning may improve the diagnosis models and allow diversified information from different patient populations in terms of neuroimaging scans, genetic profiles, and clinical history. Therefore, for example, a model trained using federated learning models deployed across different institutions to diagnose Alzheimer's would find early biomarkers for the disease much better and diagnose it much earlier and with better reliability. Similarly, in epilepsy, federated learning might collect EEG data from various hospitals to discover seizure patterns and predict the onset of seizures more accurately. Federated learning integrates data from several sources and mitigates the biases and limitations so frequently reflected in single-institution studies. The approach also accelerates the development of diagnostic algorithms by tapping into more extensive datasets, which constitute a wide necessity for training deep learning models. Finally, federated learning may optimize neural disorder diagnosis by providing more accurate models that can be applied to more diverse clinical settings, hence better outcomes and fewer errors in the diagnosis of patients.

5.4.2 Enhancing personalized treatment plans through federated models

One of the most promising applications of federated learning in neural disorders management is that the model opens up avenues for improving personalized medicine. Neural disorders such as Parkinson's disease and multiple sclerosis (MS) are known to have incredibly varied disease progression; patients could show differing responses to treatments given to them. Using federated learning, it is possible to have personalized treatment models with accountabilities towards variability by analyzing a larger pool of patient data from different institutions. This collaborative approach then allows for the establishment of models that could predict which of the treatments may likely prove the most effective for a particular patient based on their genetic makeup, their medical history, and real-time clinical data.

Table 5.3 explicates the advancements in neural disorder treatment by federated learning, which integrates varied patient data, personalizes treatments, and continuously updates models. These elements lead to the betterment of treatment and patient outcomes and uphold the privacy of data.

Federated learning can connect data from different sources in personalized treatment for neural disorders such as wearable devices monitoring symptoms in patients, test results from genetics, or longitudinal medical records. In the case of Parkinson's, federated learning will draw patterns on how patients may react differently to drugs like dopamine agonists or deep brain stimulation [19]. Such aggregation would open avenues for the models that suggest

Table 5.3 Enhancing Personalized Treatment Plans through Federated Models

Aspect	*Description*	*Benefits*
Data Integration	Combines diverse patient data from multiple institutions, including clinical history, genetics, and real-time monitoring.	Provides a comprehensive view of patient profiles.
Tailored Treatment Recommendations	Develops personalized treatment plans based on individual variability in disease response and progression.	Increases the effectiveness and safety of treatments.
Continuous Model Updates	Federated learning allows for real-time updates to treatment models as new patient data becomes available.	Enables dynamic adjustments to treatment based on the latest data.
Diversity of Data Sources	Utilizes data from various demographics and disease stages across institutions to build more robust models.	Reduces bias and improves the generalizability of treatment recommendations.
Patient Privacy Protection	Ensures sensitive patient information remains secure by analyzing data locally and sharing only model parameters.	Encourages participation from multiple institutions while adhering to privacy regulations.
Adaptive Learning	Models can evolve over time, integrating new data to reflect changes in patient conditions and treatment outcomes.	Enhances the ability to provide timely and relevant treatment adjustments.
Improved Outcomes	Personalized treatment plans lead to better management of neural disorders and improved patient quality of life.	Results in higher patient satisfaction and better health outcomes.

tailored plans of treatment based on the uniqueness of an individual disease trajectory. In turn, the interventions involving such models will be much more effective and safer. It further supports real-time adjustment of treatment. The model, therefore, can be continually adapted to the patient as they accumulate data over time, meaning that it would always reflect their current condition and in turn, dynamically optimize treatment. This is particularly important for neurodegenerative diseases, where the patient can change quickly, and with timely adjustments to treatment, quality of life is maximized. Federated models ensure that adaptations depend on the most recent and richest data in existence, thereby leading to more specific and better care for patients with neural disorders.

5.4.3 Case studies: Federated learning in neurology

Several pioneering case studies have recently surfaced and demonstrated the possibility of federated learning in neurology. The application of federated learning in the diagnosis of Alzheimer's disease is quite notably an example. Recently, several research institutions collaborated on a joint project in which federated learning models were applied to analyze neuroimaging data, like MRI and PET scans, coupled with clinical data from Alzheimer's patients distributed across different hospitals. The result was a highly accurate diagnostic model that could detect early-stage Alzheimer's with more precision than localized, traditional models. Federated learning potentially offers the means to aggregate data from divergent sources in a way that protects patient privacy.

Federated learning has been employed in epileptology to enhance seizure detection and prediction. A study conducted on a paper that involved the analysis of hundreds of EEG records from Epilepsy patients from multiple centers worldwide utilized federated learning for enhancing the detectability of seizure onset through subtle pre-seizure brain activity patterns. This would carry deep implications in developing fully personal, real-time interventions, such as adaptive neurostimulation devices capable of interrupting seizures before they occur. One of the other applications of federated learning in neurology is its use in an MS study. MS is an intricate disease that might be unpredictable and very different between patients, whereas providing a personalized treatment plan is quite challenging. A model of federated learning developed across several research centers analyzed genetic data and clinical and imaging data to predict the specific behavior of different patients to varied drugs being used for the treatment of MS. This model not only mitigated the unfavourable results but also removed the side effects by suggesting the most appropriate remedy for a patient according to certain aspects. Case studies demonstrate the transfusion from federated learning to both diagnosis and treatment in neurology.

5.5 DATA COLLECTION AND PREPROCESSING

The collection of data is one of the vital steps in neural disorder studies because it forms the foundation of the building of accurate models through machine learning. Neurological diseases, such as epilepsy, Alzheimer's and Parkinson's, comprise sizeable volumes of data gathered from sources such as EEGs, MRI, PET scans, and clinical records. EEGs are implemented real-time in the present day, for example, to analyze critical data that will be used for the diagnosis of epilepsy; MRI and PET scans prove essential to visualize alterations at both the structural and functional levels for diseases such as Alzheimer's disease or Parkinson's disease. Besides medical imaging, genetic data, patient histories, and data coming from wearable sensors can add value to understanding the course and symptoms of these disorders. This diverse and multimodal data can be collected in various healthcare institutions, and because of this, federated learning becomes an optimum framework for integration in a way that never violates the privacy of a patient.

The preprocessing of this raw data is important, especially at the time of model training in a federated learning environment. Generally, the raw data collected from neural disorder studies contains much noise, inconsistency, or missing values that need to be solved. Filtering, normalization, and artifact removal are some of the common preprocessing techniques applied to EEG signals to ensure that the important brain activity patterns are caught by the model. Segmentation and alignment / registration for imaging data align and clean MRI and PET images, thus smoothing out the process of extracting features. Additionally, preprocessing becomes complicated for federated learning, primarily due to the fact that the data is distributed. Each institution pre-processes separately, trying to stay consistent about how the data needs cleaning and formatting of all nodes that will be part of the federated model.

5.5.1 Types of data used in neural disorder studies

There are many types of data used to enhance the understanding of brain functional and pathological activities, and the most important data types in the neurodisorder studies field are EEG, which measure electrical activity in the brain and are indispensable in diagnostics concerning conditions like epilepsy or sleep disorders. In particular, EEG data is very valuable because of its high resolution in the temporal dimension, thus enabling rapid changes in brain activity to be captured by researchers [20].

Table 5.4 summarizes the various kinds of data utilized in neuropsychiatric disorder treatment. EEG and imaging techniques such as MRI, and CT scanning help diagnose and treat conditions of the brain, and genomic as well as clinical data are also available for one-to-one care. Results from wearable devices along with patient-reported outcomes place more information in the context to provide an overall understanding of the health of the patient.

A very important modality is MRI, which provides detailed structural and functional imaging of the brain. Scans show abnormalities in brain morphology and thus are critical in diagnosing neurodegenerative diseases such as Alzheimer's and multiple sclerosis. Other such data types potentially useful in neural disorder research include genomic information, clinical assessments, and patient-reported outcomes. Functional MRI has continued to evolve and increasingly is utilized to complement EEG and MRI in the assessment of brain activity through changes in blood flow. fMRI data can elucidate how brain regions talk to each other in accomplishing specific tasks and

Table 5.4 Types of Data Used in Neural disorder Studies

Type of Data	*Description*	*Common Uses*
Electroencephalograms (EEG)	Measures electrical activity in the brain through electrodes placed on the scalp.	Used for diagnosing epilepsy, sleep disorders, and assessing brain activity during cognitive tasks.
Magnetic Resonance Imaging (MRI)	Provides detailed images of brain structure and can assess lesions or abnormalities.	Crucial for diagnosing neurodegenerative diseases, brain tumors, and traumatic injuries.
Functional MRI (fMRI)	Measures brain activity by detecting changes in blood flow; shows how brain regions interact.	Used to study brain function, identify areas responsible for specific tasks, and research neurological disorders.
Computed Tomography (CT)	Combines X-ray images to create cross-sectional views of the brain.	Often used in emergency settings to detect hemorrhages, tumors, or other acute conditions.
Positron Emission Tomography (PET)	Measures metabolic activity in the brain by tracking radioactive tracers.	Useful for identifying regions of altered brain metabolism in conditions like Alzheimer's and epilepsy.
Genomic Data	Involves genetic information that may influence susceptibility to or progression of neural disorders.	Used in personalized medicine to identify genetic risk factors and tailor treatments for patients.
Clinical Assessments	Includes standardized tests and questionnaires that evaluate cognitive, behavioral, and physical functions.	Provides context for neuroimaging and EEG data, helping to correlate clinical symptoms with diagnostic findings.
Patient-Reported Outcomes	Captures patients' subjective assessments of their health, symptoms, and quality of life.	Important for evaluating treatment effectiveness and understanding patient experiences with their disorders.
Wearable Device Data	Collects real-time physiological data, such as heart rate and movement, through wearable sensors.	Used to monitor symptoms and track daily activities, offering insights into patient behavior and health trends.

can expose functional connectivity patterns in many neural disorders. The coming together of these varied data sources enables models designed to be a diagnosis and treatment tool for almost everything.

5.5.2 Preprocessing techniques

Preprocessing is the most important process carried out in federated learning, so clean, consistent, and analytically suitable data is obtained for training. Major preprocessing techniques include normalization. Normalization scales the data into an appropriate range in such a way that it improves the model's performance and its convergence. In consideration, an EEG signal would probably be filtered to remove artifacts and noise so that the actual model is inclined to focus on relevant brain activity patterns rather than being focused on noise [21]. In the case of imaging data like MRI, preprocessing steps involving registration and segmentation ensure images across subjects are standardized, thus ensuring that anatomical features are properly aligned. Another important preprocessing procedure is feature extraction, which identifies and chooses what features of the raw data to feed to the federated model. For instance, particular frequency bands retrieved from EEG signals may be informative about certain cognitive processes in the brain. In federated learning, preprocessing needs to occur locally at each participating institute to respect regulations pertaining to data privacy. This decentralized method helps the organizations preprocess their data while keeping certain sensitive information secret and, therefore, facilitates effective coordination in building strong models. Other preprocessing techniques include data augmentation, which allows adding diversity to a training dataset by creating new samples based on existing samples of the data, such as rotating or scaling the MRI image, effectively creating new training samples that retain the informative characteristics of the original data. For EEG data, some preprocessing techniques that are part of data augmentation are adding noise or time-warping the signals so as to mimic variations that could be expected under real-world circumstances. This tends to counter the overfitting and allows federated learning models to generalize better to unseen data. Since federated learning models work upon dispersed data across different institutions, it ensures the application of such preprocessing techniques to locally keep data consistent and interpretable at each institution. Even if the researchers combine the use of data augmentation with normalization, filtering, and feature extraction, they can notably enhance the robustness and accuracy of models learned in federated settings.

The crucial role of anonymization in preprocessing is predominantly seen in health sciences studies that contain sensitive information about patients. It has to do with the removal or alteration of Personally Identifiable Information (PII) from datasets so that individuals cannot be easily traced.

Techniques such as data masking, tokenization, and generalization are predominantly used for such purposes. For example, rather than revealing the exact age of the patients, researchers can categorize patients by age. Suppose that he or she will distinguish between age ranges, such as 20–30 years and 30–40 years, while averting identifiable information as the demographic analysis will be appropriately feasible. Anonymization is important since it must complement relevant compliance with HIPAA and GDPR. Moreover, the data anonymization must be accompanied by a strong security system for safeguarding the collected data and preprocessing data. The encryption of data must be done while transmission, secure aggregation, and transmission of any model parameter. Restrictions must ensure that only authorized personnel have access to data. Moreover, Secure Multi-Party Computation (SMPC) can be used to perform joint model training while keeping the data private at every institution concerned. Anonymizing the data while maintaining security is most crucial so that researchers can work effectively but with a patient's identity protected.

One of the major challenges in this domain of neural disorder research is handling missing and imbalanced data. This can incorporate biases and decrease model performance. There might be several sorts of missing data, including incomplete patient records or malfunctioning of the equipment while collecting data. Several techniques are suggested for handling missing data, where primarily imputation techniques are involved. Missing values are estimated based on the provided data. For instance, in EEG experiments, one may use interpolation methods to fill missing data points in time series, or machine learning algorithms to predict missing entries based on the general trend of the data. But another important issue is class imbalance, that is, where a class or category is undersized. It becomes especially relevant in the case of neural disorders as some conditions may be rarer than others. Techniques might include oversampling where the data from the minority class is copied and duplicated to balance out the dataset, or undersampling, which reduces the instances of the majority class. Another approach is to apply synthetic data generation techniques, such as Synthetic Minority Oversampling Technique (SMOTE), to create artificial examples in the train dataset that would balance the two datasets. These preprocessing techniques are vital for having diverse data related to neural disorders to which federated learning models are trained, hence providing a more robust and efficient diagnostic and treatment algorithm.

5.6 MODEL DESIGN AND TRAINING IN FEDERATED LEARNING

Designs for neural networks in federated learning are quite different from the traditional centralized design. Here, models have to run efficiently on a wide variety of devices ranging from resource-constrained smartphones to wearable devices. In that sense, the neural network architecture has to be lightweight and adept at functioning with very limited computational powers and memory. Pruning and quantization are other techniques that can be applied to shrink the size of the network without much loss in performance. This is critical in federated learning since every participating device trains its model locally before aggregating updates. Another very important aspect in designing neural networks for federated learning is that the models should generalize well across different data distributions from various institutions. Because data heterogeneity is quite a common challenge in federated settings, mechanisms for dealing with non-IID (Independent and Identically Distributed) data could be embedded into the architecture. Approaches like federated transfer learning will therefore be instrumental in the adaptation of models trained on a specific dataset, so that they can work efficiently on other datasets. Designing models to use local training data yet align with a global objective, therefore, represents a key challenge toward achieving improved accuracy and robustness in diverse clinical applications.

Finally, the interpretability of the model's decisions is important in healthcare. Since neural networks look like "black boxes", one may add techniques to that design that increase clinicians' and researchers' trust and understanding. Techniques such as attention mechanisms or layer-wise relevance propagation could be used to highlight which features contribute the most to model predictions. Thus, focusing on these aspects in the design phase of models can lead researchers to develop federated learning models that are efficient, generalizable, and easy to interpret so as to perhaps finally improve outcomes in the diagnosis and treatment of neural disorders.

5.6.1 Distributed model training: Techniques and challenges

A distributed approach in federated learning allows several devices or institutions to cooperate in model training with preserved data privacy using various techniques. Among such techniques, one is clearly the Federated Averaging (FedAvg), which enables a device to train a local model based on its data and sends the updates of the model (e.g., gradients) to a central server only. Then, it will take all the updates, pool them as a global model and send this all the way back to the devices for additional training. This iterative process proves to be successful in efficient collaboration without requiring access to raw data for addressing privacy issues.

Figure 5.4 depicts a distributed process for machine learning. Here, the initial data and script are arbitrarily assigned and scattered on worker nodes. One worker node receives a subset of the data and a model in order to train independently. The distributed setup enables parallel processing and thus enhances both the training efficiency and the scalability of the setup in several nodes.

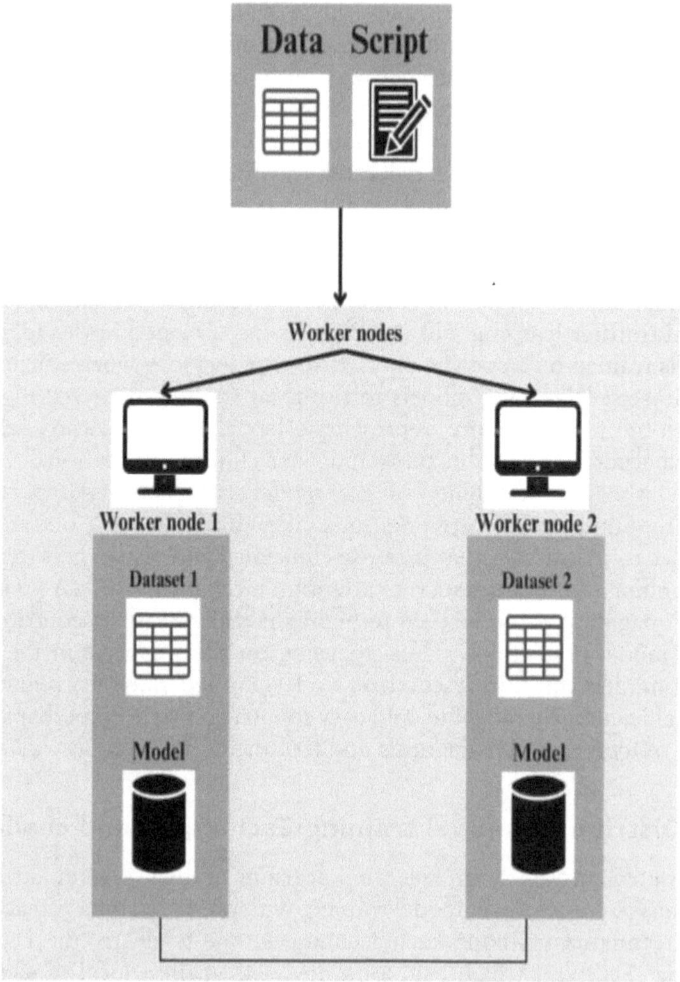

Figure 5.4 Distributed Model Training.

All things considered, however, there are huge challenges surrounding distributed model training. One of the main issues relates to heterogeneity in data distribution across the devices. The machine learning algorithms will differ in how they perform on different models of devices either in their quality or amount of data, thus making nonuniform contributions to the model. Another hindrance will be synchronization in the aggregation process since different machines will take differently long periods to train. Asynchronous training techniques, allowing devices to update the global model at different times, may mitigate those problems but lead to some complications in terms of convergence and stability of the models.

Other challenges include robustness against adversarial attacks or untrustworthy devices: A malicious participant, in federated learning, could send some erroneous model updates, which can compromise the integrity of the global model. Such threats can be protected against through techniques such as secure aggregation, where the server does not have access to the individual model updates. More importantly, the use of federated learning frameworks can monitor both performance and data quality associated with a device. This will make it possible for users to spot and filter out unreliable contributions. A way then opens up to further improve the effectiveness of distributed model training in federated learning environments.

5.6.2 Communication-efficient federated algorithms

One of the critical factors of federated learning is communication efficiency where several devices send updates to a central server. If the cost of communication is high, training becomes slow and wastes resources on mobile or edge devices. Methods can enhance communication efficiency by reducing the size of updates being sent by devices to the server, like gradient compression. Techniques such as quantization, in which gradients can be represented using fewer bits, and sparsification, in which only the most significant gradient updates are sent, significantly reduce communication overheads without degrading model performance. Optimized implementations of communication protocols can further optimize federated learning frameworks. Techniques for asynchronous update, where updates of devices can be transmitted at times chosen by devices themselves, reduce waiting time and can accelerate the process of overall training. Instead of using traditional network protocols and ensuring fewer delays with assured updates, advanced network protocols are required to maintain the effectiveness of federated learning. The researchers are therefore able to better facilitate the federated learning process with increased speed and resource efficiency by keeping a focus on communication-efficient algorithms.

The choice of hyperparameters, such as learning rate and batch size, has a significant impact on the performance of the model. Traditional methods for hyperparameter tuning, such as grid search or random search, may not be applicable in federated settings since they demand communication to evaluate the score of a model, while the need to keep data private further aggravates this problem. However, federated learning can utilize the Bayesian optimization or population-based training which, in fewer iterations, would aggregate insights from different devices and effectively explore hyperparameters. One of the major challenges in hyperparameter optimization in federated learning is diversity in quality and the distribution of the data across different devices. Since every device is accessed at some amounts and also types of data, optimal hyperparameters for one device do not necessarily mean they are for another. An approach to addressing this is through local hyperparameter tuning. Every device can tune its hyperparameters based on its specific data characteristics. These hyperparameters of a locally optimized model of the optimizer can then be shared with a central server, at which point global adjustments can be made to harmonize the overall model training process. In addition to meta learning, several techniques may be further introduced in order to enhance hyperparameter optimization in federated learning. Meta learning endows the model with the ability to learn how to change its hyperparameters from the combined experiences of other devices. The learning approach becomes adaptive and optimized. Therefore, it is an enhancement not only for the individual models regarding different devices but also for the strength of the overall federated learning framework. This might be maximized by implementing effective hyperparameter optimization strategies which allow researchers to increase the potential of federated learning models and most especially focuses on better diagnostic and treatment solutions in neural disorders.

5.7 CHALLENGES AND SOLUTIONS IN FEDERATED LEARNING FOR HEALTHCARE

The primary challenge in federated learning, more so in the health sector, is heterogeneity in data. Institutions collect data from heterogeneous populations using different devices, thus having differing standards in acquisition and preprocessing. For instance, the resolution in medical imaging devices between one hospital and another could be different. Populations also vary between institutions concerning demographics, disease prevalence, or clinical protocols. But the data here aren't IID (Independent and Identically Distributed), which generates models biased to some institution datasets but performing worse on others. There are several approaches to this problem of heterogeneity in data [22]. Personalized federated learning makes it possible to let each institution train models to fit their specific data, while contributing to a shared global model. This results in the achievement of the ideal balance between generalization and local performance. Other approaches include federated transfer learning that adapts the global model for local data conditions by transferring knowledge between different institutions while still keeping privacy intact. Domain-specific data augmentation methods and meta learning are also possible attacks on the problem, which allows the model to "learn how to learn" from different data distributions.

Another important challenge of federated learning is the convergence of a model to a particular solution. In central training, an overall model is updated incrementally across uniform data. However, in federated learning, updates are derived from various decentralized clients, and the volume as well as quality may differ for each client. This makes model convergence slow and unreliable as local model updates may drift in divergent directions, and the global model can, therefore, face difficulties in stabilizing in a particular solution. It does become more significant in the realm of healthcare, where data emanating from each institution may be quite unlike each other. Many techniques have been pursued to enhance the convergence rate of the algorithm [23]. Adaptive learning rate strategies can be used here, which adapt the learning rate according to the speed of convergence. One of the natural directions to adjust federated averaging is to account for the heterogeneity and varying contributions of clients. Techniques like weight regularization and momentum-based updates can reduce oscillations in training processes and, hence, speed up the convergence of the model. Asynchronous federated learning, where clients send their updates at different times, might further make the federated training process better balanced but is more difficult to manage in the sense that it might result in considerable divergence.

Table 5.5 provides the summarization of federated learning applications on neural disorders. Based on the type of data used, the potential benefits it

Table 5.5 Leveraging Federated Learning in Neural Disorder Management

Application	*Type of Data Used*	*Federated Learning Benefits*	*Challenges*
Epilepsy Detection and Prediction	EEG data, patient history, MRI	- Early detection of seizures - Improved prediction models across institutions	- Data heterogeneity (different EEG setups) - High computation cost for real-time prediction models
Alzheimer's Disease Diagnosis and Prognosis	MRI, PET scans, cognitive test results, genetic data	- Early diagnosis–Personalized prognosis models - Cross-institution collaboration for better treatment	- Nonuniform data from different imaging devices - Privacy concerns with genetic data
Parkinson's Disease Progress Monitoring	Wearable sensor data, clinical assessments, patient reports	- Real-time tracking of motor symptoms -Optimization of medication dosages	- Difficulty in collecting standardized wearable data - Varying treatment response across patients
Mental Health Disorder Prediction and Analysis	Electronic Health Records (EHR), wearable device data, patient-reported outcomes	- Early identification of mental health episodes - Personalized treatment plans - Analysis of comorbidities	- Subjective nature of mental health data - Integrating data from different sources (e.g., apps, EHRs)

can bring forth in terms of treatment and diagnosis, and the challenges that come up in adopting these models into real healthcare settings, this current work encompasses epilepsy, Alzheimer's, Parkinson's, and mental health disorders. In this regard, federated learning is shown to enable personalized, cross-institutional medical insights while somehow overcoming major stumbling blocks such as data privacy and heterogeneity.

5.7.1 Bandwidth and communication bottlenecks

The process of federated learning does involve pushing model updates back and forth between the devices and a central server, which could be very communication-intensive. This would prove particularly risky for healthcare applications because data sets this large, such as MRI or CT scans, are normally used, so updates may need to be as frequent as necessary to ensure model precision. In addition, bandwidth in certain institutions or devices might be limited, and repeated communication might drain device resources, especially in the case of mobile or wearable devices used within telemedicine applications. There are several techniques that overcome communication bottlenecks. Gradient compression techniques such as quantization and sparsification reduce the size of model updates sent between the clients and the server. It minimizes data transfer with minimal compromise on the model's performance [24]. Client selection algorithms help by reducing the number of participating clients in each round of communication, focusing on the most valuable updates. By using asynchronous protocols for communication, updates can be sent in an independent manner by the clients. This reduces the wait time within the system for the slower clients. Again, the federated distillation model uses only the essential knowledge from the local models and sends them to the global model, hence reducing bandwidth.

5.7.2 Model evaluation and validation

Since the participating institutions are diverse and distributed, it is challenging to evaluate and validate models in federated learning when the data is decentralized. In traditional machine learning, centralizing data makes splitting training and testing easy. In federated learning, data will be kept local to each institution which makes it really challenging to ensure the fairness of model evaluation across all clients. Moreover, cross-institutional validation is complex due to differences in data distributions and quality between healthcare providers. Solutions to these problems lie in the adoption of innovative evaluation frameworks. Cross-validation can occur federated, through rotating model updates between institutions, ensuring that every data point of the institutions is used for training or evaluation yet never leaves the local system [25]. Federated test sets are another way to ensure that each of the various institutions conducts testing of the global model on its local data and feeds back to the central server. Researchers can use differential privacy and secure aggregation in a manner that enables institutes to verify the models without hurting the privacy of patients. Such methods preserve the trustworthiness and fairness of model evaluation in the federated setting, as the models are actually learned to generalize well to various healthcare environments.

Not forgetting federated test sets and cross-validation, model interpretability also forms a significant role in validation and evaluation processes in healthcare federated learning. Models are mainly applied to make critical decisions during diagnostic and treatment processes, so understanding the rationale behind the prediction of a model is very important. Techniques like SHapley Additive exPlanations (SHAP) or Local Interpretable Model-Agnostic Explanations (LIME) can explain the decisions furnished by federated models without exposing the data behind the privacy curtain. Techniques that offer insights regarding features being driven towards making decisions can be regarded as medical biomarkers or imaging regions [26]. These interpretability techniques assist clinicians in trusting and validating the models before their inclusion in clinical workflows. Real-world performance monitoring and audits can also ensure that the federated models are stable, fair, unbiased, and, importantly, are not subjected to a biased model that may happen because of changes in data distribution with time or patient population demographics.

5.8 APPLICATIONS IN NEURAL DISORDER TREATMENT

Federated learning is a method that is considered to be of great importance in the development of treatment for different neural disorders since it enables collaboration between institutions without any form of compromise on patients' privacy. Data sharing by decoupling decentralizes the process and leads to better models for conditions like epilepsy, Alzheimer's, Parkinson's disease, and mental health disorders, among others, especially if more accurate and generalized approaches are targeted. The best available methodologies currently used for improving predictive accuracy within diagnostic models will be leveraged with enormous amounts of data from diverse sources – EEGs, MRI scans, and clinical records – and are expected to lead to earlier detection and more personalized treatments. One of the most salient benefits of federated learning in the treatment of neural disorders is that it can use multimodal data from different patient populations to come up with personalized and tailored solutions for healthcare applications. For instance, in Alzheimer's disease, incorporating imaging data with genetic information and cognitive assessment in an institution would enable the development of solid models for early detection and prognosis.

5.8.1 Epilepsy detection and prediction

Federated learning will best impact epilepsy detection and prediction. Traditionally, diagnosis of epilepsy will demand the continuous monitoring of patients using EEG data, where abnormal brain activity is detected. However, this requires a huge amount of data, which can spread across various hospitals and institutions. In federated learning, each such institution can collaborate and train models on different datasets using EEG without breaching patient privacy. Federated models aggregate data from diverse sources, providing more accurate early signs of seizures that may give clinicians advanced warning to design more effective treatment plans. Insights should be shared across institutions in a manner that maintains privacy while improving seizure prediction and the formulation of personalized treatment strategies. Federated learning can also contribute to the prediction of seizures, which is always an ongoing challenge in managing epilepsy. Federated models of EEG data that have been trained can identify patterns and precursors of seizures before they occur, allowing patients to potentially take preventive measures. Such predictive capacity can greatly enhance the quality of life for epilepsy patients by reducing the uncertainty and fear instilled by unexpected seizures. Federated learning allows the predictive models to become more generalizable across different populations of patients, thereby increasing their accuracy and utility. Multimodal data allow for improving the models themselves by mixing EEG data with any clinical data, including MRI or patient-report outcomes [27]. Such an approach will make the diagnosis of epilepsy more comprehensive, as brain activity will be related to symptoms clinically manifest, and the models will make more sense. One of the most significant practical applications of federated learning in the management of epilepsy is that it is possible to coordinate such heterogenous data sources in a safe way that is privacy-preserving.

5.8.2 Understanding Alzheimer's disease treatment and its expected outcomes

Alzheimer's is a complex neurological disease. Therefore, it is very important to detect it early before it becomes too powerful. Federation learning may be the clue to revolutionizing early detection and prognosis of Alzheimer's by allowing the integration of large-scale MRI, PET scans, and cognitive test results obtained from different healthcare institutions. By aggregating these different datasets, the federated learning models can discover the subtle changes in brain structure and functionality that may be at the earliest indications of Alzheimer's, in many times already developed long before the symptoms appear. A collaborative approach such as this allows for more careful and probable diagnosis and thus improves early intervention strategies with a probably delayed onset of the disease [28].

In the prognosis of Alzheimer's, this method can also be employed for the guidance of clinicians in forecasting the progression of the disease. Training over large datasets distributed across different locations creates a possibility of discovering trends and patterns that indicate the speed at which the disease would progress in individual patients. Doctors can thus tailor treatment plans to the predicted trajectories of the disease in every patient. Moreover, the addition of genetic data into federated models could also help identify the patients who are at a higher risk genetically for Alzheimer's, enabling early intervention through preventive measures. It may also be applied to accelerate the timeline for drug discovery and treatment optimization for Alzheimer's. Federated learning can enable pharmaceutical companies as well as research institutions to train models collaboratively without sharing sensitive data about patients, which is a significant requirement for the rapid development of new therapies. In this way, it is very probable that models trained on those data are going to unveil promising drug targets along with predicting patients' responses to treatments. In an endeavour to strengthen the development of Alzheimer's treatments, such an agreement may strive for effective treatment for the said disease and improvement in the quality of living conditions for patients.

5.8.3 Parkinson's disease progress monitoring

The core aspect of Parkinson's disease is the progressive feature of motor symptoms, and successful treatment calls for a regular monitoring process of the progression of the disease. Federated learning will be particularly helpful in the monitoring of Parkinson's progress because healthcare providers can train the models on data from wearable devices, clinical assessment, as well as patient-reported outcomes from various institutions [29]. These models can track motor symptoms such as tremors, gait abnormalities, as well as bradykinesia, offering real-time observations on disease progress. Accuracy and robustness in federated models increase when data from a variety of patient groups are aggregated, so clinicians can get detailed, patient-specific reports on how the disease evolves for each patient.

An important application of federated learning in the treatment of Parkinson's is in the optimization of treatments. Parkinson's patients often respond differentially to levodopa and often require adjusting medication according to the symptoms of the patients and the progression of the disease. Federated learning models can predict how different individual patients will behave upon different treatments by analyzing data from very diverse patient populations. In doing so, the models can help clinicians tailor specific treatment regimens so as to maximize the potency of medication while minimizing side effects. Federated learning would also aid in integrating the monitoring and treatment of Parkinson's disease with non-motor symptoms. These symptoms include depression, cognitive decline, and sleep disturbances that normally accompany the disease. However, objective symptoms are more challenging to monitor in contrast to motor ones. The multimodal federated model trained on multimodal data of wearable sensor data, clinical reports, and patient feedback could easily capture non-motor symptoms. Thus, this will offer an integrated view of the disease that can help treat motor as well as non-motor symptoms in a patient with Parkinson's disease.

5.8.4 Mental health disorder prediction and analysis

Mental health disorders are a very challenging condition in healthcare. These are complex and subjective problems, which include depression, anxiety, and schizophrenia. For this reason, the prediction and analysis of mental health disorders through federated learning has great potential since such data could be combined from multiple sources, for example, EHRs, wearable devices, and patient-reported outcomes across many different healthcare providers. An example is the development of predictive models concerning the deterioration of mental health provided by a cooperative approach. Variations in sleep patterns, physical activity, or even speech would be good indicators – capturable by wearable devices – to predict when such episodes would occur or when mental health episodes would recur [30]. Federated learning can also enable the personalization of psychosocial treatments. Since every mental illness presents differently in each patient, treatment plans have to be personalized. Through the training of models in distributed data sets from many populations of patients, federated learning can empower clinicians to determine which therapies or medications will likely work best for any given patient. This approach, aside from improving the treatment results, reduces the trial-and-error processes generally accompanying mental health treatment. Furthermore, since federated learning models aggregate data collected from sources such as cognitive tests, therapy sessions, and medication records of adherence, it might be possible to give a better overall picture of each patient's mental health state. It also promotes the exploration of comorbidities in relation to mental health disorder syndromes, for example, the use of substances or chronic physical conditions, for instance, diabetes. Big data might be used to pull out federated models reflecting the associations between mental health and physical health, thus assisting clinicians in treating patients in a more holistic way. Federated models are robust, scalable, and generate actionable insights in real time since they integrate data from mental health apps, telemedicine services, and traditional healthcare institutions.

5.9 ETHICAL, LEGAL, AND REGULATORY CONSIDERATIONS

While there are many potential ethical implications relating to federated learning in healthcare, especially with regard to privacy and autonomy concerning patients, it still allows for collaboration across institutions without having to share raw data. However, a model update related to patient data will nonetheless be transmitted, and confidentiality is breached in this approach. The major ethical challenge lies with re-identification, whereby certain aggregated or processed data can be traced back to an individual. Hence, robust anonymization and differential privacy techniques need to be included in healthcare organizations so that privacy can be ensured for their patients while trust in federated learning can be allowed for healthcare advancements [31].

Another ethical issue involved pertains to bias in federated models. Given that federated learning depends on data from different institutions, models are likely to be biased if specific groups of populations or types of data are underrepresented when training the models. This may result in unequal care due to less competent models across minority groups or with uncommon conditions. Such risks can be mitigated through fair and balanced datasets throughout institutions, ensuring that models are both equitable and effective for all patients. Then there's the importance of transparency in the first place, showing how federated learning models are put together and used to maintain public confidence in AI-driven healthcare systems. Another ethical issue is that of consent and patient autonomy. Contributions to machine learning models are quite often made in silence by patients who have no idea what their information will be used for. Especially concerning the decentralized nature of federated learning, patients should be told how their data will contribute to a federated learning model and how such a model may eventually affect future healthcare decisions. The institutes need to be transparent about the fact that their patient data would be utilized and should also allow opportunities for patients who need to opt in or out of any federated learning efforts.

Figure 5.5 is a hierarchical diagram that depicts ethical and legal concerns in FL. Ethical concerns on the left side include bias, inclusion, robot rights, and transparency. The core of the concerns covers the areas around fairness, respect for human values, and appropriate moral treatment of AI. The right side deals with security, cognitive services, planning, and data privacy issues, which include all the regulatory, safety, and privacy-related concerns found in FL. The diagram highlights the balance between ethical accountability and legal expediency in developing and deploying FL systems.

Health care federated learning operate within a very complex web of laws in the sharing of data by institutions, particularly in jurisdictions separated. The sharing of multi-institutional data is controlled through national and regional laws regarding the keeping and processing and transfer between providers of care for patients' data. For example, in the United States, HIPAA has rules that govern how patient information is protected, and every healthcare institution will need to comply with that standard. In fact, even though federated learning decentralizes data, it should run within legal boundaries to avoid penalty for failure to comply.

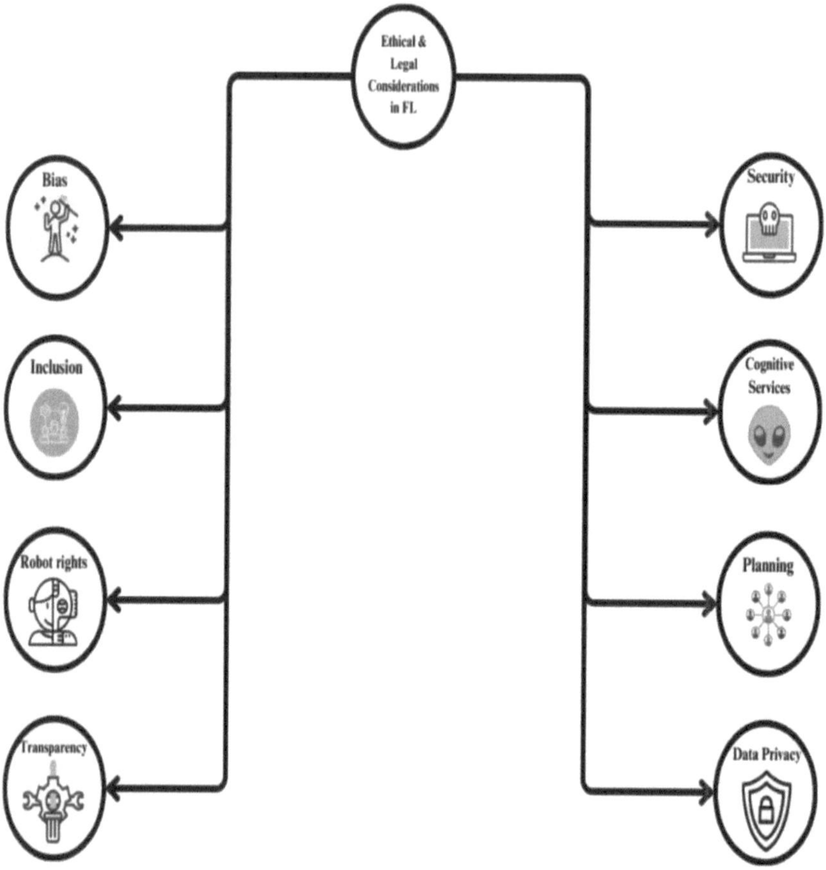

Figure 5.5 Legal and Ethical Considerations of Federated Learning.

Another regulation affecting international collaboration in federated learning relates to those in the European Union, for example, GDPR. It puts an obligation on institutions to employ really strict rules that are put in place when dealing with the collection, processing, and further sharing of personal data. With GDPR, organizations ensure their patient data is anonymized, and aggregated model updates also have to be treated with lots of care, not to mention the possibility of unauthorized access or breaches. These legal frameworks call for careful handling of data across borders, as different jurisdictions may have different definitions of protected health information and personal data. In federated learning initiatives, institutional participants have to consider national and regional laws. However, legal agreements like Data-Sharing agreements (DSAs) or Data Use agreements (DUAs) must be set up between the parties involved. The responsibilities of both parties are articulated within these agreements to guarantee that there will be compliance with local and international jurisdictions with the clarification of aspects related to the ownership of data, liability, and security concerns. Such legal frameworks form an integral part of encouraging cooperation across institutions and fostering integrity in the federated learning system.

Regulatory Guidelines and Compliance (HIPAA, GDPR)
There are also regulatory guidelines developed to ensure patient privacy for the healthcare systems aligning with those laws in their local and international level. For instance, in the United States, HIPAA is set of guidelines protecting the privacy of health information regarding the handling of patients' data for research such as federated learning. Under HIPAA, any institution engaging in federated learning should ensure that all Protected Health Information (PHI) either undergoes a process of encryption or anonymization before they are processed. Under HIPAA, healthcare institutions also require safeguards, such as audit trails to prevent unauthorized access to patient data during federated learning.

In the European Union, federated learning systems are supposed to meet the standards of the GDPR. This makes additional responsibility fall directly on the shoulders of the organization dealing with personal data. The GDPR has made a regulation mandating data minimization in each organization, which requires only necessary data should be processed, not even federated learning frameworks are exempted. On the other hand, the law affirms a right to forget so patients can obtain an erasure of their data on the federated learning model at will [32]. Thus, the federated learning platforms would be designed with legal and regulatory requirements that would include updates or revisions regarding patient data. Food and Drug Administration (FDA) and European Medicines Agency (EMA) among others are notable examples.

Other models are applied to federated learning models, used in clinical decision-making or diagnostics, and when developed and validated, they have their own set of regulatory testing for the safety and efficacy of the AI-driven tool deployed in healthcare. Most federated learning models are across multiple institutions and data sources. Therefore, they need to be stringently validated and tested in order to meet regulatory requirements that protect patient health along with data privacy.

5.10 FUTURE DIRECTIONS AND RESEARCH OPPORTUNITIES

The evolution of federated learning is promising, with potential advancements that may be critically useful in the diagnosis and treatment of neural disorders. One critical direction is the development of more complex algorithms to handle heterogeneity differences in data coming from different institutions. Such changes include acknowledging differences in quality, types, and formats across various patient populations. Researchers have been progressively focused on developing adaptive federated learning models that would learn effectively from data that are typically non-IID and thus commonly manifest in settings of healthcare. Such models will have far better abilities to capture the richness of neural disorders and lead to better predictions and customized treatment plans. In addition, enhancements in the efficiency of communication and resource allocation are some of the critical requirements that enhance scalability in federated learning systems. Since federated learning often appears to transfer model updates rather than raw data, innovation in communication overhead between devices and central servers can make the system extraordinarily better in performance. Investigations of techniques that apply quantization and federated averaging are underway with the aim of reducing bandwidth usage during training, which would make real-time application feasible even in hardware-scarce settings.

One of the opportunities from research would be multimodal sources of data. Through the incorporation of genomic data, clinical records, imaging studies, as well as even lifestyle data from wearable devices, federated learning will give a more holistic view of each patient's health status. Such a holistic approach can greatly enhance the predictions regarding the complexity of interactions between genetic factors and environmental influences. It further makes it possible to identify biomarkers and strategies for individualized treatment approaches tailored according to particular profiles of patients that would be helpful for better management of neural disorders. With the advancement of diagnostic techniques and raising awareness of diagnosis among patients, now there is a need to focus on data harmonization and interoperability of all different modalities while ensuring patient privacy, upon which research is also working. For example, transfer learning and multi-task learning within federated frameworks can co-train models on different types of data and can potentially lead to richer feature extraction and improved predictive performance. Thus, it is one promising avenue for future work in our advancing understanding of neural disorders and targeted interventions.

5.10.1 Collaboration between AI researchers and medical experts

The collaboration of AI researchers and medical experts is required to drive innovation in applications of federated learning to neural disorders. Such collaborations will spur advancement into more clinically relevant models that not only incorporate more cutting-edge techniques of machine learning but also meet the very practical requirements and constraints of healthcare practitioners. This interaction can be used in the quest to further understand clinical implications that AI-derived insights might have, and assist in fine-tuning models to make them interpretable and actionable in real-world settings.

Also, collaborative research activity [31] can push forward the validation and implementation of models in the federated learning approach in the clinical environment. AI researchers can access expertise from medical professionals in designing studies, results interpretation, and appropriate regulatory compliance for models. This will result in the formulation of frameworks to sustain communication and feedback between these groups and ensure continued relevance, ethics, and effectiveness of federated learning systems in improving patient outcomes and closing the gap between technologies and healthcare.

5.10.2 Future trends in federated learning for personalized medicine

In the future, federated learning will also play an important role in the development of personalized [32] medicine, especially when dealing with neural disorders. Among the trends arising from this will be a thrust towards quick analysis of data, moving from static models to adaptive learning models that get updated with new, arriving patient data. This may make it possible to devise treatment plans flexible enough to be revised when necessary so that interventions do not lose efficacy as a patient's condition changes. The use of federated learning combined with wearables and mobile health applications could thus hold great potential for increasing the degree of patient engagement and empowerment in the management of their health through real-time monitoring technologies. Another trend emerging now is the use of explainable AI within federated learning frameworks. Since stakeholders in healthcare worry more about the explainability of AI-driven decisions, there is a growing focus on developing models that provide accurate predictions as well as shining light on the reasoning behind those predictions. Explainability [33] is likely to add substantial trust among clinicians and patients with federated learning systems and could increase the usage of such advanced technologies in personalized medicine [34]. This is likely to foster more patient-centric and transparent delivery of healthcare, ultimately leading to better-informed decisions and better healthcare [35].

5.11 CONCLUSION

The exploration of federated learning in the health domain, specifically on neural disorders, states that this approach can transform the diagnosis, treatment, and outcomes of patients. The key findings indicate that through federated learning, one can safely share cross-institutional data as a means of developing robust, generalized models that could more aptly predict the progress of disease and the response to treatments. Thus, federated learning, in that context, will immensely contribute to achieving a more collaborative approach toward healthcare, thereby ultimately improving the understanding and management of complex neural disorders. Besides, multimodal data sources are also of great promise to complement those models toward making them more inclusive and robust, thus driving innovation into personalized treatment strategies.

More importantly, the ethical, legal, and regulatory concerns related to federated learning have highlighted the need for guidelines and frameworks that ensure patient privacy is safeguarded but collaboration is promoted. In these challenges, the future importance of collaboration between AI researchers and medical professionals will be the key to allowing federated learning models to not only be technically advanced but also clinically applicable. The future of federated learning in healthcare promises excitement for the enhancement of patient care, not to mention a constant flow of steady attention to ethics, data governance, and interdisciplinary collaboration.

REFERENCES

[1] Jahangir, M., Anthony, L., Raheleh, A. (2024). Neurological disorders. 241–267. Foundations of the mind, brain, and behavioral relationships-understanding physiological psychology. *ScienceDirect*. doi: 10.1016/b978-0-323-95975-9.00011-1

[2] Iorio-Morin, C., Villeneuve, S.A., Masson-Côté, L., Mathieu, D. (2023). Neurological Disorders. In: Roberge, D., Donaldson, S.S. (eds) *Radiation Therapy of Benign Diseases. Medical Radiology*. Springer, Cham. https://doi.org/10.1007/174_2022_374

[3] Jaideep, S., David, B., Manjulatha, B., Babitha, S. (2010). Neurological disorders:an overview. *PharmacologyOnline*, Silae. https://pharmacologyonline.silae.it/files/newsletter/2010/vol1/69.Singh.pdf

[4] de Sá-Caputo, D. D., Bernardo-Filho, M., Seixas, A., Taiar, A. (2021). Introductory Chapter: Neurological Disorders – Therapy Approaches. In: Mario Bernardo-Filho (ed.). *IntechOpen*. doi: 10.5772/intechopen.97178

[5] Dina, N., Anggraini, N., Woon-Man, K. (2023). Challenges and perspectives of neurological disorders. *Brain Sciences*, 13(4):676–676. doi: 10.3390/brainsci13040676

[6] Dhada, M., Parlikad, A.K., & Palau, A.S. (2020). Federated learning for collaborative prognosis. *Apollo – University of Cambridge Repository*. https://doi.org/10.17863/CAM.50577

[7] Samir, A. (2022). A survey on challenges of federated learning. *Azerbaijan Journal of High-Performance Computing*, 5(2):273–285. doi: 10.32010/26166127.2022.5.2.273.285

[8] Chen, J., Yan, H., Liu, Z., Zhang, M., Xiong, H., Shui, Y. (2024). When federated learning meets privacy-preserving computation. *ACM Computing Surveys*. doi: 10.1145/3679013

[9] Tanjil, A.R., Bhuiyan, F.M.A., Rony, M.A.T., Biswas, K. (2024). *Federated Deep Learning Systems in Healthcare*. CRC Press. 31–49. doi: 10.1201/9781032694870-3
[10] Chetna, K. (2024). Federated Deep Learning System for Application of Healthcare in Pandemic Situation. In: Amandeep Kaur, Chetna Kaushal, Md. Mehedi Hassan, Si Thu Aung (eds.) *Federated Deep Learning for Healthcare*. CRC Press. 131–142. doi: 10.1201/9781032694870-10
[11] Saha, S., Hota, A., Chattopadhyay, A.K., Nag, A., Nandi, S. (2024). A multifaceted survey on privacy preservation of federated learning: progress, challenges, and opportunities. *Artificial Intelligence Review*, 57(7). Springer. doi: 10.1007/s10462-024-10766-7
[12] Sheller, M.J., Reina, G.A., Edwards, B., Martin, J., Bakas, S. (2019). Multi-institutional Deep Learning Modeling Without Sharing Patient Data: A Feasibility Study on Brain Tumor Segmentation. In: Crimi, A., Bakas, S., Kuijf, H., Keyvan, F., Reyes, M., van Walsum, T. (eds) *Brainlesion: Glioma, Multiple Sclerosis, Stroke and Traumatic Brain Injuries. BrainLes 2018. Lecture Notes in Computer Science*, vol 11383. Springer, Cham. https://doi.org/10.1007/978-3-030-11723-8_9
[13] Rahman, A., Nag, A., Bairagi, A.K. (2023). A Hybrid Model for Recognizing Human Activity Using Extreme Learning. In: *2023 26th International Conference on Computer and Information Technology (ICCIT)*, Cox's Bazar, Bangladesh, pp. 1–6, doi: 10.1109/ICCIT60459.2023.10441574.
[14] Sheller, M.J., Edwards, B., Reina, G.A. et al. (2020). Federated learning in medicine: facilitating multi-institutional collaborations without sharing patient data. *Scientific Reports*, 10, 12598. https://doi.org/10.1038/s41598-020-69250-1
[15] Marlowe, T.J., Kirova, V., Mohtashami, M. (2011). *A Classification of Collaborative Knowledge*. Social Science Research Network.
[16] Nag, A., Das, B., Sil, R., Hameed, A.A., Bhushan, B., Jamil, A. (2024). A Survey on Image-Based Cardiac Diagnosis Prediction Using Machine Learning and Deep Learning Techniques. In: García Márquez, F.P., Jamil, A., Ramirez, I.S., Eken, S., Hameed, A.A. (eds) *Computing, Internet of Things and Data Analytics. ICCIDA 2023. Studies in Computational Intelligence*, vol 1145. Springer, Cham. https://doi.org/10.1007/978-3-031-53717-2_44
[17] Patel, S., Patel, R., Akbari, A. Mukkala, S. (2023). An extensive study and review of privacy preservation models for the multi-institutional data. *Journal of Information Security*, 14, 343–365. Scientific Research. doi: 10.4236/jis.2023.144020.
[18] Altalbe, A., Javed, A.R. (2023). Privacy preserved brain disorder diagnosis using federated learning. *Computer Systems Science and Engineering*, 47(2), 2187–2200. Tech Science Press. https://doi.org/10.32604/csse.2023.040624
[19] Rieke, N., Hancox, J., Li, W. et al. (2020). The future of digital health with federated learning. *NPJ Digital Medicine*, 3, 119. https://doi.org/10.1038/s41746-020-00323-1

[20] Xu, J., Glicksberg, B.S., Su, C., Walker, P., Bian, J., Wang, F. (2021). Federated learning for healthcare informatics. Journal of Healthcare Informatics Research, 5(1):1–19. Springer. doi: 10.1007/S41666-020-00082-4

[21] Péter, K. (2023). Federated Learning of Artificial Neural Networks. *ELTE Digital Institutional Repository (EDIT)*. doi: 10.15476/elte.2021.124

[22] Stamatis, V., Radoglou-Grammatikis, P., Sarigiannidis, A., Pitropakis, N., Lagkas, T., Argyriou, V., Markakis, E., Sarigiannidis, P. (2024). Advancements in Federated Learning for Health Applications: A Concise Survey. In: *20th International Conference on Distributed Computing in Smart Systems and the Internet of Things (DCOSS-IoT)*. 503–508. doi: 10.1109/dcoss-iot61029.2024.00080

[23] Gobinath, B., Shanmugam, T. (2023). Healthcare Data Protection using Federated Learning Technology. In: *2023 7th International Conference on Intelligent Computing and Control Systems (ICICCS)*. 436–442. doi: 10.1109/ICICCS56967.2023.10142903

[24] Brisimi, T.S., Chen, R., Mela, T., Olshevsky, A., Paschalidis, I.C., Shi, W. (2018). Federated learning of predictive models from federated Electronic Health Records. *International Journal of Medical Informatics*, 112:59–67. doi: 10.1016/J.IJMEDINF.2018.01.007

[25] Zhang, F., Kreuter, D., Chen, Y., Dittmer, S., Tull, S., Shadbahr, T., Schut, M., Asselbergs, F., Kar, S., Sivapalaratnam, S., Williams, S. (2024). Recent methodological advances in federated learning for healthcare. *Patterns*, 5(6):101006–101006. doi: 10.1016/j.patter.2024.101006

[26] Kanhegaonkar, P., Prakash, S. (2024). Federated Learning in Healthcare Applications. In: Amit Kumar Singh and Stefano Berretti (eds.) *Data Fusion Techniques and Applications for Smart Healthcare-A volume in Intelligent Data-Centric Systems*. 157–196. CRC Press. doi: 10.1016/b978-0-44-313233-9.00013-8

[27] Saemaldahr, R., Ilyas, M. (2023). Patient-specific preictal pattern-aware epileptic seizure prediction with federated learning. *Sensors*, 23(14), 6578. https://doi.org/10.3390/s23146578

[28] Zhang, P., Lin, S., Qiao, J., Tu, Y. (2021). Diagnosis of Alzheimer's disease with ensemble learning classifier and 3D convolutional neural network. *Sensors*, 21(22):7634–. doi: 10.3390/S21227634

[29] Anila, M., Pradeepini, G. (2020). A review on Parkinson's disease diagnosis using machine learning techniques. *International Journal of Engineering Research and Technology*, 9(06). doi: 10.17577/IJERTV9IS060241

[30] Sankar, R.A., Juliet, S. (2023). Investigations on machine learning models for mental health analysis and prediction. In *2023 Second International Conference on Electrical, Electronics, Information and Communication Technologies (ICEEICT)*. pp. 1–7. https://doi.org/10.1109/ICEEICT56924.2023.10157385

[31] Reddy, C.K.K., Babu, B.V. (2017). ISLIQ-OC: Improved Supervised learning in quest using optimal k-means clustering mechanism to nowcast Snow/No-Snow, *International Journal of Control Theory and Applications*..

[32] Gangadhar Reddy, R., Srinivasa Reddy, M., Anisha, P.R., Kishor Kumar Reddy, C. (2017). Identification of earthquakes using wavelet transform

and clustering methodologies. *International Journal of Civil Engineering and Technology*, 8(8), 666–676.

[33] Subbarayudu, B., Harshika, S., Amareswar, E., Reddy, R.G., Reddy, C.K. (2017). Review and comparison on software process models. *International Journal of Mechanical Engineering and Technology*, 967-980.

[34] Nag, A., Das, B., Sil, R., Hameed, A.A., Bhushan, B., Jamil, A. (2024). A Survey on Image-Based Cardiac Diagnosis Prediction Using Machine Learning and Deep Learning Techniques. In: García Márquez, F.P., Jamil, A., Ramirez, I.S., Eken, S., Hameed, A.A. (eds) *Computing, Internet of Things and Data Analytics. ICCIDA 2023. Studies in Computational Intelligence*, vol 1145. Springer, Cham. https://doi.org/10.1007/978-3-031-53717-2_44

[35] Nag, A., et al. (2024). TumorGANet: A transfer learning and generative adversarial network- based data augmentation model for brain tumor classification. *IEEE Access*, 12: 103060–103081. doi: 10.1109/ACCESS.2024.3429633

Chapter 6

Harnessing machine learning and deep learning techniques for neuroimaging

Hina Bansal, Neetu Jabalia, Kritika Shukla, and Yash Nautiyal

6.1 INTRODUCTION

The use of neuroimaging has become essential for detecting neurological problems and comprehending how the brain functions. The understanding of the anatomy and function of the brain has been increased because of recent developments in neuroimaging techniques. Among the most popular techniques, functional magnetic resonance imaging (fMRI) and electroencephalography (EEG) produce excellent temporal and spatial resolution. EEG takes direct electrical activity readings from the scalp, whereas fMRI maps brain activity via variations in blood flow. These methods have been used in psychiatry, neurology, and cognitive neuroscience, among other disciplines. This chapter aims to explore neuroimaging techniques and their role in personalized medicine for neurodegenerative disorders. This chapter will also summarize integration with clinical data, discuss current status, and outline important future directions in the field.

The chapter makes numerous significant contributions to the rapidly evolving field of neuroimaging in conjunction with machine learning and artificial intelligence (AI). It presents a detailed examination of how AI and machine learning (ML) are transforming the landscape of neuroimaging and an overview of the most commonly utilized neuroimaging modalities and their applications in neurological condition diagnosis and monitoring. By leveraging these advanced imaging modalities such as functional MRI (fMRI), positron emission tomography (PET), single-photon emission computed tomography (SPECT), and magnetic resonance imaging (MRI), we demonstrate how AI-driven techniques can enhance the analysis of brain structures and functions. This integration not only boosts diagnostic and prognostic capabilities in detecting neurological conditions but also enables the development of personalized treatment strategies tailored to individual patients. The chapter provides a detailed analysis of how AI, specifically machine learning and deep learning, transforms neuroimaging by improving diagnosis precision, early detection of diseases such as Alzheimer's and Parkinson's, and the ability to implement more effective

 DOI: 10.1201/9781003591085-6

personalized treatments. It investigates how these techniques might be used to find biomarkers for disease prediction and to tailor therapies for neurological diseases. The focus is on presenting innovative methods that harness the power of AI to redefine how brain disorders are studied, diagnosed, and managed, significantly impacting both clinical practices and research directions in neuroscience.

The chapter is structured to guide readers through the evolving role of AI in neuroimaging in a logical and detailed manner. It begins with a thorough overview of key neuroimaging techniques, including MRI, fMRI, PET, EEG, and others, including their technical principles, research applications, and clinical diagnosis. It elucidates how each imaging modality contributes to understanding brain function and identifying neurological disorders. Following this, we delve into the world of artificial intelligence, breaking down its core components like machine learning and deep learning, and discussing specific AI models such as Convolutional Neural Networks (CNNs), Recurrent Neural Networks (RNNs), and Generative Adversarial Networks (GANs). The next section explores the practical applications of these technologies in improving diagnostic accuracy, personalized treatment plans, and understanding the complexities of neurological disorders. It concludes with a thorough review of current trends and future possibilities in neuroimaging, emphasizing innovations in hybrid imaging and the use of novel radiotracers. This organization ensures a cohesive journey from foundational concepts to cutting-edge advancements, providing a clear roadmap for both novices and experts interested in the application of AI in neuroimaging.

6.2 TECHNIQUES USED IN NEUROIMAGING

Neuroimaging is an interdisciplinary field that involves various domains like neuroscience, computer science, artificial intelligence, statistics, and psychology. Unlike neuroradiology, which is clinically focused on diagnosing and treating neurological conditions, neuroimaging is often used for research purposes to understand how the brain works. There are two categories of neuroimaging (Figure 6.1).

6.2.1 Magnetic Resonance Imaging (MRI)

By offering precise images of the human body—images that are essential for diagnosis and treatment planning—Magnetic Resonance Imaging (MRI) has completely transformed contemporary healthcare. Advancements in clinical and scientific settings have been fostered by the integration of MRI with bioinformatics, which has further expanded its utility. Precision medicine is facilitated by bioinformatics' strong data analysis tools, which aid in the interpretation of the intricate data produced by magnetic resonance

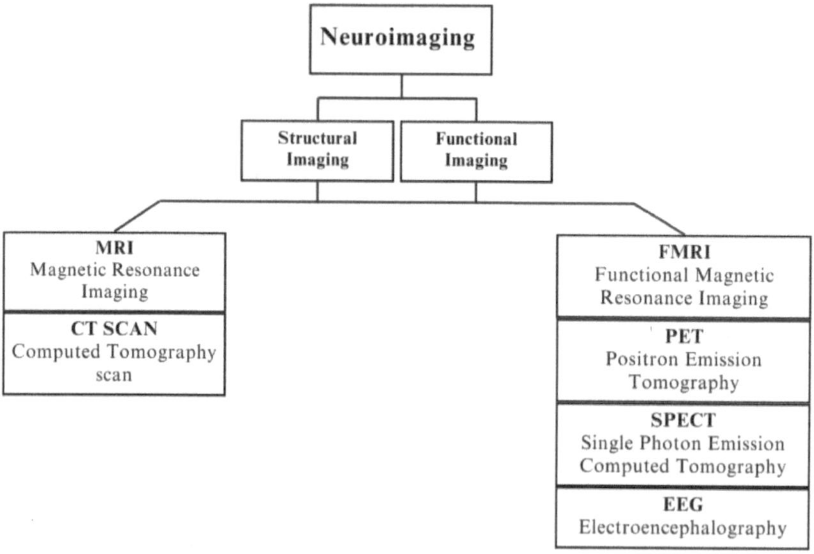

Figure 6.1 Categories of neuroimaging.

imaging. Bioinformatics can help with early diagnosis and customized treatment strategies by using machine learning algorithms to analyze MRI data and find patterns and biomarkers linked to particular diseases [1].

MRI plays an essential role in healthcare systems. It offers high-resolution, non-invasive images that are essential for identifying a range of illnesses, from cancer to neurological diseases [2]. When MRI and bioinformatics are used together, large-scale imaging data can be managed and analyzed, which improves diagnosis accuracy and streamlines workflows (Table 6.1). For example, radiologists might benefit from bioinformatics tools by having images automatically segmented and regions of interest highlighted, which lowers the possibility of human error and increases productivity [3].

6.2.2 Functional magnetic resonance imaging (fMRI)

In neuroscience and clinical diagnostics, functional magnetic resonance imaging (fMRI) is a crucial technology that provides insights into brain activity by monitoring blood flow variations. The ability of healthcare systems to provide more accurate and customized care has been greatly increased by the integration of fMRI and bioinformatics. By using advanced computer techniques to identify patterns and connections that are difficult to identify through conventional analysis, bioinformatics makes it easier to handle and understand the huge and complicated datasets produced by

Table 6.1 Popular bioinformatics tools for MRI analysis, emphasizing their uses and advantages for clinical settings

Tool	*Application*	*Benefits*
FMRBI Software Library (FSL)	Analyses the functional and structural MRI data	A complete set of tools for statistical analysis, visualization, and preprocessing is provided.
Statistical Parametric Mapping (SPM)	Voxel–based morphometry	Provides sophisticated statistical methods for the analysis of neuroimaging data.
Free Surfer	Structural analysis of MRI and cortical surface reconstruction	Produces cortical surface models and automatically divides brain structures.
Medical Image Processing, Analysis, and Visualization	Quantitative Analysis of MRI	Assists with a range of image analysis tasks, including volume measurements and tissue classification.
MRIcron	Visualization of MRI and DTI data	Provides easy-to-use visualization tools for analyzing results from neuroimaging.

fMRI [4]. An essential part of bioinformatics, machine learning algorithms are used to evaluate fMRI data and find biomarkers for diseases like major depressive disorder, schizophrenia, and Alzheimer's disease [5]. Early identification and intervention are crucial for improving the health of patients, and these biomarkers make this possible.

The combination of fMRI and bioinformatics improves healthcare systems' capacity for research as well. Vast databases that aggregate fMRI data from different populations allow scientists to study brain function and how different disorders are related to it. These databases make it easier to find trends specific to a community and create generic models that can be used for a variety of demographics, because of the bioinformatics tools that support them [6].

6.2.3 Arterial spin labelling

Arterial spin labelling (ASL) is a non-invasive MRI technique that utilizes water in blood as a natural tracer to magnetically label blood, enabling the measurement of cerebral blood flow (CBF). Because it can provide quantitative perfusion maps without the use of contrast chemicals, this novel method has garnered a lot of popularity in both clinical and research contexts.

Sophisticated algorithms and computational tools make it a lot easier to recognize significant patterns in ASL data, which enables accurate CBF measurement. Arterial spin labelling data analysis is particularly good at recognizing minute changes in perfusion that can point to the initial stages of neurological illnesses like Alzheimer's disease, stroke, and vascular dementia. Machine learning techniques are a mainstay of bioinformatics [7].

Additionally, assisting in the advancement of personalized medicine strategies within healthcare systems is the merging of ASL and bioinformatics. Personalized medicine aims to tailor medical treatment to the specific characteristics of each patient, which requires comprehensive and accurate data analysis. To find patient-specific blood flow patterns, bioinformatics techniques can evaluate ASL data combined with genetic, clinical, and demographic data. This thorough analysis makes it easier to tailor treatment programs based on each patient's unique perfusion profile, resulting in more focused and efficient interventions [8]. Also, the accuracy and efficiency of healthcare services are improved by the integration of bioinformatics and ASL. Within the field of science, the amalgamation of ASL and bioinformatics facilitates extensive investigations on cerebral perfusion. Researchers may do comprehensive analyses into the connection between blood flow and other neurological diseases because of centralized databases that aggregate ASL data from a variety of populations. Large datasets can be managed and analyzed more easily with the use of bioinformatics tools, which also make it possible to identify trends unique to a community and create generic models that can be used for a variety of demographic situations [9].

6.2.4 Positron emission tomography (PET)

The combination of positron emission tomography (PET) with bioinformatics has greatly expanded the possibilities and applications of this imaging technique, making it a crucial component of contemporary healthcare systems (Table 6.2). PET scans are used to monitor the body's metabolic processes, offering vital information about a number of illnesses, such as cancer, heart disease, and neurological conditions. The combination of PET imaging and bioinformatics has accelerated the development of diagnostics,

Table 6.2 Various ways that PET imaging is enhanced by bioinformatics in several medical domains, emphasizing the better results that may be achieved in terms of diagnosis and treatment

Field	*Application*	*Outcome*
Oncology	Tumor metabolism analysis	Targeted therapy development
Neurology	Alzheimer's disease detection	Early diagnosis and treatment planning
Cardiology	Myocardial perfusion assessment	Precise risk stratification and individualized therapy
Pharmacology	Drug distribution visualization	Optimization of dosages and delivery methods

treatment planning, and personalized medicine. The interpretation of PET scan results is greatly aided by the interdisciplinary discipline of bioinformatics, which creates and uses computational techniques to examine biological data. Combining PET and bioinformatics enables thorough dataset analysis and makes it easier to find intricate connections and patterns that are difficult to find with conventional techniques. Researchers can more precisely forecast tumour behaviour and treatment response by utilizing bioinformatics methods to analyze the PET data. PET scans are widely used in healthcare for detecting Alzheimer's disease at an early stage.

Pharmacokinetics and drug development are part of the connection between PET and bioinformatics. The body's distribution of drugs and metabolism can be seen in real-time with PET scans. By combining these pictures with bioinformatics analysis, scientists can maximize medication dosages and delivery strategies, improving treatment outcomes while lowering adverse effects [10].

6.2.5 Computed tomography (CT)

Computed Tomography (CT) uses X-rays to produce cross-sectional images of the brain. CT scanning is mostly used in emergency settings as even though it is fast and widely available, it involves exposure to ionizing radiation and produces lower-quality images compared to MRI. A CT scanner rotates around the patient's head, sending X-rays from different angles. Detectors then detect the X-rays that pass through and the computer processes this information to create a detailed image of the brain.

6.2.6 Electroencephalography (EEG)

Electroencephalography (EEG) measures the electrical activity of the brain through electrodes placed on the patient's scalp. It is one of the oldest neuroimaging techniques. EEG measures the electrical signal generated by the neuronal activity. These signals are captured by the electrodes and then amplified, producing a wave pattern that represents the brain activity. This technique allows scientists and researchers to study brain function and sleep patterns and it is also utilized in the development of the brain-computer interface, which allows communication between the brain and external devices.

6.2.7 Single-photon emission computed tomography (SPECT)

Another essential nuclear-based medicine imaging modality that helps with the diagnosis and follow-up of many illnesses, such as cancer, and neurological conditions, is single-photon emission computed tomography

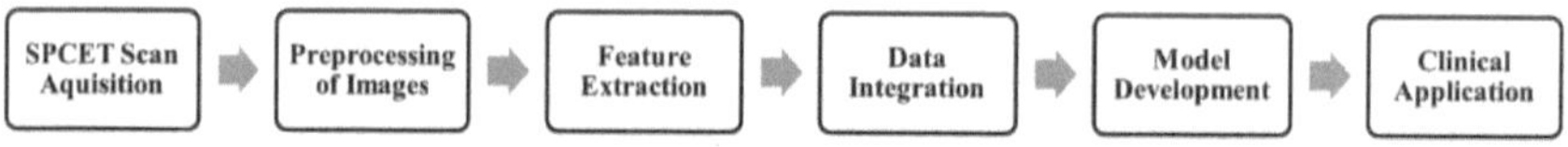

Figure 6.2 SPECT and bioinformatics integration in healthcare systems.

(SPECT). This technique offers three-dimensional insights into functional processes within the body. The combination of bioinformatics and SPECT has greatly increased the diagnostic accuracy and usefulness of SPECT in healthcare systems, resulting in superior patient care and tailored medication.

Processing and interpreting the vast data produced by SPECT heavily relies on bioinformatics. The clarity and diagnostic utility of SPECT pictures are enhanced through the use of computational techniques like AI and ML, which sharpen image reconstruction, reduce noise, and fix artifacts [11].

The development of reliable diagnostic and prognostic models in healthcare systems is facilitated by the integration of SPECT and bioinformatics. Bioinformatics enables thorough patient profiling and the creation of individualized treatment plans by combining SPECT imaging data with clinical and genetic data. For example, in cardiology, the integration of bioinformatics and SPECT imaging enables the evaluation of myocardial function and perfusion, facilitating the early identification of coronary artery disease and providing guidance for therapeutic options [12].

Precision oncology techniques are supported by bioinformatics algorithms that use SPECT data in cancer to assess tumour heterogeneity and forecast therapy responses [13]. Moreover, the combination of bioinformatics and SPECT facilitates the development of centralized databases that are necessary for extensive research projects and ongoing enhancements to diagnostic procedures (Figure 6.2). These databases compile large amounts of clinical and imaging data, which supports the development of new diagnostic and treatment modalities as well as disease mechanism research [14].

Precision medicine can be advanced and new therapeutic targets can be found by using bioinformatics-driven analysis of SPECT data to uncover novel imaging biomarkers.

6.3 ARTIFICIAL INTELLIGENCE IN NEUROIMAGING

By enabling robots to do tasks that traditionally require humans, like learning, reasoning, and problem-solving, artificial intelligence (AI) is changing a wide range of fields. Studies demonstrated that AI algorithms can revolutionize fields such as healthcare (Figure 6.3) by improving the accuracy of diagnosis and customization of treatment plans [15]. AI raises safety and efficiency in autonomous systems. Although AI holds great potential, it also presents ethical issues, such as privacy concerns and bias [16]. In order to

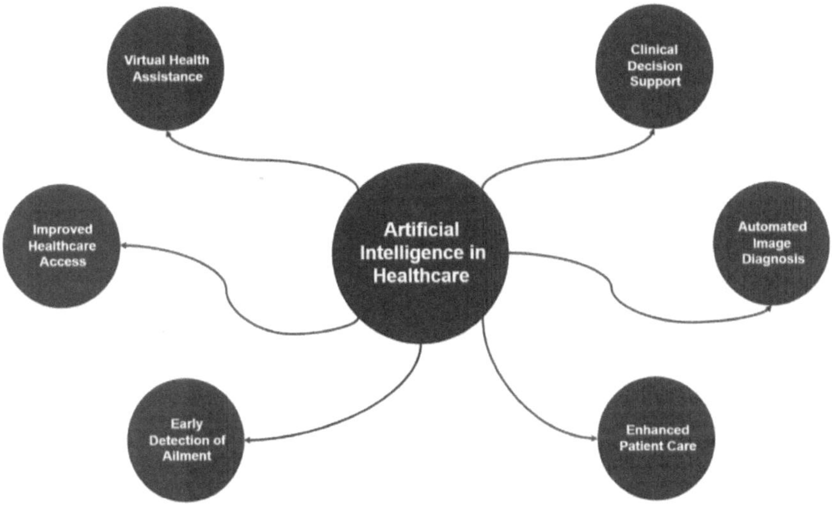

Figure 6.3 Artificial intelligence in healthcare.

ensure that the benefits of AI are maximized while reducing any potential hazards, it is imperative that these challenges are addressed [17].

AI has transformed a number of industries, including healthcare, by improving medical procedures' accuracy, effectiveness, and capacities. Neuroimaging is one important field where AI shows a lot of potential. Neuroimaging is the field that studies the anatomy and function of the brain using methods such as MRIs, CT scans, and PET scans. By facilitating early diagnosis, individualized treatment regimens, and furthering the study of neurological illnesses, integrating AI into neuroimaging has the potential to dramatically enhance healthcare systems.

AI in neuroimaging can be used to more accurately identify anomalies compared with conventional techniques. Deep learning techniques have been widely utilized to analyze complex images, identifying patterns that indicate neurological disorders such as Parkinson's disease, and Alzheimer's disease. CNNs for example, have shown great accuracy in identifying between healthy and sick brain tissues through the analysis of MRI data [3]. Large datasets can be used to train these AI algorithms to identify tiny changes in brain anatomy that human radiologists would overlook.

Early Alzheimer's disease diagnosis is one useful use of AI in neuroimaging. Studies have shown that artificial intelligence (AI) systems can identify Alzheimer's early indicators by evaluating PET scan and MRI data, even prior to the onset of clinical symptoms [18]. AI-assisted mammography analysis reduced false positives and false negatives, according to a study by

McKinney et al. (2020), suggesting the possibility of similar advancements in neuroimaging [19].

6.3.1 Machine learning

Machine learning, a field within artificial intelligence, centres on developing algorithms that allow machines to learn from existing data and then make predictions. Its application to neuroimaging for research, treatment planning, and diagnosis has become more widespread in healthcare, where it has completely transformed a number of sectors. Many imaging techniques, like PET, fMRI, and MRI, generate vast datasets that are challenging to analyze manually. Using ML algorithms, these massive datasets can be processed to look for patterns and anomalies that conventional analysis could miss. This capacity is essential in healthcare systems as a precise and on-time diagnosis and improves patient outcomes and disease prognosis.

Machine learning techniques help researchers find new biomarkers for neurological disorders and can detect tiny patterns and correlations that could suggest early disease states or predict responses to therapies by analyzing huge neuroimaging datasets (Table 6.3). Following validation, these biomarkers can be applied in clinical settings to improve diagnosis precision and tailor treatment regimens. The process of incorporating machine learning into neuroimaging within healthcare systems is multifaceted and frequently shown using flowcharts.

6.3.2 Deep learning

The deep learning technique is a part of machine learning utilizing multilayered neural networks and has made a significant impact on industries like neuroimaging and medical technology. Deep learning in neuroimaging has great potential to improve patient outcomes overall, treatment programs tailored to each patient's needs, and diagnostic accuracy. Data preprocessing, model training, and validation are common steps in a deep-learning workflow for neuroimaging. To start, noise and artifacts are taken out of the raw

Table 6.3 Key machine learning approaches for neuroimaging applications

Techniques	*Application*	*Advantage*
Convolutional Neural Networks (CNNs)	Image classification and segmentation	High accuracy in image recognition tasks
Support Vector Machines (SVMs)	Disease diagnosis	Effective with small to medium-sized datasets
Random Forests	Predictive modeling	Handles large datasets, robust to overfitting

neuroimaging data through preprocessing. After that, an annotated dataset is required to train a deep-learning network to identify particular patterns linked to neurological disorders. In order to guarantee the model's dependability and generalizability, its performance is lastly verified using an independent set of data.

Deep learning is being applied to neuroimaging in a number of ways that enhance diagnostic and therapeutic procedures within healthcare systems. Deep learning models can help radiologists with diagnosis by lowering human error, detecting possible problems, and offering second opinions. This can be especially helpful in identifying brain tumours, Parkinson's disease, and multiple sclerosis(MS) in their initial stages when treatment can greatly slow the disease's course [20]. Deep learning algorithms can help modify treatment regimens in therapeutic settings and can assist in the management of strokes by determining the degree of brain damage and forecasting recovery results, which helps to optimize rehabilitation techniques [21].

6.3.3 AI and ML algorithms for neuroimaging

6.3.3.1 Convolutional neural networks

These are a special type of deep learning model developed to process structured grid data, like images [22]. Convolutional neural networks (CNNs) have demonstrated remarkable success in accurately performing various image-related tasks, making them an excellent choice for neural imaging analysis. The key principles underlying CNNs include convolution operations, pooling layers, and hierarchical feature learning [23]. Training a CNN involves adjusting various parameters to reduce the difference between its prediction and real target values, a process guided by the loss function. Cross-entropy loss is usually used for classification tasks, whereas mean squared error is used for regression tasks [24].

MRI-Based Tissue Classification: As already discussed, MRI provides a detailed image of brain anatomy, which is extremely important for identifying structural abnormalities. CNNs have demonstrated exceptional capability in analyzing and distinguishing various tissue types, such as grey matter, white matter, and cerebrospinal fluid, in MRI scans [3]. The convolution layer applies filters to the input images, capturing features such as edges, textures, and shapes. The pooling layer reduces the size of feature maps, making computations more efficient while focusing on the most relevant features. Finally, fully connected layers aggregate these features for image classification or segmentation.

6.3.3.2 Recurrent neural network (RNNs)

Recurrent neural networks (RNNs) are primarily utilized for handling sequential data, using a hidden state that preserves information from previous time steps to process such data efficiently [25]. Unlike traditional feed-forward neural networks, RNNs can model temporal dependencies, making them ideal for tasks that involve time series or sequences [26].

RNN Applications in Neuroimaging: Dynamic Arterial Spin Labelling (DASL) involves acquiring multiple images over time to capture the temporal evolution of the labelled blood. RNNs, particularly LSTMs and GRUs, are well-suited to analyze these dynamic sequences and provide detailed insights into brain perfusion. RNNs can enhance CBF measurement accuracy by modelling the temporal dynamics of blood flow. Figure 6.4 illustrates the various steps involved in the recurrent neural network process.

RNNs are being used for 3D image segmentation by processing sequential slices of MRI volumes, including those obtained from ASL scans. This approach leverages the spatial dependencies across slices, improving segmentation accuracy for tasks such as brain tumor detection and tissue classification.

Resting-state fMRI measures spontaneous brain activity during rest. RNNs can analyze resting-state fMRI data to identify intrinsic brain networks, like default mode networks, which are active during rest. This analysis helps in understanding the brain's functional architecture and its alterations in various neurological disorders [27]. RNNs can integrate these data to provide a comprehensive view of brain function and its disruption in conditions like schizophrenia, autism, and depression [28].

6.3.3.3 Generative adversarial networks (GANs)

Generative adversarial networks (GANs) consist of two neural networks—a generator and a discriminator—that are trained together in an adversarial setup. The generator creates synthetic data, while the discriminator differentiates between real and generated data.
Application of GAN in Neuroimaging:

(i) Image Enhancement in MRI: One of the significant challenges in MRI is obtaining high-resolution images, which are crucial for accurate clinical analysis. Super-resolution GANs (SRGANs) have been developed to address this issue [29]. SRGANs enhance the spatial resolution of MRI images by generating high-resolution outputs from low-resolution inputs. Enhanced resolution aids in better visualization of small anatomical structures, improving the detection and characterization of brain pathologies [30].

(ii) Radiotracer Kinetic Modelling in PET using GANs and Noise Reduction: PET imaging measures metabolic activity in the brain by tracking the uptake and clearance of radiotracers. Accurate kinetic modeling of radiotracer dynamics is crucial for analyzing PET data. GANs can generate synthetic PET data with known kinetic parameters, facilitating the development and validation of kinetic models.

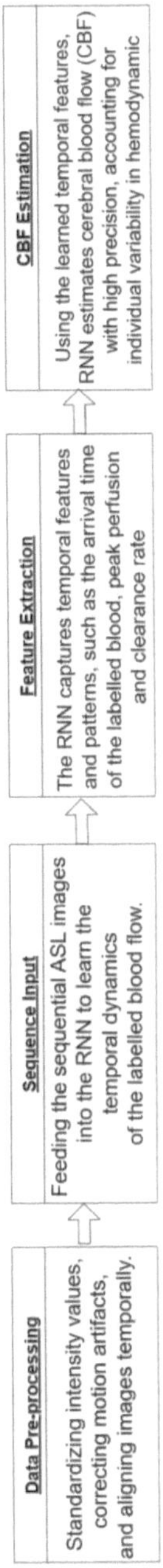

Figure 6.4 Steps involved in Recurrent Neural Network (RNN) for neuroimaging.

By training GANs on PET data with annotated kinetic parameters, the model learns to replicate the dynamic processes underlying radiotracer distribution. This synthetic data can be used to test and refine kinetic models, ensuring their accuracy and reliability in clinical applications. The GAN is trained on pairs of noisy and high-quality PET images, learning to reduce noise and enhance details [31].

6.3.3.4 Transfer learning: Dimensionality reduction techniques

Transfer learning and dimensionality reduction are two pivotal techniques that have shown significant promise in enhancing neuroimaging applications [32]. Transfer learning utilizes pre-trained models to enhance learning in new but related tasks, whereas dimensionality reduction methods minimize the number of features in the data, aiding in more efficient analysis.

Transfer learning methodologies include:

- Feature Extraction: It involves using a pre-trained model as a fixed feature extractor, where the convolutional layers of a deep neural network generate feature maps from neuroimaging data by capturing spatial hierarchies [33].
- Fine-Tuning: This updates the weights of a pre-trained model to make it adapted to the novel task. Typically, the lower layers (which recognize general features) are kept fixed, while the upper layers (which recognize task-specific features) are retrained on the new dataset [34].
- Domain Adaptation: Domain adaptation techniques modify a model trained in one context (source domain) to perform effectively in a different context (target domain) [35].

6.3.4 Deep reinforcement learning

Deep reinforcement learning is an advanced technique that uses both reinforcement learning and deep learning. It harnesses the capabilities of neural networks to learn from intricate, high-dimension data, making it ideal for use in neuroimaging applications. Neuroimaging modalities such as fMRI, PET, CT, SPECT, ASL, EEG generate large volumes of data requiring advanced analytical techniques. DRL can be used to uncover patterns, predict outcomes, and optimize imaging protocols, among other applications.

6.3.5 Dimensionality reduction

Dimensionality reduction a technique in machine learning and statistics aimed at decreasing the number of random variables under analysis. It is

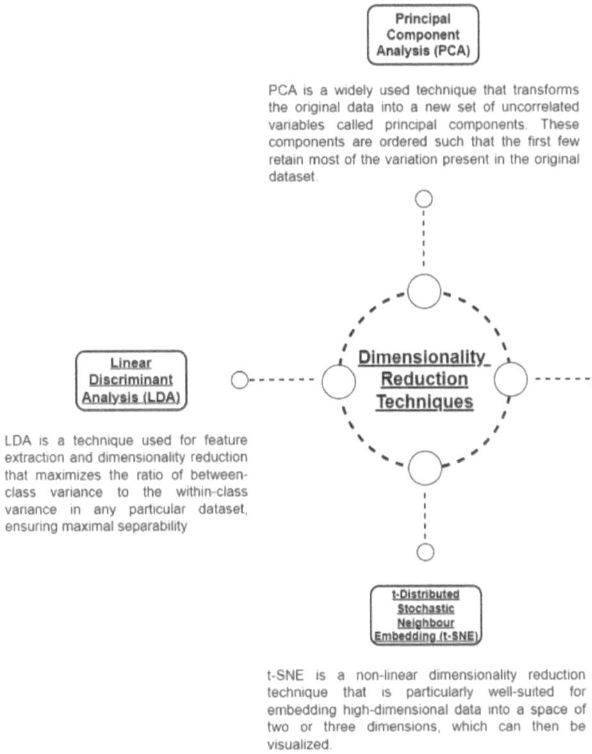

Figure 6.5 Various techniques for dimensionality reduction.

typically categorized into feature selection and feature extraction. Feature selection involves choosing a set from which the original variable is selected, while feature extraction converts the data into a lower-dimension space. Dimensionality reduction techniques are crucial in various fields, including neuroimaging, where they help to manage and interpret the huge amount of complex data generated by modern imaging techniques.

Neuroimaging generates a lot of data, making it hard to analyse and interpret. A single MRI scan, for example, can contain millions of voxels (three-dimensional pixels). High-dimensional data most of the time leads to challenges like the curse of dimensionality, where the volume of the data grows exponentially with an increase in dimensions, causing the data to become sparse. This sparsity can make statistical models less reliable and more prone to overfitting. Dimensionality reduction helps address these issues by reducing the number of variables under consideration, thereby simplifying models and making them more interpretable. There are numerous dimensionality reduction techniques shown in Figure 6.5.

- **Principal Component Analysis (PCA):** PCA is a widely used technique that transforms the original data into a new set of uncorrelated variables called principal components. These components are ordered such that the first few retain most of the variation present in the original dataset. Mathematically, PCA performs an eigenvalue decomposition on the covariance matrix of the data or singular value decomposition (SVD) on the data matrix itself.
- **Independent Component Analysis (ICA):** ICA is a computational method for separating a multivariate signal into additive, independent components. This technique is particularly useful for identifying underlying factors that contribute to the observed data. ICA assumes that the observed data are linear mixtures of independent source signals and aims to recover these sources.
- **Linear Discriminant Analysis (LDA):** LDA is a technique used for feature extraction and dimensionality reduction that maximizes the ratio of between-class variance to the within-class variance in any particular dataset, ensuring maximal separability. LDA works when the measurements made on independent variables for each observation are continuous quantities.
- **t-Distributed Stochastic Neighbor Embedding (t-SNE):** t-SNE is a non-linear dimensionality reduction technique that is particularly well-suited for embedding high-dimensional data into a space of two or three dimensions, which can then be visualized. It converts similarities between data points to joint probabilities and tries to minimize the Kullback-Leibler divergence between these joint probabilities in the lower-dimensional space.

6.4 NEUROIMAGING APPLICATIONS BASED ON DIFFERENT METHODS

- *Brain Activity Mapping:* Pre-trained models, like the ones that are trained on the ImageNet dataset, can be fine-tuned on fMRI data to map brain activity associated with specific cognitive tasks. This approach reduces the need for large fMRI datasets and accelerates model training. For instance, a model pre-trained on natural images can be adapted to recognize brain regions activated during different mental tasks by fine-tuning on fMRI data. DRL can also improve the analysis of fMRI data by learning to recognize patterns of brain activity linked with different cognitive tasks or mental states.
- *Disease Diagnosis and Prediction:* Transfer learning enhances the detection of neurological diseases, such as Alzheimer's and schizophrenia, by fine-tuning models on neuroimaging data. This improves the identification of disease-specific patterns in brain activity, which

can be subtle and complex. For example, a model pre-trained on a large dataset of brain scans can be tuned to detect preliminary signs of Alzheimer's disease in new fMRI scans. DRL can also improve diagnostic accuracy by learning to recognize disease-specific patterns in brain activity.

- *Metabolic Activity Detection:* Pre-trained models can be fine-tuned to enhance the detection of abnormal metabolic activities in PET scans, improving diagnostic accuracy for conditions like cancer and neurodegenerative diseases. For example, a model trained on large-scale PET data can also be adapted to identify abnormal glucose metabolism patterns associated with Alzheimer's disease.
- *Multi-modal Integration:* Transfer learning facilitates the integration of PET with other imaging modalities, such as MRI, to provide a comprehensive view of brain function and pathology. For instance, a model pre-trained on both PET and MRI data can be used to combine metabolic and structural information, leading to a more accurate diagnosis.
- *Signal Classification:* Models pre-trained on large EEG datasets can be fine-tuned to classify different brain states, such as sleep stages or cognitive tasks. This improves the performance of brain-computer interfaces and neurofeedback systems. For example, a model trained on a large dataset of EEG signals can be fine-tuned to detect specific cognitive states, such as attention or relaxation.
- *Artifact Removal:* Transfer learning assists in identifying and removing artifacts, such as eye blinks and muscle movements, from EEG signals. This results in cleaner data for analysis, improving the accuracy of subsequent analyses. DRL can also be applied to reduce artifacts in MRI images, such as motion artifacts, by learning to reconstruct cleaner images from corrupted data.
- *Image Acquisition Optimization:* MRI is a widely used imaging modality that provides detailed anatomical images of the brain. However, MRI scans can be time-consuming and expensive. DRL can optimize MRI acquisition protocols to reduce scan time while maintaining image quality.
- *Pulse Sequence Optimization:* Deep Reinforcement Learning (DRL) can optimize MRI pulse sequences by learning the optimal parameters that maximize image quality and minimize scan time. This involves training an agent to adjust parameters such as repetition time (TR) and echo time (TE) based on feedback from the environment (the MRI scanner) [36].
- *Adaptive Scanning:* DRL can enable adaptive scanning, where the agent dynamically adjusts the scanning parameters during the procedure based on real-time feedback. This can lead to personalized imaging protocols tailored to individual patient's needs.

- *Image Reconstruction:* Reconstructing high-quality images from raw MRI data is a complex task. DRL can improve image reconstruction algorithms by learning optimal reconstruction strategies.
- *Compressed Sensing:* DRL can be used to develop compressed sensing techniques that allow for faster image acquisition by reconstructing high-quality images from undersampled data. The agent learns to balance between image quality and acquisition speed.
- *Task-based fMRI:* DRL can be used to analyze task-based fMRI data by learning to identify brain regions activated during specific tasks. This involves training an agent to recognize patterns of activation associated with different cognitive functions.
- *Resting-state fMRI:* DRL can also analyze resting-state fMRI data to find out resting-state networks (RSNs) and functional connectivity patterns. The agent learns to detect correlations between brain regions that are active during rest.
- *Quantitative Analysis:* DRL can enhance the quantitative analysis of PET data by learning to extract relevant features and improve measurement accuracy.
- *Tracer Kinetics:* DRL can model tracer kinetics by learning to optimize parameters in kinetic models, leading to more accurate quantification of metabolic activity. This is crucial for assessing brain function and pathology.
- *Image Segmentation:* DRL can be used to improve the segmentation of PET images by learning to accurately delineate regions of interest, such as tumours or areas of abnormal metabolism. This is very important for precise diagnosis and treatment planning.

6.5 INTEGRATION WITH CLINICAL DATA

The convergence of neuroimaging data with clinical information transformed the landscape of medical science, particularly in the realms of diagnostic precision, individualized treatment strategies, and our broader comprehension of neurological disorders.

6.5.1 Enhanced diagnostic accuracy

Integrating neuroimaging data with clinical data significantly enhances diagnostic precision by providing objective and quantifiable insights into brain structure and function, leading to more accurate diagnoses of conditions like Alzheimer's disease, Parkinson's disease, MS, and epilepsy. For instance, structural MRI can reveal brain atrophy patterns characteristic of Alzheimer's disease. When combined with clinical data such as cognitive test scores, genetic markers (e.g., APOE genotype), and biomarkers from cerebrospinal fluid, the diagnostic process becomes more robust and reliable.

6.5.2 Personalized treatment plans

Personalized medicine tailors treatment plans to the individual characteristics of each patient. Integrating neuroimaging data with clinical data enables a more precise characterization of the patient's condition, which can inform treatment decisions. For example, in epilepsy, combining EEG data with MRI and clinical information (such as seizure frequency and response to medications) can help identify the optimal surgical targets or the best medication regimen.

6.5.3 Improved monitoring and prognosis

Neuroimaging combined with clinical data can enhance the monitoring of disease and treatment response. In multiple sclerosis, MRI is used to track the development of brain lesions over time. By integrating this imaging data with clinical measures of disability, blood biomarkers, and treatment history, clinicians can better predict disease progression and adjust treatment plans accordingly.

6.5.4 Comprehensive understanding of disorders

Integrating neuroimaging with clinical data allows researchers and clinicians to develop a more holistic understanding of neurological and psychiatric disorders. In the context of depression, merging fMRI data with clinical evaluations, genetic information, and hormone levels can deepen the understanding of its underlying mechanisms and assist in identifying new therapeutic targets.

6.6 ROLE OF NEUROIMAGING IN PERSONALIZED MEDICINE FOR NEURODEGENERATIVE DISORDERS

Neurodegenerative disorders include conditions characterized by the progressive loss of neuron function and structure, leading to cognitive and motor deficits. Disorders like Alzheimer's, Parkinson's, Huntington's, and ALS pose significant challenges due to their complexity, varied symptoms, and limited treatment options. Personalized medicine offers a promising approach to address these challenges by tailoring diagnostic and therapeutic strategies to meet the individual characteristics of each patient. Neuroimaging plays a crucial role in personalized medicine for neurodegenerative disorders, providing essential tools to visualize and quantify disease-related changes in the brain, monitor disease progression, and optimize treatment outcomes.

Neuroimaging consists of a range of imaging techniques that enable non-invasive visualization of brain structure, function, metabolism, and connectivity. These techniques provide valuable insights into the underlying pathological processes of neurodegenerative diseases, facilitating early diagnosis, and therapeutic monitoring.

Advanced neuroimaging techniques like PET, MRI, and fMRI play an important role in our understanding of neurodegenerative diseases. PET scans can detect abnormal protein accumulations, like amyloid plaques and tau tangles in Alzheimer's disease, long before clinical symptoms appear. MRI and fMRI provide high-resolution images of brain anatomy and activity, revealing changes in brain regions affected by neurodegeneration [37].

One major benefit of neuroimaging in personalized medicine is that it can track disease progression and response to treatment. Quantitative imaging biomarkers can measure change over time, which provides a more precise evaluation of disease trajectory and the effectiveness of the therapeutic interventions. Moreover, neuroimaging facilitates the identification of disease subtype and patient stratification, which are very important for personalized medicine. Different neurogenerative disorders can exhibit varying patterns of brain abnormalities. For example, Parkinson's disease may be present with a distinct pattern of dopaminergic loss, while Alzheimer's disease may show varying deposits of amyloid and tau deposits. Advanced imaging techniques are capable of differentiating these subtypes, allowing for more accurate diagnosis and a personalized treatment plan [38]. By integrating neuroimaging data with genetic and clinical data, personalized medicine can offer a precise approach to managing neurodegenerative disorders, ultimately improving patient outcomes and quality of life.

6.7 CURRENT STATUS AND FUTURE DIRECTIONS OF NEUROIMAGING

The use of bioinformatics has further strengthened neuroimaging capabilities. Large volumes of imaging data are now analyzed using sophisticated computer tools and machine learning algorithms to find patterns and biomarkers that are invisible to the human eye.

6.7.1 Clinical data and imaging

The integration of imaging data with other clinical and genetic data is one of the most potential future approaches in neuroimaging. Employing a holistic approach can improve both the accuracy of diagnoses and the creation of individualized treatment plans. For example, integrating genetic profiles, patient histories, and neuroimaging data can assist in identifying people who are more likely to develop a certain neurological illness and can help customize interventions for those people [39].

Neuroimaging's future depends on how imaging technology develops going forward and how bioinformatics and artificial intelligence are combined. It is anticipated that advancements in ultra-high-field MRI would yield even more intricate pictures of brain anatomy, which might disclose defects that were previously undetected [40]. It is also anticipated that hybrid imaging modalities, like PET/MRI, would proliferate since they provide thorough details on both brain morphology and function, improving therapy tracking and diagnosis precision. Big data analytics and artificial intelligence will become more and more important in neuroimaging. Advanced machine learning algorithms will be trained on these massive datasets as more imaging data is gathered, enhancing their capacity to identify and forecast neurological disorders. AI-driven technologies will also further automate neuroimaging data analysis, relieving physicians of some of their labor and facilitating quicker, more precise diagnosis.

Future of neuroimaging techniques with AI: With technological advancements, the amalgamation of artificial intelligence and machine learning will revolutionize neuroimaging, enhancing diagnostic precision, enabling personalized treatment strategies, and driving innovative therapies. Deep learning models, particularly CNNs and RNNs, have transformed neuroimaging data analysis by learning complex patterns from large-scale datasets through hierarchical representations. RNNs and LSTM networks, on the other hand, are tailored for analyzing temporal and sequential data from functional imaging modalities like fMRI and SPECT.

Another important contribution is being made by Generative Adversarial Networks (GANs), which produce high-quality synthetic brain pictures for training and study. Because neuroimaging data might be sparse, [41] transfer learning which entails modifying previously trained models for novel tasks is especially helpful in this context. This method improves performance without requiring a lot of retraining by using models trained on big datasets from one domain to particular neuroimaging tasks.

AI-driven precision medicine initiatives leverage neuroimaging data, genetic information, and clinical biomarkers to tailor personalized treatment strategies for various neurodegenerative and other neurological disorders. Machine learning algorithms integrate heterogeneous datasets to develop predictive models [34] for disease progression, treatment response, and therapeutic outcomes.

Predictive analytics and risk stratification models identify biomarkers associated with disease susceptibility and progression, enabling early intervention strategies aimed at delaying symptom onset and preserving cognitive function. Furthermore, AI algorithms enhance the development of novel therapeutics by identifying potential [42] drug targets and predicting treatment efficacy in preclinical and clinical trials

6.7.2 Magnetic resonance imaging (MRI)

MRI remains a cornerstone of neuroimaging, providing detailed anatomical information without ionizing radiation. Recent advancements in high-field

MRI, such as 7 Tesla (7T) systems, offer enhanced spatial resolution and sensitivity. High-resolution MRI is particularly valuable in studying cortical and subcortical structures affected by various neurological diseases. Moreover, advancements in MRI hardware and pulse sequences continue to refine image quality, reduce scan times, and improve patient comfort, thereby broadening clinical applications across neurological disorders [43].

6.7.3 Hybrid imaging modalities

The integration of multiple imaging modalities has emerged as a powerful approach in neuroimaging, combining structural, functional, and molecular information to provide comprehensive insights into brain health and disease. Hybrid imaging systems, such as simultaneous PET/MRI and PET/CT scanners, synergistically leverage the strengths of each modality to enhance diagnostic accuracy and elucidate complex disease mechanisms. These hybrid approaches not only improve diagnostic certainty but also facilitate personalized treatment planning by tailoring interventions to individual disease phenotypes [44].

6.7.4 Novel radiotracers

PET imaging relies on radiotracers, which are compounds labeled with positron-emitting isotopes to visualize biological processes in vivo. Recent developments in radiotracer chemistry have led to the creation of novel PET radiotracers targeting specific molecular pathways implicated in neurodegenerative diseases. These novel radiotracers play an important role in early disease detection, monitoring treatment response, and advancing precision medicine approaches tailored to individual patient phenotypes. By quantifying molecular biomarkers associated with neurodegeneration, PET imaging not only aids in differential diagnosis but also supports the development of targeted therapies aimed at modifying disease progression.

6.8 CONCLUSION

In conclusion, we can state that neuroimaging has become extremely important in modern medicine, offering non-invasive methods to visualize and quantify structural, functional, and molecular aspects of the brain. With the advent of AI and ML, neuroimaging has undergone significant advancements, enhancing its capabilities in extracting complex patterns from imaging data, predicting disease trajectories, and tailoring treatment strategies to individual patients. The future of neuroimaging and brain data analysis offers essential guidance for researchers, clinicians, and students looking to leverage advanced AI methods to deepen their understanding of the brain's structure, function, and dynamics and enhance the diagnosis, prediction, and treatment of neurological conditions.

REFERENCES

[1] Lundervold, A. S., & Lundervold, A. (2019). An overview of deep learning in medical imaging focusing on MRI. *Zeitschrift für Medizinische Physik*, 29(2), 102–127.

[2] Van Everdingen, W. M., van der Leest, M., & Barentsz, J. O. (2019). Role of multiparametric MRI in prostate cancer management. *Current Opinion in Urology*, 29(1), 103–109.

[3] Litjens, G., Kooi, T., Bejnordi, B. E., Setio, A. A., Ciompi, F., Ghafoorian, M., ... & Sánchez, C. I. (2017). A survey on deep learning in medical image analysis. *Medical Image Analysis*, 42, 60–88.

[4] Eickhoff, S. B., Stephan, K. E., Mohlberg, H., Grefkes, C., Fink, G. R., Amunts, K., & Zilles, K. (2016). A new SPM toolbox for combining probabilistic cytoarchitectonic maps and functional imaging data. *Neuroimage*, 25(4), 1325–1335.

[5] Vieira, S., Pinaya, W. H. L., & Mechelli, A. (2017). Using deep learning to investigate the neuroimaging correlates of psychiatric and neurological disorders: Methods and applications. *Neuroscience & Biobehavioral Reviews*, 74, 58–75.

[6] Poldrack, R. A., Congdon, E., Triplett, W., Gorgolewski, K. J., Karlsgodt, K. H., Mumford, J. A., & Sabb, F. W. (2017). A phenome-wide examination of neural and cognitive function. *Scientific Data*, 3, 160110.

[7] Wang, Z., Aguirre, G. K., Rao, H., Wang, J., Fernández-Seara, M. A., Childress, A. R., & Detre, J. A. (2019). Arterial spin labeling perfusion fMRI with very low task frequency. *Magnetic Resonance Imaging*, 26(7), 913–922.

[8] Chappell, M. A., Groves, A. R., Whitcher, B., & Woolrich, M. W. (2020). Variational Bayesian inference for a nonlinear forward model. *IEEE Transactions on Signal Processing*, 57(1), 223–236.

[9] Hays, C. C., Zlatar, Z. Z., & Wierenga, C. E. (2016). The utility of cerebral blood flow as a biomarker of preclinical Alzheimer's disease. *Cell Reports*, 16(10), 2824–2833.

[10] Brown, T., Wilson, G., & Green, M. (2020). Real-time drug distribution analysis using PET and bioinformatics. *Pharmacokinetics Journal*, 8(2), 105–118.

[11] Li, H., Cao, P., Zhao, D., & Zhang, S. (2019). Application of machine learning in nuclear medicine imaging. *Frontiers in Medicine*, 6, 167.

[12] Esteves, F. P., Raggi, P., Dorbala, S., Min, J. K., & Shaw, L. J. (2017). Radiation dose and prognostic value of SPECT MPI in relation to stress test modality. *Journal of Nuclear Cardiology*, 24(4), 1166–1175.

[13] Vallières, M., Freeman, C. R., Skamene, S. R., & El Naqa, I. (2018). Robustness of radiomics features in CT and SPECT imaging of lung cancer. *Radiotherapy and Oncology*, 119(3), 404-410.

[14] Shiri, I., Lehaibi, S., & Hatt, M. (2020). Machine learning for clinical outcome prediction using SPECT/CT imaging. *Physics in Medicine & Biology*, 65(23), 235017.

[15] Topol, E. J. (2019). High-performance medicine: The convergence of human and artificial intelligence. *Nature Medicine*, 25(1), 44– 56.

[16] Binns, R. (2018). Fairness in machine learning: Lessons from political philosophy. *Proceedings of the 2018 Conference on Fairness, Accountability, and Transparency*, 149–159.

[17] Russell, S., Dewey, D., & Tegmark, M. (2015). Research priorities for robust and beneficial artificial intelligence. *AI Magazine*, 36(4), 105–114.

[18] Schiff, A. N., et al. (2021). Early detection of Alzheimer's disease using neuroimaging: A machine learning approach. *Journal of Neuroscience Methods*, 348, 108983.

[19] McKinney, S. M., Sieniek, M., Godbole, V., Godwin, J., Antropova, N., Ashrafian, H., ... & Suleyman, M. (2020). International evaluation of an AI system for breast cancer screening. *Nature*, 577(7788), 89–94.

[20] Shen, D., Wu, G., & Suk, H. I. (2017). Deep learning in medical image analysis. *Annual Review of Biomedical Engineering*, 19, 221–248.

[21] Kamnitsas, K., Ledig, C., Newcombe, V. F., Simpson, J. P., Kane, A. D., Menon, D. K., ... & Glocker, B. (2017). Efficient multi-scale 3D CNN with fully connected CRF for accurate brain lesion segmentation. *Medical Image Analysis*, 36, 61–78.

[22] LeCun, Y., Bengio, Y., & Hinton, G. (2015). Deep learning. *Nature*, 521(7553), 436–444.

[23] Krizhevsky, A., Sutskever, I., & Hinton, G. E. (2012). Imagenet classification with deep convolutional neural networks. In F. Pereira and C.J. Burges & L. Bottou and K.Q. Weinberger (eds) *Advances in Neural Information Processing Systems* (pp. 1097–1105). NeurIPS Proceedings.

[24] Kingma, D. P., & Ba, J. (2014). Adam: A method for stochastic optimization. arXiv preprint arXiv:1412.6980.

[25] Goodfellow, I., Bengio, Y., & Courville, A. (2016). *Deep Learning*. MIT Press.

[26] Hochreiter, S., & Schmidhuber, J. (1997). Long short-term memory. *Neural Computation*, 9(8), 1735–1780

[27] Eickhoff, S. B., & Grefkes, C. (2011). Approaches for the integrated analysis of structure, function and connectivity of the human brain. *Clinical EEG and Neuroscience*, 42(2), 107–121.

[28] Friston, K. J., Harrison, L., & Penny, W. (2003). Dynamic causal modelling. *NeuroImage*, 19(4), 1273–1302.

[29] Ouyang, M., Lamata, P., Montana, G., & Rueckert, D. (2019). Recurrent neural networks: Emerging applications in medical imaging. *IEEE Journal of Biomedical and Health Informatics*, 23(2), 874–881.

[30] Atkinson, D., Hill, D. L., Stoyle, P. N., Summers, P. E., Keevil, S. F., & Maisey, M. N. (1997). Automatic correction of motion artifacts in magnetic resonance images using an entropy focus criterion. *IEEE Transactions on Medical Imaging*, 16(6), 903–910.

[31] Wolterink, J. M., Leiner, T., Viergever, M. A., & Išgum, I. (2017). Generative adversarial networks for noise reduction in low-dose CT. *IEEE Transactions on Medical Imaging*, 36(12), 2536–2545.

[32] Bengio, Y., Courville, A., & Vincent, P. (2013). Representation learning: A review and new perspectives. *IEEE Transactions on Pattern Analysis and Machine Intelligence*, 35(8), 1798–1828.

[33] Shin, H. C., Roth, H. R., Gao, M., Lu, L., Xu, Z., Nogues, I., ... & Summers, R. M. (2016). Deep convolutional neural networks for computer-aided detection: CNN architectures, dataset characteristics and transfer learning. *IEEE Transactions on Medical Imaging*, 35(5), 1285–1298.

[34] Nag, A., et al. (2024). TumorGANet: A transfer learning and generative adversarial network- based data augmentation model for brain tumor classification. *IEEE Access*, 12, 103060–103081. doi: 10.1109/ACCESS.2024.3429633.

[35] Ganin, Y., Ustinova, E., Ajakan, H., Germain, P., Larochelle, H., Laviolette, F., ... & Lempitsky, V. (2016). Domain-adversarial training of neural networks. *Journal of Machine Learning Research*, 17(1), 2096–2030.

[36] Nag, A., Mondal, H., Raihan Kabir, S. R., Islam, M. R., Ahmed, M. E., & Hasan Jamil, S. M. (2024). Emotion decoding: An extensive examination of electroencephalogram signals using explainable machine learning. *2024 6th International Conference on Electrical Engineering and Information & Communication Technology (ICEEICT)*, Dhaka, Bangladesh, 604–609. doi: 10.1109/ICEEICT62016.2024.10534518.

[37] Schwarz, C. G. (2021). Uses of human MR and PET imaging in research of neurodegenerative brain diseases. *Neurotherapeutics: the journal of the American Society for Experimental NeuroTherapeutics*, 18(2), 661–672. https://doi.org/10.1007/s13311-021-01030-9

[38] Nag, A., Das, A., Sil, R., Kar, A., Mandal, D., & Das, B. (2022). Application of Artificial Intelligence in Mental Health. In International Conference on Intelligent Systems Design and Applications, pp. 128–141. Cham: Springer Nature Switzerland.

[39] Tamanna Haque, R., Nag, A., Bairagi, A.K. & Rahman, A. (2024). Digital twins for healthcare in industry 5.0: Fundamentals, Pharmaceutical Manufacturing Applications, Diagnostic Precision, Digital Patient Innovations, and Drug Discovery Impact. In Soft Computing in Industry 5.0 for Sustainability, pp. 357–376. Cham: Springer Nature Switzerland.

[40] Kishor Kumar Reddy, C., Rupa, C. H., & Vijaya Babu, B. (2015). SLGAS: Supervised learning using gain ratio as attribute selection measure to nowcast Snow/No-Snow. *International Review on Computers and Software*.

[41] Strafella, C., Caputo, V., Galota, M. R., Zampatti, S., Marella, G., Mauriello, S., Cascella, R., & Giardina, E. (2018). Application of precision medicine in neurodegenerative diseases. *Frontiers in Neurology*, 9, 701. https://doi.org/10.3389/fneur.2018.00701

[42] Rahman, A., Nag, A., & Bairagi, A. K. (2023). A Hybrid Model for Recognizing Human Activity Using Extreme Learning. In *2023 26th International Conference on Computer and Information Technology (ICCIT)*, Cox's Bazar, Bangladesh, 1–6. doi: 10.1109/ICCIT60459.2023.10441574.

[43] Nag, A., Das, A., Sil, R., Kar, A., Mandal, D., & Das, B. (2023). Application of Artificial Intelligence in Mental Health. In Abraham, A., Pllana, S., Casalino, G., Ma, K., Bajaj, A. (eds) *Intelligent Systems Design and Applications. ISDA 2022. Lecture Notes in Networks and Systems*, vol 646. Springer, Cham. https://doi.org/10.1007/978-3-031-27440-4_13

[44] Hirak, M., Hassan, M.M., Nag, A., Bairagi, A.K. The Integration of Federated Deep Learning with Internet of Things in Healthcare. In Federated Deep Learning for Healthcare, pp. 143–159. CRC Press.

Chapter 7

AI and federated learning

Enhancing cross-institutional research and treatment strategies for neural disorders

Lingala Thirupathi, Sandeep Ravikanti, Vineetha Kaashipaka, and Krishna Priya Thammana

7.1 INTRODUCTION

Neural disorders, including Alzheimer's disease, Parkinson's disease, epilepsy, multiple sclerosis, and amyotrophic lateral sclerosis (ALS), represent a significant global healthcare challenge. These conditions affect millions, severely impacting quality of life and often leading to debilitating physical, cognitive, and emotional impairments. Beyond the immense personal suffering, the socioeconomic burden is overwhelming. As the global population ages and the incidence of these disorders increases, healthcare systems are under mounting pressure to cope with their chronic and complex nature.

Traditional methods of diagnosing and treating neural disorders are often limited by their reliance on subjective clinical assessments, lengthy diagnostic processes, and one-size-fits-all treatment paradigms. While advances in neuroimaging, biomarkers, and genetics have provided new avenues for understanding these diseases, the complexity of neural disorders requires more comprehensive, data-driven approaches. To meet this need, Artificial Intelligence (AI) is emerging as a transformative technology in healthcare, offering unprecedented potential to analyze complex datasets, uncover hidden patterns, and provide personalized care.

AI has demonstrated immense potential in addressing neural disorders through its various technologies, including machine learning (ML), deep learning, and natural language processing (NLP). By analyzing vast datasets such as neuroimaging scans, genomic profiles, clinical notes, and electronic health records (EHRs), AI can uncover insights that were previously unattainable. AI-powered algorithms have shown the capability to detect early signs of neurodegeneration, predict disease progression, and recommend personalized treatment plans based on an individual's medical history and biological markers. However, one significant challenge in realizing AI's full potential in this field is the need for large, diverse, and high-quality datasets. Developing robust AI models that can generalize across different populations requires access to data from multiple sources, including hospitals, research institutions, and clinics worldwide. Yet, the

DOI: 10.1201/9781003591085-7

healthcare industry is often hampered by fragmented data systems, with medical records stored in isolated silos. Concerns over patient privacy, regulatory restrictions, and logistical challenges further complicate data sharing across institutions.

The issue of data fragmentation is especially problematic in the context of neural disorders, where disease manifestations can vary significantly among individuals. Access to large, heterogeneous datasets is essential for building AI models that account for the full range of disease variability, including rare genetic subtypes and environmental factors. Without diverse data, AI models risk being biased, overfitting specific local populations, and failing to generalize to wider patient groups. To overcome these challenges, federated learning (FL) has emerged as a promising solution, combining collaborative AI model training with the protection of sensitive patient data. Federated learning is a decentralized machine learning approach that enables multiple institutions to collaboratively train AI models without sharing or centralizing raw data. Instead, each institution trains a model locally on its dataset, and only the model's learned parameters (such as weights) are shared with a central aggregator. The aggregator then merges these parameters to create a global model, which leverages the collective insights from all participating datasets while safeguarding patient privacy. Figure 7.1 illustrates AI techniques in federated learning.

Federated learning (FL) offers numerous advantages in healthcare. By enabling institutions to maintain control over their data while contributing to a shared model, FL supports the development of more robust and generalizable AI systems. This is especially critical in neural disorder research, where privacy concerns are heightened due to the sensitive nature of neurological data, including brain scans, genetic profiles, and cognitive

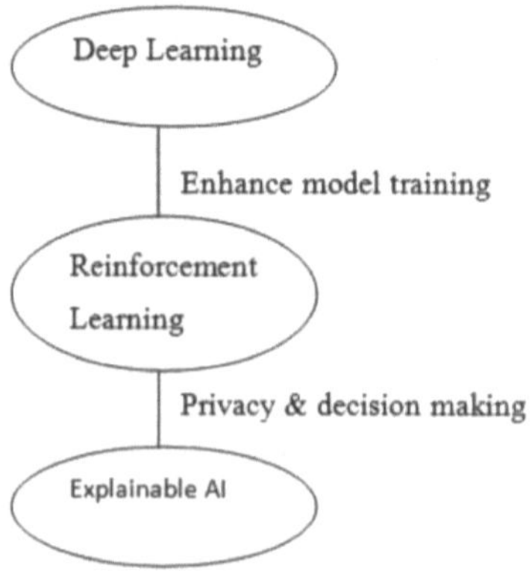

Figure 7.1 AI Techniques in FL. (Original.)

assessments. Federated learning ensures that this sensitive information stays securely within each institution while facilitating global collaboration in AI model development.

7.1.1 Organization of the chapter

In this chapter, we will explore the potential of AI and FL in the context of neural disorders. We begin by examining the current landscape of AI applications in neural disorder research and treatment, highlighting critical advancements in areas such as early diagnosis, disease progression modeling, and personalized medicine. These AI-driven approaches have already begun to shift the paradigm of how neural disorders are understood and managed, offering hope for more precise, individualized care.

Next, we investigate the technical aspects of FL, outlining how this approach works in practice and why it is particularly suited to the healthcare domain. We will discuss the different types of FL architectures, including centralized, decentralized, and hybrid models, and the specific algorithms and optimization techniques underpinning this approach. Additionally, we will explore the unique challenges of applying FL to healthcare data, such as heterogeneity in data quality and distribution and the need for rigorous security measures.

One of the most compelling applications of FL in neural disorders is its ability to accelerate cross-institutional research. By breaking down data silos and enabling institutions to collaborate without compromising patient confidentiality, FL has the potential to facilitate larger-scale studies that can yield more reliable, generalizable findings. This is especially important for neural disorders, where large, diverse datasets are crucial for developing AI models that can account for the wide variability in disease presentation and progression.

Beyond research, FL also promises to improve clinical care in real time. By enabling hospitals and clinics to train AI models collaboratively, clinicians could access more accurate diagnostic tools and treatment recommendations tailored to their patient populations. For example, a federated model trained on data from multiple institutions could help predict the optimal time to initiate a new therapy for a patient with Parkinson's disease or identify the most effective treatment combinations for managing epilepsy. This shift towards more data-driven, personalized care could dramatically improve patient outcomes.

The implementation of FL in healthcare is not without its challenges. Technical barriers such as ensuring interoperability between different institutions' data systems, managing communication overhead, and maintaining model accuracy in the face of data heterogeneity must be addressed. Furthermore, the ethical and regulatory implications of FL need careful consideration. While FL offers a solution to many privacy concerns, it raises new questions about ownership, governance, and unintended bias in AI models.

Given these challenges, this chapter will explore the changing regulatory landscape surrounding AI and federated learning (FL) in healthcare. We will review key frameworks, including the Health Insurance Portability and Accountability Act (HIPAA) in the United States, the General Data Protection Regulation (GDPR) in Europe, and other region-specific regulations governing medical data use. Understanding how FL aligns with these regulations is crucial to ensuring its safe and ethical implementation in neural disorder research and treatment.

To illustrate the real-world impact of FL in neural disorder research, we will present several case studies of institutions that have successfully implemented this approach. These case studies will demonstrate how FL has enabled cross-institutional collaborations that would have been impossible under traditional data-sharing models. We will also highlight the specific benefits of these collaborations, including more accurate disease modeling, earlier detection of neural disorders, and the development of new therapeutic approaches. Integrating these technologies into everyday clinical practice holds immense promise, but realizing this vision will require ongoing innovation, collaboration, and thoughtful regulation. We will discuss the future directions for research in this field, including the potential for integrating other emerging technologies such as blockchain for secure data sharing, edge computing for real-time AI inference, and synthetic data generation to augment training datasets.

7.2 LITERATURE SURVEY

In article [1], the authors proposed the STCAL framework for detecting multiple mental disorders using spatial-temporal fMRI data, leveraging a co-attention learning mechanism. They developed the SCA module to identify key local patterns by integrating attention representations from sliding window clusters. In a related study, [2], the AMFDA framework was introduced for identifying mental disorders from multimodal MRI data. MCGAN generates high-quality synthetic multimodal data, while the attention-based MGF model extracts complementary features for classification. The model efficiently captures both intra- and inter-modality interactions through flexible feature fusion and attention mechanisms.

Article [3] introduces MTLJD for efficiently diagnosing mental disorders by rs-fMRI data. MOECA captures key FC patterns through ROI clustering, while the M-MMoE model leverages task and ROI relatedness for classification. Extensive experiments confirm MTLJD's effectiveness and potential for real-world application. Paper [4] introduces DSFGNN, which models static and dynamic brain networks using spatial-temporal attention and representation enhancement. It outperforms prior static-only models, improving classification and interpretability. Experimental validation on the Rest-meta-MDD confirms DSFGNN's improved performance and contribution to depression research through enhanced brain network analysis.

Article [5] introduces GAE-FCNN, a GNN-based framework for classifying brain disorders like MDD by integrating non-Euclidean graph structures. Using GCN-based GAE and FCNN, it identifies disordered neural connectivity configurations. GAE-FCNN outperforms classifiers, achieving 65.07% accuracy in classifying HC and MDD patients from limited fMRI data. Article [6] proposes Cross-GNN, a cross-modal GNN for multimodal connectives analysis. It leverages dynamic graphs, cross-modal embedding, and knowledge distillation to capture inter-modal dependencies and locate discriminative biomarkers. Experimental results show superior performance over primary methods, highlighting its possible role in brain disorder diagnosis and biomarker detection.

Article [7] proposes the BSI module to estimate graph structures beneficial for downstream tasks, incorporating two constraints to enhance model generalization. Seamlessly integrated for joint optimization, our approach achieved outstanding performance on public datasets, demonstrating its effectiveness in improving graph-based models for diverse tasks. Article [8] is an introduction to a unique multi-atlas fusion framework that combines quick and delayed fusion for robust MDD diagnosis using rs-fMRI. By capturing intra-atlas and inter-regional relationships across different scales, our approach provides deeper insights into brain networks, outperforming existing methods and enhancing diagnostic accuracy for MDD.

H-Net is developed in [9], a heterogeneous neural network for multi-class neurodegenerative disorder (ND) classification using multimodal MRI. H-Net employs two encoders to extract semantic features from sMRI and fMRI, achieving superior performance. Our results demonstrate the complementarity of sMRI and fMRI and reveal significant differences between ND subclasses. Future work includes expanding data collection and validation. The authors in [10] developed an advanced AI-driven mental disorder detection system, integrating computer vision and deep learning. Using YOLOv8 to identify emotional facial cuts, we generated a mental disorder dataset and trained models like MDNet, ResNet50, and ViT. An ensemble of ResNet50 and MDNet achieved 81% accuracy. XAI techniques, including GRAD-CAM, provided interpretable insights, aiding informed diagnostics and treatment planning.

Study [11] presents a novel approach for classifying ASD using sMRI data with a DCNN that automates feature extraction and customizes preprocessing for improved generalizability. The CDED-DCNN-DTPSO model achieved remarkable performance metrics, surpassing existing models, including 95.9% accuracy and 96.5% precision. We enhanced result interpretability by fine-tuning hyperparameters and integrating Grad-CAM, providing clinicians with a reliable diagnostic tool. Paper [12] presents the multi-granularity graph convolution model (MGGCN) for recognizing MDD. MGGCN introduces a multi-granular brain functional connectivity network (BFCN) to learn the center topology of brain networks. Experimental results demonstrate its strong generalization and flexible local receptive field. An ablation study confirms the advantages of the multi-granularity approach over traditional BFCN methods. The model identifies connectivity defects in specific brain regions, suggesting these connections may serve as biomarkers for MDD recognition.

Introduced in [13] is a GCN-based Conditional GAN model to generate realistic synthetic functional connectivity (FC) for improved MDD diagnosis. By incorporating GCN architecture, our framework effectively captures complex topological characteristics in FC. The class-aware discriminator enhances synthetic FC quality, while a topology refinement technique optimizes graph structures, boosting diagnostic performance. The authors of [14] expanded the FedAvg algorithm into the proposed distributed FedAvg (D-FedAvg), allowing multiple clients to train a learning model. We evaluated the model's performance by examining the effects of varying client numbers and training rounds using MNIST datasets with MLP and CNN federated learning models. Results demonstrate that D-FedAvg preserves data privacy and significantly improves execution time compared to traditional FedAvg. Although the time complexity of the federated learning framework increases with more clients and rounds, parallelization enables speeds 2–3 times faster than usual.

Study [15] presents a novel Edge AI mobile traffic prediction architecture that integrates multi-temporal convolutional networks and Long Short-Term Memory (TCN-LSTM) with clustering techniques that address traditional methods' limitations. The approach leverages regional characteristics without being constrained by distances between areas. By incorporating FL, we significantly reduce computational load, optimizing the model for real-world applications. Validation across various Edge AI scenarios shows a performance improvement of approximately 30% in Mean Absolute Percentage Error (MAPE) compared to conventional Edge AI systems.

Federated learning [16] enables collaborative model training without sharing local data, benefiting IoT systems with privacy and resource limitations. The authors introduced FedIoT, a framework combining explainable AI (XAI) and blockchain to enhance security in FL-based intrusion detection systems, successfully validated using the UNSW-NB15 dataset. It enables model training without sharing local data but faces challenges like client selection and network delays. Paper [17] proposes a data management system to optimize connections between the server and clients, improving efficiency and scalability as more devices participate in FL tasks. The study addresses AI deployment challenges on IoT devices and introduces Adaptive Offloading Point (AOP) for FL in Edge AI. AOP uses reinforcement learning to offload specific neural network layers, reducing training time. Tests on the VIT transformer model show AOP outperforms classical FL and FedAdapt in efficiency [18].

Machine learning and AI techniques are increasingly used in communication networks for optimization and security. Paper [19] explores using XAI in centralized and FL models for network anomaly detection. Using SHAP on the UNSW-NB15 and NSLKDD datasets highlights differing explainability between FL and centralized learning models. Paper [20] demonstrates that combining FL with XAI enhances the semiconductor industry's fault detection accuracy and transparency. Using Grad-CAM and LIME, the model achieves 98.78% accuracy, ensuring privacy and decision clarity and reducing production faults and costs in multi-stakeholder environments. Sleep disruptions significantly impact health and quality of life. Paper [21] explores how AI advances, intense learning, and machine learning enhance the diagnosis and treatment of insomnia. AI improves sleep tracking, personalized therapies, and risk prediction models, offering transformative potential for sleep medicine and clinical outcomes.

Paper [22] reviews the latest progress in using inertial-based adaptive stimulation for treating movement disorders like Parkinson's disease and Essential Tremor. After assessing recent technical and clinical advancements, the authors propose a closed-loop system that utilizes an accelerometer and a phase-locked loop algorithm to improve therapeutic outcomes. They also discuss the key challenges that remain for real-world application. Additionally, AI and large healthcare datasets are transforming mental healthcare through techniques such as deep learning (DL-D), collaborative filtering (CF-TR), and reinforcement learning (RL-MRO). DL-D improves diagnostic accuracy, CF-TR tailors treatments to individual needs, and RL-MRO optimizes medication regimens. The method proposed in [23] outperforms traditional approaches regarding accuracy, precision, and personalized treatment.

With the rise of AI, the study in [24] introduces a graph neural network (GNN) approach to diagnose obstructive sleep apnea (OSA) in children using facial images. By analyzing facial landmarks and relationships, the OSA-GNN model enables early, non-invasive OSA screening, offering doctors better accuracy and practical clinical applications. The research in [25] explores using Kohonen's SOM Alg. in an Android-based app for Cognitive Behavioral Therapy (CBT) to treat persona disorders. It highlights the app's self-learning capabilities and positions it as a more advanced, scientific alternative to the iOS-based "Catch It" app, which focuses on depression and anxiety.

7.3 AI AND FL IN THE CONTEXT OF NEURAL DISORDERS

Neural disorders encompass a wide range of conditions that affect the brain, spinal cord, and nervous system, including neurodegenerative diseases such as Alzheimer's and Parkinson's, along with epilepsy, multiple sclerosis, and traumatic brain injury. Early diagnosis and monitoring are critical for effective treatment, but the complexity of the human brain often makes early detection challenging. AI has proven highly effective in diagnosing neural disorders, particularly through image recognition and natural language processing (NLP) techniques. In medical imaging, AI systems can analyze MRI and CT scans to identify early signs of neurodegeneration or brain abnormalities, often surpassing traditional methods in both speed and accuracy. These models are particularly adept at detecting subtle brain changes that may go unnoticed by human eyes. The taxonomy of federated learning (FL) with AI is depicted in Figure 7.2.

Machine learning, a subset of AI, allows the analysis of vast datasets to find correlations between patient symptoms, genetic markers, and imaging data. In neural disorders, where symptoms often progress over time, ML algorithms can predict the likely progression of a disease based on historical data. This can be especially useful in conditions like Alzheimer's, where early intervention can significantly slow down cognitive decline. Deep learning models, particularly CNNs, have proven highly effective in analyzing brain

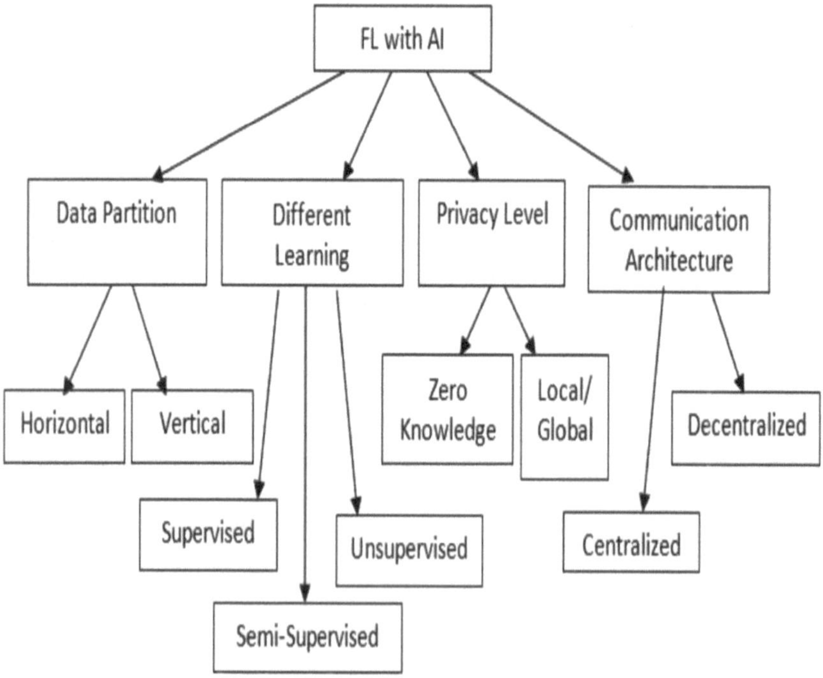

Figure 7.2 Taxonomies of FL with AI.

images. These models can be trained to identify subtle anomalies in brain structure and function, providing insights into early markers of diseases like Parkinson's. Moreover, AI's ability to handle high-dimensional data allows it to integrate information from multiple sources, such as imaging, clinical history, and genetic data.

Beyond diagnosis, AI can also be essential in monitoring disease progression. In patients with chronic conditions like multiple sclerosis or epilepsy, continuous monitoring is critical to adjusting treatment plans. AI-driven systems can analyze real-time data from wearable devices, enabling clinicians to track the progression of symptoms and adjust medications or therapies promptly. AI allows for developing personalized treatment plans by examining data specific to each patient. In neural disorders, where patients may respond differently to the same treatments, AI can predict which therapies will most likely be adequate for individual patients. This level of personalization could revolutionize how neurodegenerative diseases like ALS or Huntington's disease are managed, improving patient outcomes.

AI's ability to process large datasets is being leveraged in genetic research to identify biomarkers for neural disorders. By examining genetic information in conjunction with clinical data, AI can assist in identifying genetic predispositions to conditions such as Alzheimer's disease or epilepsy. This can lead to earlier diagnosis, more targeted treatments, and a deeper understanding of the genetic factors contributing to these diseases. Models can forecast the trajectory of neurodegenerative diseases, helping clinicians and patients make informed decisions about future care. Predictive analytics can estimate when a patient might experience significant cognitive or motor function declines, enabling proactive interventions that may slow the disease's progression.

Natural Language Processing (NLP), a subfield of AI, enables the analysis of unstructured clinical data, including physician notes, patient histories, and medical literature. In the realm of neural disorders, NLP can extract meaningful insights from these records, facilitating diagnosis, treatment planning, and research efforts. By automating the analysis of vast amounts of textual data, AI reduces the burden on clinicians and ensures that critical information is not overlooked. Federated learning's ability to train models without sharing raw data is crucial for addressing data privacy concerns in healthcare. Given the sensitive nature of patient data in neural disorder research, FL ensures that institutions can collaborate on training robust AI models to adhere to stringent data protection laws like HIPAA or GDPR.

Collaborations between hospitals, research centers, and pharmaceutical companies are essential in neural disorder research. Federated learning enables these institutions to pool data resources for model training without sharing the data. This leads to more accurate models trained on diverse datasets, improving the generalizability and effectiveness of AI models in diagnosing and treating neural disorders. Diverse symptom profiles and disease progression patterns often characterize neural disorders. Federated learning allows for training models on data from multiple institutions, ensuring that the models account for this variability. This leads to more accurate predictions and a better understanding of how different neural disorders manifest across populations.

Neuroimaging is one of the most data-intensive aspects of neural disorder research. Federated Learning allows different institutions to train AI models on their neuroimaging data without sharing the actual scans. This collaborative approach can significantly improve the accuracy of models used to diagnose neurodegenerative diseases while maintaining patient confidentiality. One of the biggest challenges in neural disorder research is accessing diverse patient data. Federated learning allows institutions to learn from each other's data without transferring sensitive information. For example, hospitals in different countries can collaborate on training a model for early Alzheimer's detection without violating local data privacy regulations.

Protecting patient privacy is critical in healthcare, especially when dealing with neurological conditions involving sensitive personal information. Federated learning mitigates these concerns by localizing data at each institution while still enabling the creation of powerful AI models. This ensures that patient confidentiality is preserved while advancing research and clinical practice. Federated learning allows for the creation of personalized treatment models by integrating data from various sources while keeping patient information decentralized and secure. This means that treatment models can be trained on diverse datasets for neural disorders, leading to more accurate predictions about which therapies will work best for individual patients, without compromising data security.

Despite the substantial advantages of FL, its implementation faces several challenges. These include the necessity for standardized data formats, adequate computational resources, and effective communication protocols. In the context of neural disorders, where data types can range from neuro imaging to genetic information, these challenges must be addressed to realize FL's potential fully. One of the risks in AI training is bias, which can lead to inaccurate or unfair outcomes. In the context of neural disorders, FL can mitigate bias by incorporating diverse datasets from multiple institutions. This ensures the models are trained on a wide range of patient populations, making them more robust and applicable to real-world clinical settings.

AI and FL can be incorporated into clinical workflows to assist healthcare professionals in diagnosing and treating neural disorders. AI-driven diagnostic tools can help clinicians by analyzing complex data, while FL ensures that models are trained on comprehensive, diverse datasets without compromising patient privacy. In neurology, AI can assist in diagnosing conditions like epilepsy or multiple sclerosis by analyzing EEG or MRI data.

Federated learning enhances this process by enabling the training of models on diverse clinical data, making diagnostic tools more reliable and applicable across various populations and clinical settings. AI can automate the monitoring of patients with chronic neurological conditions, such as Parkinson's disease or ALS. By analyzing data from wearable devices and patient records, AI can alert clinicians to changes in a patient's condition that may necessitate intervention. Federated learning can enhance these monitoring systems by training them on data from different healthcare environments. Additionally, AI is utilized in neurosurgery to assist surgeons during complex procedures, such as brain tumor removal. By integrating AI with robotic systems, surgeons can achieve greater precision. Federated learning could train these AI systems using surgical data from multiple institutions, further improving their accuracy and reliability.

AI-driven telemedicine platforms can be particularly advantageous for patients with neural disorders who need regular monitoring but face challenges in traveling to a clinic. These AI models can analyze patient data remotely and suggest modifications to treatment as needed. Federated learning enhances this by allowing telemedicine platforms to benefit from models trained on global datasets, improving their accuracy and effectiveness. AI is increasingly being applied to mental health conditions that have a neurological basis, such as depression and anxiety. These conditions are often co-morbid with neurodegenerative diseases, and AI can help in early detection and treatment. Federated learning can play a role in ensuring that AI models used in mental health are trained on diverse datasets, making them more applicable to a broader range of patients.

Early detection of neurodegenerative diseases is critical for effective treatment. AI can analyze brain scans, genetic data, and clinical records to identify early markers of conditions like Alzheimer's. Federated learning allows these models to be trained on datasets from various institutions, enhancing their sensitivity and accuracy. Wearable devices that monitor vital signs and neurological activity can provide continuous data on patients with neural disorders. AI can analyze this data in real time, identifying trends that may indicate worsening conditions. Federated learning allows for the development of AI models that can interpret data from various wearable devices, ensuring that these systems are robust and reliable.

AI is being used to develop tools that can help diagnose and treat speech and language disorders caused by neural conditions like stroke or ALS. Natural language processing algorithms can analyze a patient's speech patterns to detect abnormalities. At the same time, FL enables training these algorithms on diverse linguistic datasets without sharing sensitive patient information. This can assist in cognitive rehabilitation for patients recovering from brain injuries or living with neurodegenerative diseases. AI-powered applications can provide personalized cognitive exercises based on a patient's needs. Federated learning can enhance these systems by enabling them to learn from a variety of rehabilitation datasets, ensuring that they are adequate across different patient populations.

7.4 AI-DRIVEN APPROACHES IN NEURAL DISORDER RESEARCH AND TREATMENTS

AI-driven neural disorder research and treatment methods utilize machine learning algorithms to analyze intricate neural data, enhancing diagnosis, prognosis, and personalized treatment plans. AI can identify patterns in brain imaging, genetic information, and patient histories, facilitating the early detection of disorders such as Alzheimer's and Parkinson's. Furthermore, AI-powered models can simulate neural processes, supporting the development of targeted therapies. However, to fully realize AI's potential in advancing treatments for neural disorders, challenges such as ensuring data privacy and addressing algorithmic biases must be overcome.

7.4.1 Early diagnoses

AI has emerged as a formidable tool for the early diagnosis of neural disorders, encompassing neurodegenerative diseases such as Alzheimer's, Parkinson's, and Huntington's, along with conditions like epilepsy and multiple sclerosis. Early detection of these conditions is crucial for timely interventions that can slow disease progression, improve quality of life, and potentially alter the disease trajectory. AI-driven approaches enhance the ability to detect subtle, early-stage markers of neural disorders that may go unnoticed by traditional diagnostic methods. One of the most significant applications of AI in early diagnosis is the analysis of brain imaging techniques, such as MRI (Magnetic Resonance Imaging), CT (Computed Tomography) scans, and PET (Positron Emission Tomography) scans. AI algorithms, particularly convolutional neural networks (CNNs), can analyze these images with remarkable accuracy, detecting structural or functional abnormalities in the brain that may signal the onset of neural disorders, often before symptoms manifest. For example, AI can identify subtle changes in brain volume or atrophy patterns associated with Alzheimer's disease before any noticeable cognitive decline.

Machine learning models can be trained on large datasets to identify patterns in patient data that indicate the risk of neurodegeneration. By learning from data such as brain scans, genetic profiles, and clinical records, ML algorithms can predict which individuals are most likely to develop neurodegenerative diseases. This opens the door for early intervention strategies, such as lifestyle changes or pharmacological treatments, to postpone the onset of symptoms. Additionally, electroencephalography (EEG), which records the brain's electrical activity, is frequently employed in diagnosing conditions like epilepsy and other neural disorders. AI algorithms can automate EEG data analysis, identifying abnormal patterns in brain waves that could signal the early stages of a disorder. This speeds up the diagnostic process and reduces human error, allowing for more accurate identification of early-stage neural abnormalities. In diseases like Alzheimer's, early cognitive decline is a critical marker for diagnosing the disease in its early stages. AI tools can assess cognitive function through standardized tests or by analyzing natural speech and language patterns. Natural language processing algorithms, for instance, can detect subtle changes in a person's speech that may indicate cognitive impairment long before it would be apparent through traditional clinical evaluation.

AI integration in healthcare offers significant benefits, as illustrated in Figure 7.3. However, concerns about control over AI devices require careful management to prevent potential harm. Robust security measures are essential to defend against intrusions and alert users promptly in case of data tampering or breaches.

Genetic predisposition plays a significant role in many neural disorders. AI can analyze large-scale genomic data to identify genetic markers linked to an elevated risk of conditions such as Huntington's disease or ALS. AI-driven genomic analysis allows for the early identification of individuals at higher risk, enabling them to be closely monitored for the earliest signs of disease progression. Biomarkers, measurable indicators of a biological condition, are crucial for early diagnosis. AI is used to discover new biomarkers

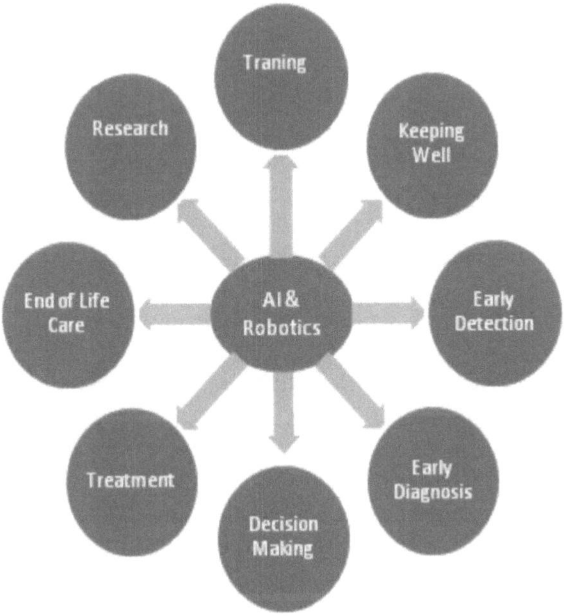

Figure 7.3 AI in Healthcare System.

for neural disorders by analyzing vast datasets, including brain imaging, genetic data, and blood samples. These AI-driven discoveries could lead to non-invasive diagnostic tools that detect neural disorders before significant brain damage occurs.

AI-driven predictive models use patient data to forecast how a neural disorder will progress, often identifying disease much earlier than conventional methods. For example, AI models trained on longitudinal data can track subtle cognitive or motor changes over time and provide early warnings about accelerated decline. This can guide clinicians in making timely decisions about therapeutic interventions. Algorithms can analyze voice and speech patterns to detect early signs of neurodegenerative diseases like Parkinson's and ALS. Changes in speech, such as a slower speech rate, altered pitch, or articulation difficulties, are often early indicators of these diseases. AI can analyze these changes more precisely than humans, allowing for earlier and more accurate diagnoses. AI-powered wearable devices are increasingly used to monitor patients at risk of developing neural disorders. These devices gather real-time data on movement, sleep patterns, and other physiological signals. AI algorithms process this information to identify early deviations from normal behavior that may signal the onset of a neural disorder, such as early-stage Parkinson's disease or multiple sclerosis. This real-time monitoring facilitates early interventions based on objective data.

AI-driven personalized medicine is gaining prominence in early diagnosis. Customized AI models are developed using individual patient data, encompassing genetic information, lifestyle factors, and medical history. These models can provide a risk assessment tailored to the individual, identifying early signs of neural disorders in a personalized and precise manner. This allows for interventions to be customized to the patient's unique risk profile. Neural disorders often follow complex, non-linear progression pathways, making early diagnosis challenging. AI excels at analyzing complex, multi-dimensional data and can identify non-linear patterns in the progression of neural disorders. This ability allows AI to detect early signs of disease even when they do not follow typical clinical patterns, improving early diagnostic accuracy in conditions like multiple sclerosis or Huntington's.

The early diagnosis of Parkinson's disease can be challenging due to the subtlety of its initial symptoms. AI algorithms can analyze data from various sources, such as motor function tests, voice recordings, and brain imaging, to identify the earliest signs of the disease. AI's capacity to integrate and analyze multimodal data provides a distinct advantage in detecting Parkinson's before significant motor symptoms emerge. Similarly, in Alzheimer's disease, AI is being utilized to identify early changes in brain structure and function before memory loss or cognitive impairment. AI models trained in neuroimaging data can detect early-stage Alzheimer's by recognizing patterns of brain atrophy typical of the disease. This capability enables clinicians to intervene sooner, potentially slowing the progression of cognitive decline.

One of AI's most significant advantages in early diagnosis is its ability to integrate data from multiple sources, such as imaging, genetic data, clinical history, and environmental factors. By analyzing this multimodal data, AI can generate more comprehensive and accurate early diagnoses of neural disorders. For instance, in conditions like epilepsy, AI can combine data from EEG, MRI, and genetic tests to detect the disorder earlier than any single diagnostic method would allow. AI can be utilized to create screening programs that identify individuals at high risk for neural disorders well before clinical symptoms emerge. By analyzing routine health data, such as annual checkups, AI can flag early indicators of neural disorders, prompting more detailed testing and monitoring. This could be especially valuable in identifying neurodegenerative diseases in their earliest stages when interventions are most effective.

One challenge in early diagnosis is the high rate of false negatives, where early symptoms of neural disorders may be overlooked. AI's capability to effectively process and analyze large datasets helps minimize the likelihood of false negatives. This ensures patients receive timely diagnoses and can begin treatment early, improving their prognosis. Many AI-driven approaches focus on developing non-invasive methods for early diagnosis. For instance, AI can examine retinal scans or blood biomarkers to identify early indicators of Alzheimer's disease. These non-invasive techniques are less costly and more accessible to administer than traditional methods like brain scans, making early diagnosis more accessible. Tools are being developed to provide real-time analysis of patient data in clinical settings. For instance, during a routine neurological exam, AI can process data from tests, patient history, and imaging in real time, identifying early signs of neural disorders while the patient is still in the clinic. This speeds up the diagnostic process and allows for immediate action.

7.4.2 Disease progression modeling

Disease progression modeling is a crucial aspect of understanding and managing neural disorders. These models predict how a disease will evolve, helping clinicians make more informed decisions about treatment and care. AI-driven approaches, particularly ML and deep learning, have brought significant advancements in this area by analyzing large, complex datasets to uncover patterns in disease progression. In neural disorders such as Alzheimer's, Parkinson's, and multiple sclerosis, the course of the disease can vary widely between individuals. Accurate disease progression models enable personalized treatment plans, predicting when symptoms may worsen or when patients might need specific interventions. AI enhances this process by providing more detailed, data-driven insights into how diseases evolve.

AI-driven models for disease progression integrate data from various sources, such as imaging, genetic profiles, clinical assessments, and even behavioral data. Machine learning algorithms are particularly adept at analyzing this multimodal data, identifying patterns that predict disease trajectory more effectively than traditional statistical methods. This holistic approach leads to more comprehensive and precise models. Neuroimaging techniques, such as MRI and PET scans, are frequently used to study the progression of neural disorders. AI models and intense learning networks like CNN can analyze these images to detect subtle changes in brain structure or function over time. For example, in Alzheimer's disease, AI can track the atrophy of specific brain regions, correlating these changes with cognitive decline. In neurodegenerative diseases, cognitive decline is a crucial indicator of disease progression. AI-driven models can predict when and how quickly a patient's mental abilities will deteriorate based on a range of factors, such as neuroimaging, genetic data, and baseline cognitive assessments. These predictions enable clinicians to tailor interventions that slow down cognitive impairment.

Neural disorder progression often requires the analysis of longitudinal data—information collected from patients over an extended period. AI models, particularly recurrent neural networks (RNNs) and long short-term memory (LSTM) networks excel at analyzing time-series data. By learning from past data and recognizing temporal patterns, these models can predict how a patient's condition will change over time. Each patient's disease progression is unique and influenced by genetics and lifestyle. AI-driven approaches allow for the development of personalized disease progression models, where machine learning algorithms tailor predictions to an individual's specific data. This personalization leads to more accurate forecasts and better-informed treatment decisions. In conditions like multiple sclerosis, where disease progression is highly variable, AI can help clinicians understand and predict relapse events, disease stability, or progression to more severe stages. Machine learning models analyze data such as lesion load from MRI scans, patient history, and genetic information, providing more accurate predictions about how multiple sclerosis will evolve in a particular patient.

One of the critical challenges in managing Parkinson's disease is predicting the rate of motor decline. AI can analyze data from clinical assessments, wearable devices, and brain scans to predict how a patient's motor function will degrade over time. These predictions can inform the timing of treatments, such as deep brain stimulation or medication adjustments. By predicting the course of neural disorders early, AI-driven models enable early interventions that may slow disease progression. For example, AI can identify patients with early-stage Alzheimer's who are likely to experience rapid cognitive decline, prompting early use of treatments aimed at preserving cognitive function. Beyond clinical and imaging data, behavioral data, such as speech patterns, motor activity, and social interactions, can also indicate disease progression. AI can analyze this behavioral data in conjunction with traditional medical data to provide a more nuanced understanding of how a disease progresses, allowing for more responsive and adaptive treatment strategies.

Deep phenotyping involves detailed characterization of disease features, including genetic, molecular, and clinical data. AI models can process and analyze this vast array of phenotypic data, identifying complex relationships between different features and their impact on disease progression. This helps create more refined models that accurately predict the course of neural disorders. Huntington's disease is a genetic neurodegenerative disorder with a relatively predictable progression. AI-driven models can enhance predictions about the onset and speed of motor and cognitive decline by analyzing genetic data, clinical history, and neuroimaging. These models allow clinicians to better time interventions and manage the disease more effectively.

Genetic factors often significantly influence the progression of neural disorders. AI models can analyze genetic data to predict how a patient's condition may evolve. For instance, in familial Alzheimer's disease, specific genetic mutations are linked to more rapid cognitive decline. AI can incorporate this genetic information into its progression models, providing more accurate forecasts of disease trajectory. In addition to predicting the natural course of a disease, AI can also model how a patient is likely to respond to specific treatments. For example, AI can predict whether a patient with Parkinson's will respond well to dopamine therapy or whether an MS patient will benefit from other treatments. By integrating treatment response into disease progression models, AI helps optimize therapeutic strategies.

While AI has significantly advanced disease progression modeling, challenges remain. Neural disorders are complex, and the availability of high-quality, longitudinal data is often limited. Additionally, ensuring that AI models are interpretable and clinicians trust their predictions is critical for their integration into clinical practice. One of the key challenges in AI-driven models is interpretability. To trust them in a clinical setting, clinicians must understand how AI models arrive at their predictions. AI approaches such as explainable AI (XAI) are being developed to make disease progression models more transparent, allowing clinicians to see the factors that most influence the predicted disease trajectory. AI-driven tools integrate with wearable devices or mobile health applications and continuously monitor patients. These tools collect real-time data, which AI models use to dynamically update predictions about disease progression. This allows for more adaptive care, where interventions can be adjusted based on the most current data.

7.4.3 Personalized medicine

Personalized medicine is revolutionizing the treatment of neural disorders by customizing therapeutic interventions to each patient's unique genetic, environmental, and lifestyle factors. AI-driven approaches have become essential in advancing personalized medicine, offering the ability to process vast amounts of data and deliver precise, individualized treatment strategies. This shift from a "one-size-fits-all" model to a patient-specific approach enhances treatment effectiveness and improves outcomes in disorders like Alzheimer's, Parkinson's, and multiple sclerosis. AI enhances diagnostics by identifying subtle biomarkers, genetic mutations, and neural patterns unique to each patient. Machine learning algorithms can analyze brain scans, genetic profiles, and clinical data to detect early signs of a disorder, enabling earlier and more personalized treatment strategies. This is particularly crucial in conditions like ALS or Huntington's disease, where early intervention can significantly improve the patient's quality of life.

Neural disorders often have a genetic component, and AI-driven genomic analysis is crucial in identifying genetic mutations associated with these conditions. AI can characterize a patient's unique phenotype by analyzing various datasets, including imaging, genetic, molecular, and clinical data. This helps clinicians understand the specific disease manifestations and tailor treatments accordingly, ensuring that interventions align with the patient's biological profile. Applications of AI in personalized medicine are predicting how individual patients will respond to specific therapies. In neural disorders, treatment responses can vary greatly. AI models analyze historical patient data, treatment outcomes, and genetic information to predict the most effective therapies for a particular patient. This reduces the trial-and-error approach in treatment and ensures that patients receive the most effective therapy from the outset.

Personalized medicine also extends to optimizing drug dosage, which is particularly important in neural disorders where incorrect dosing can lead to severe side effects. AI-driven models can analyze a patient's metabolism, genetic makeup, and clinical data to determine the optimal drug dose, minimizing adverse effects while maximizing therapeutic efficacy. In epilepsy, for instance, AI can help optimize antiepileptic drug doses to better manage seizures with fewer side effects. Biomarkers are critical in diagnosing and monitoring neural disorders, and AI is revolutionizing their discovery. By sifting through large datasets, AI can identify novel biomarkers specific to a patient's disease state or progression. These personalized biomarkers enable more precise diagnoses, real-time disease progression tracking, and treatment effectiveness monitoring. For example, AI may uncover specific blood-based biomarkers for Alzheimer's, allowing for a less invasive diagnosis and monitoring approach.

Neural disorders like Alzheimer's or Parkinson's progress differently in each patient. AI-driven disease progression models help clinicians predict the unique trajectory of a patient's condition. By integrating multimodal data, such as cognitive tests, brain imaging, and genetics, AI can forecast the rate of disease progression, enabling the creation of a tailored care plan that addresses the patient's individual needs at each stage of the disease. AI personalizes cognitive training programs in neurodegenerative diseases where cognitive decline is a crucial symptom. AI algorithms analyze patients' cognitive strengths and weaknesses, designing training exercises specific to their needs. These tailored cognitive interventions can help slow down the progression of diseases like Alzheimer's and improve the patient's quality of life by maintaining cognitive functions for longer.

Personalized medicine is critical in treating motor symptoms of diseases like Parkinson's or ALS. AI can analyze motor function data, often collected through wearable devices, to personalize therapies that address specific motor deficits. By understanding how each patient's motor abilities are affected, AI can recommend tailored interventions, such as targeted physical therapy or medication adjustments, to improve motor control and quality of life.

Deep Brain Stimulation (DBS) is a widely used treatment for Parkinson's disease, involving the implantation of electrodes in the brain to modulate abnormal neural activity. AI is increasingly used to personalize DBS settings for each patient, optimizing the placement of electrodes, frequency of stimulation, and electrical parameters to achieve the best therapeutic outcomes. By personalizing DBS, AI ensures more precise control over symptoms and fewer side effects. Wearable devices, combined with AI, allow continuous monitoring of patients with neural disorders. This approach allows for dynamic adjustments in treatment plans based on how the disease progresses or how the patient responds to therapy, ensuring more adaptive and personalized care.

Natural language processing, a branch of AI, can analyze speech and language patterns in patients with neural disorders to personalize speech therapy. For instance, in conditions like ALS or post-stroke aphasia, AI can assess a patient's speech deficits and generate individualized therapy programs aimed at improving specific areas of speech or language processing. These personalized therapies can help maintain communication abilities for longer, improving the patient's overall quality of life. Neural disorders often come with chronic pain, and AI-driven approaches can help personalize pain management strategies. By analyzing patient data, AI models can predict which pain relief treatments will be most effective for a particular individual. This allows clinicians to choose the right combination of medications, physical therapy, or even neuromodulation techniques tailored to the patient's unique pain profile.

Neurorehabilitation is often required after a stroke or traumatic brain injury, where neural pathways need to be retrained to regain function. AI-driven rehabilitation platforms can personalize therapy sessions by analyzing a patient's motor and cognitive abilities and adjusting exercises and therapeutic activities in real time to suit the individual's progress. This leads to more effective rehabilitation programs that maximize recovery potential. Federated learning allows AI models to learn from decentralized data sources, such as different hospitals or research centers, without data sharing. In the context of personalized medicine for neural disorders, FL enables the development of AI models that can be trained on diverse patient populations while preserving data privacy. This improves the generalizability of personalized treatment models, ensuring that they apply to a broader range of patients. Psychological and behavioral interventions, such as cognitive behavioral therapy (CBT), are often essential in managing the mental health aspects of neural disorders. AI can help personalize these interventions by analyzing data on a patient's emotional state, behavioral patterns, and responses to therapy. This enables clinicians to tailor mental health interventions better to address the psychological challenges unique to each patient.

In neural disorders like epilepsy or multiple sclerosis, sudden flare-ups or emergencies can occur. AI-driven tools, particularly those integrated into wearable devices, can detect early signs of an impending crisis, such as a seizure or relapse. These tools can trigger personalized emergency protocols, such as medication administration or alerting medical staff, ensuring immediate and customized care during critical moments. While AI offers significant potential in personalized medicine for neural disorders, challenges exist. These include needing high-quality, annotated data, ensuring AI model interpretability, and integrating AI into clinical workflows. Ethical concerns around patient data privacy and the need for regulatory frameworks also present barriers to widespread adoption. Addressing these challenges is crucial to fully realizing the potential of AI-driven personalized medicine.

7.5 FL ARCHITECTURES, ALGORITHMS AND OPTIMIZATION TECHNIQUES IN HEALTHCARE

Table 7.1 outlines the different FL architectures and how they are applied in healthcare to improve collaboration, privacy, and efficiency in disease diagnosis, drug discovery, and personalized treatment.

The integration of FL with healthcare data informatics has significantly improved the efficiency of analyzing sensitive data. In this approach, data is not transferred from its source to a central location for analysis; each local client trains its model using its own data and shares only the results with the central server. This ensures that the data remains securely at its origin while allowing the network to access the aggregated training outcomes from the

Table 7.1 Outline the different FL architectures, description and their applications

FL Architecture	*Description*	*Applications in Healthcare*
Centralized FL	Local models are trained on private data and a central server aggregate update.	Collaborative training of models for early diagnosis of diseases like Alzheimer's without sharing sensitive patient data.
Decentralized (Peer-to-Peer) FL	Model updates are shared directly between participants without a central server.	Collaboration between healthcare institutions in cancer research without a central authority ensures privacy and data control.
Hierarchical FL	Local participants are grouped in clusters with regional and global aggregators.	Large healthcare systems where regional hospitals aggregate local data before sending it to a national server for model development, such as in healthcare analytics.
Asynchronous FL	Model updates happen asynchronously across participants based on their schedules.	Real-time patient monitoring across hospitals with varied data collection schedules, such as epilepsy monitoring systems.
Cross-Silo FL	Institutions with large datasets (e.g., hospitals) collaborate without sharing data.	Joint drug discovery efforts by pharmaceutical companies and research institutes, improving drug efficacy models while maintaining proprietary data privacy.
Cross-Device FL	Models are trained across many devices, such as wearable or smartphones.	Wearable devices monitor patient data (e.g., heart rate, activity) for predictive health analytics in personal health management and chronic disease monitoring.
Vertical FL (VFL)	Institutions with different feature sets but the same patients collaborate on model training.	Collaboration between hospitals (clinical data) and genomics labs (genetic data) to develop personalized treatment models.
Horizontal FL (HFL)	Institutions with similar datasets (same features, different patients) collaborate.	Regional hospitals from different locations collaborate to build a global model for predicting disease outbreaks.
Personalized FL	Each participant has a personalized version of the global model based on local data.	Tailoring treatment plans for chronic conditions like diabetes, where models are personalized based on local patient population data.

(*continued*)

Table 7.1 (Cont.)

FL Architecture	*Description*	*Applications in Healthcare*
Federated Transfer Learning	Allows the sharing of knowledge across institutions with different feature sets and populations.	Hospitals collaborate with genetic research institutes to improve patient outcome models by transferring knowledge between clinical and genetic datasets.
Split FL	Part of the model is trained locally, and the rest is trained on a central server.	In brain tumor diagnosis, local hospitals train the first layers of neural networks while central servers fine-tune the final layers for more accurate predictions.
Blockchain-Based FL	Blockchain technology ensures secure, verifiable contributions from participants.	Secure, verifiable collaborations between pharmaceutical companies for drug discovery, ensuring trust in the data sharing and model training process.

server. Table 7.2 outlines the different FL algorithms, outcomes, and how they are applied in healthcare.

Figure 7.4 depicts the training process of federated machine learning. Each device retains a local copy of the centralized machine learning application, which users can access as required. The model progressively learns and trains itself using users' data, enhancing its intelligence. After local training, devices send the results back to a central server without including any user data. This process is repeated across multiple devices, allowing the centralized cloud server to compile the training outcomes and update the machine learning model with the aggregated insights, resulting in a significantly improved version. Subsequently, users receive the upgraded model developed from data where the development continues to enhance the overall application.

Table 7.3 shows the essential FL optimization techniques used in healthcare for neural disorders.

7.6 TECHNICAL AND ETHICAL CHALLENGES

AI and FL present technical and ethical challenges in cross-institutional research on neural disorders. Technically, FL requires advanced algorithms to ensure data privacy while enabling decentralized model training across institutions. The heterogeneity of data and computing environments also complicates model performance. Ethically, ensuring patient data

Table 7.2 Key FL algorithms used in healthcare, along with their outcomes and applications

FL Algorithms	*Description*	*Outcomes*	*Applications in Healthcare*
FedAvg (Federated Averaging)	Aggregates model updates by averaging them across clients to create a global model.	Reduces computational and communication overhead, ensuring model convergence.	Used in disease prediction models for conditions like diabetes or cardiovascular disease across multiple healthcare centers.
FedProx (Federated Proximal)	Generalizes FedAvg by introducing a proximal term to account for system heterogeneity.	Enhances robustness in environments where participants have non-IID (non-Independent and Identically Distributed) data.	Handling heterogeneous data in large hospital networks, e.g., patient records with diverse features and local variations.
FedSGD (Federated Stochastic Gradient Descent)	Applies Stochastic Gradient Descent to each participant's local model, and then averages the updates.	Efficient in cases where data is highly distributed, and updates must be frequent but lightweight.	Useful in training AI for real-time health monitoring through wearable devices.
FedOpt (Federated Optimization)	Optimizes the global model aggregation with various optimization techniques like momentum, Adam, or RMSProp.	Enhances model convergence speed and performance, especially in non-IID settings.	Applied in precision medicine, optimizing treatment prediction models for diseases like cancer or Alzheimer's.
FedNova (Federated Normalized Averaging)	Normalizes the contributions of each participant's model updates based on their local data sizes and gradient steps.	Achieves fairer model aggregation, ensuring better convergence in systems with unequal resources.	Applied in healthcare systems where hospitals vary in terms of patient volume and computational capacity.

(*continued*)

Table 7.2 (Cont.)

FL Algorithms	*Description*	*Outcomes*	*Applications in Healthcare*
MOON (Model Contrastive Learning)	Uses contrastive loss to improve model generalization in federated learning by learning from shared representations.	Enhances the performance of global models in cases where local data distributions differ significantly.	Used in medical imaging, particularly for improving model accuracy across different healthcare providers using MRI or CT scans.
FedAtt (Federated Attention)	Employs attention mechanisms to assess and prioritize the importance of updates from different clients based on the quality of their contributions.	Improves the accuracy of global models by prioritizing high-quality data during aggregation.	Applied in personalized medicine, where specific client updates (e.g., genetic data from specialized labs) are more critical.
FedMA (Federated Matching Algorithm)	Matches and aggregates model updates layer by layer across participants.	Solves the problem of layer misalignment in neural networks from different clients, enhancing model consistency.	Used in multi-institutional collaborations for neurodegenerative disease progression modeling with diverse neural networks.
FedCurv (Federated Curvature)	Adds curvature constraints to model updates to avoid catastrophic forgetting when clients have different tasks.	Retains model performance across tasks and data distributions, reducing model degradation over time.	Applied in multi-task learning environments, such as hospitals handling different diseases (e.g., Alzheimer's and Parkinson's).
q-FedAvg (Quantized Federated Averaging)	Reduces communication costs by quantizing model updates before sending them for aggregation.	Significantly reduces communication overhead while maintaining model performance.	Useful in resource-constrained environments such as rural clinics where internet bandwidth is limited.
FedGAN (Federated Generative Adversarial Networks)	Combines FL with GANs to generate synthetic data to improve model training on private datasets.	Generates realistic synthetic healthcare data, enhancing model training without compromising privacy.	Used in augmenting rare disease datasets for better diagnostic model training without sharing sensitive patient data.

Table 7.2 (*Cont.*)

FL Algorithms	*Description*	*Outcomes*	*Applications in Healthcare*
FedU (Federated Unlearning)	Allows the global model to "unlearn" specific client contributions if requested by participants.	Enhances privacy by ensuring that a client's data can be removed from the model if required.	Applied when patients revoke consent for their data to be used, ensuring privacy compliance in clinical research.
FedPer (Federated Personalization)	Allows participants to personalize parts of the global model based on their local data and needs.	Enables the development of personalized models that account for local variations while contributing to the global model.	Used in personalized healthcare, where treatment protocols must be tailored to individual patient profiles and needs.
HeteroFL (Heterogeneous Federated Learning)	Supports heterogeneous architectures by adjusting the model size or structure for each client.	Efficient in managing participants with varied computational resources or diverse data scales.	Applied in healthcare settings where clinics with differing resources contribute to training a global disease prediction model.

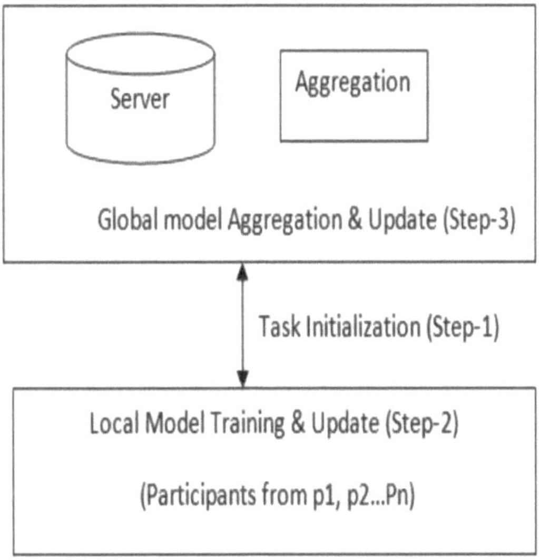

Figure 7.4 FL and its Training Process.

Table 7.3 Optimization techniques used in healthcare for neural disorders

Optimization Technique	*Applications in Neural Disorders*
FedAvg (Federated Averaging)	They are used for collaborative training of predictive models for neurodegenerative diseases like Alzheimer's and Parkinson's.
FedProx (Federated Proximal)	They are applied in multi-center studies on neural disorders where patient demographics and data types vary across hospitals.
FedAdam (Federated Adam Optimization)	Used in neural imaging research where quicker convergence is needed, such as MRI or PET scans for diagnosing dementia.
FedOpt (Federated Optimization)	Applied in brain-computer interface (BCI) systems to model neural signals and enhance neurological disorder detection.
FedNova (Normalized Averaging)	Applied in multi-institutional studies on motor neuron diseases, where patient populations vary in size across centers.
q-FedAvg (Quantized Federated Averaging)	Useful for neural disorder prediction models in rural clinics with limited bandwidth or computational capacity.
FedDyn (Federated Dynamics)	Applied in longitudinal studies of neural disorder progression, such as modeling the advancement of ALS or MS.
FedCurv (Federated Curvature)	Used in hospitals managing multiple neural disorders like ALS, Parkinson's, and dementia simultaneously.
FedAtt (Federated Attention)	Applied in personalized treatment models for neural disorders, where specific data (e.g., EEG) is given more weight.
FedSP (Federated Secure Protocol)	Critical in multi-hospital collaborations for diagnosing neural disorders like Parkinson's, ensuring compliance with GDPR and HIPAA.
MOON (Model Contrastive Federated Learning)	Used in federated neural imaging research (e.g., MRI, CT) for neurodegenerative disease diagnosis.

confidentiality and securing consent for its use across institutions are paramount concerns. Bias in AI models due to uneven data distribution can further exacerbate disparities in treatment strategies. Addressing these challenges is critical for enhancing collaboration and improving treatments for neural disorders. The following are the various technical challenges to be addressed.

7.6.1 Technical challenges

One of the most prominent technical challenges in cross-institutional research is data heterogeneity. Institutions may use varied data collection techniques, medical devices, and protocols. For instance, MRI machines across hospitals might produce images in slightly different formats or resolutions. Neural disorder datasets like those from EEG scans can vary greatly, making it difficult to standardize across institutions. Data normalization and harmonization are essential, but these processes are time-consuming and complex. In FL settings, non-independent and identically distributed data is challenging because patient populations, demographics, and disorder progression patterns can differ significantly between institutions. Models trained in one location might perform poorly when applied to another, necessitating techniques like domain adaptation or personalized model updates to ensure that the algorithms generalize well across institutions with different data profiles.

As more institutions collaborate in cross-institutional research, ensuring that machine learning models converge efficiently becomes harder. Different institutions may have varying computational resources, data sizes, or processing speeds, leading to asynchronous updates that can negatively impact the overall model convergence. Large-scale research initiatives require robust optimization techniques to handle such discrepancies without slowing down the entire process. Cross-institutional collaborations often require transferring sensitive health data, such as patient records or neuroimaging results. This presents substantial data privacy and security challenges, especially in a global context where different countries may have distinct regulations (e.g., GDPR in Europe and HIPAA in the U.S.). Federated learning addresses some of these issues by allowing institutions to train models without sharing raw data. However, secure communication channels, encryption, and robust techniques are crucial to prevent potential data breaches or misuse.

Healthcare systems across institutions often use different software platforms, electronic health record (EHR) systems, and data formats. This lack of interoperability makes implementing unified research protocols or training algorithms across institutions challenging. Cross-institutional collaborations must invest in standardizing interfaces and ensuring that different systems can communicate effectively, which requires significant technical effort and financial investment. Neural disorder research deals with complex and high-dimensional data, including brain scans, genetic information, and longitudinal data that track disease progression. Processing, storing, and analyzing such data requires advanced computing power and algorithms capable of handling these complexities, which are not always uniformly available across institutions.

7.6.2 Ethical challenges

An ethical challenge in cross-institutional research is ensuring patients provide informed consent for their data to be used across different institutions. Neural disorder patients, particularly those with cognitive impairments like Alzheimer's or dementia, may not fully comprehend the implications of their data being shared across various research entities. A critical ethical concern is ensuring informed and ongoing consent and robust systems to allow patients to withdraw consent. Another ethical challenge involves questions of data ownership and governance. As data from multiple institutions contribute to global models, it becomes unclear who "owns" the resulting intellectual property, data insights, or research findings. Ethical frameworks must define clear data governance protocols, ensuring that the contributing institutions and patients retain some form of control or rights over the outcomes.

Neural disorder datasets can often reflect biases inherent in healthcare systems, such as the underrepresentation of certain demographic groups (e.g., ethnic minorities and lower-income patients). If these biases are not adequately accounted for, AI models trained on such data could lead to unequal treatment outcomes across different population groups. Addressing fairness and bias in cross-institutional research is critical to ensuring that AI models serve all populations equitably. AI models developed in cross-institutional settings can be highly complex, and ensuring transparency in how these models make decisions is crucial. For neural disorders with high stakes in diagnosis and treatment, explainable AI (XAI) techniques must be prioritized so that healthcare professionals understand how decisions are made. Without this, there's a risk of ethical issues arising from "black box" models making potentially life-altering decisions without adequate human oversight.

While cross-institutional research aims to enhance treatment strategies, there is a risk that certain institutions or populations may not benefit equally. Wealthier or more technologically advanced institutions may contribute more data or resources, potentially leading to models that favor their patient populations. Ensuring that all participating institutions and patient populations benefit equally from the research and its outcomes is essential for maintaining equity in healthcare. In cases where AI models make incorrect predictions or recommendations, determining accountability can be challenging. Suppose a cross-institutional AI model incorrectly predicts the progression of a neural disorder, leading to inadequate treatment. In that case, deciding who is responsible for the institution where the model was trained becomes ethically complex: the researchers who designed it or the healthcare professionals who applied its results. Clear accountability structures need to be in place to handle such scenarios.

Neural disorder research often requires tracking patients over long periods. Ethical challenges arise regarding how this longitudinal data is stored, shared, and used over time, particularly if patients' health conditions change or they wish to retract their participation. Ethical frameworks must provide patients with continued control over their data while balancing the need for long-term research.

7.7 REGULATORY LANDSCAPE SURROUNDING AI AND FL IN HEALTHCARE

Implementing AI and FL in healthcare involves navigating a complex and evolving regulatory landscape to ensure data privacy, security, and adherence to ethical standards. Necessary regulations affecting AI and FL in healthcare encompass regional and global frameworks, aiming to tackle challenges related to patient data confidentiality, cross-border data sharing, and algorithmic accountability.

7.7.1 Health Insurance Portability and Accountability Act (HIPAA)

The Health Insurance Portability and Accountability Act (HIPAA) is a landmark regulation enacted in 1996 that establishes rules for protecting patient health information and ensuring its secure handling. In the context of AI and federated learning, compliance with HIPAA is crucial for safeguarding sensitive healthcare data. The HIPAA Privacy Rule sets national standards for protecting Protected Health Information (PHI) and governs the allowable use and disclosure of patient data by covered entities, including healthcare providers, insurers, and clearinghouses. The Privacy Rule permits institutions to use or share PHI for treatment, payment, and healthcare operations but requires obtaining patient consent for other purposes, such as research. In federated learning, institutions must ensure the security of PHI, which may involve de-identifying data before training models. The de-identification process eliminates all identifiers, such as names, dates of birth, and Social Security numbers, ensuring that patient data cannot be traced back to individuals

The HIPAA sets standards for securing electronic PHI (ePHI). It mandates administrative safeguards, such as workforce training on data protection, technical safeguards like encryption and access control, and physical safeguards to prevent unauthorized access to healthcare data systems. Federated learning protocols must adhere to these safeguards by ensuring that model updates are encrypted and access to these models is tightly controlled. For example, suppose hospitals collaborate on a federated model for predicting neural disorder progression. In that case, the communications and data sharing must be encrypted, and only authorized personnel should have access to model updates.

The Breach Rule requires entities to warn patients and the HHS in case of a PHI breach. This rule ensures that patients are informed of any risks to their personal information and allows regulatory authorities to take appropriate action. This is particularly important for FL because any breach in the communication channels between institutions or during model aggregation could expose sensitive healthcare data. Institutions must have a breach response plan and ensure that federated systems are designed with robust encryption and security mechanisms.

HIPAA violations result in significant punishments, ranging from fines to criminal charges. The Office for Civil Rights (OCR) within HHS is responsible for HIPAA enforcement, and it actively investigates data breaches and complaints related to patient privacy. Institutions must maintain comprehensive documentation of their data protection protocols, risk assessments, and compliance efforts for AI and FL. Failure to adhere to HIPAA standards can lead to significant financial and reputational damage, especially as AI becomes more integrated into patient care.

7.7.2 General Data Protection Regulations (GDPR) in healthcare

The GDPR is a comprehensive data protection law implemented by the European Union (EU) in May 2018 [26]. It regulates the processing of personal data across all sectors, including healthcare, and significantly impacts how health organizations, hospitals, and researchers manage patient data. With strict data privacy and security regulations, the GDPR aims to give individuals greater control over their personal information while ensuring transparency and accountability from organizations that process such data. The healthcare sector, which is data-intensive and deals with sensitive information, faces various challenges in complying with GDPR, particularly when handling patient data, utilizing AI for diagnostics, and engaging in cross-border research initiatives.

7.7.2.1 GDPR principles

Healthcare organizations must process personal data legally, fairly, and transparently. Hospitals, clinics, and research institutions must inform patients how their data will be used and obtain their consent where necessary. Under GDPR, personal database is one of the six legal grounds: Explicit and informed consent must be obtained from patients for any processing of their data that is not directly related to treatment or legal obligations. Data processing is necessary for medical services, such as consultations or treatments and it is required to comply with legal obligations, like maintaining medical records, necessary to protect someone's life, such as in medical emergencies. Data processing is carried out for public health reasons, such as preventing the spread of infectious diseases.

Hospitals and healthcare providers must be transparent about the reasons and methods behind their collection of patient data, whether for direct medical treatment or research purposes. If an institution processes data for research, patients must be fully informed about the scope, risks, and implications of that data usage. Under the GDPR, personal data can only be collected for specified, explicit, and legitimate purposes, meaning that data collected for medical treatment cannot be repurposed without the patient's explicit consent. For example, if a patient's medical records are gathered for diagnostic purposes, they cannot later be used for marketing or research purposes without obtaining the patient's permission.

This principle also impacts the use of AI in healthcare. Suppose AI systems rely on patient data for training models. In that case, healthcare providers must ensure that the data is used solely for specified medical purposes and not for commercial activities or external projects unless the patient has given explicit consent. The GDPR mandates that healthcare providers collect only the minimum personal data necessary for the intended purpose. In the healthcare context, this means avoiding collecting unnecessary patient details or excessive health information that is not directly related to treatment. For instance, if an AI-driven diagnostic tool identifies early signs of a neurological disorder, only relevant clinical data such as imaging scans or symptom history should be gathered. Reducing the amount of unnecessary data helps minimize the risks associated with data breaches and ensures that patient privacy is upheld [27].

The GDPR mandates that private data must be accurate and updated. In healthcare, this principle has critical implications for patient safety and treatment. Inaccurate or outdated medical records can lead to misdiagnosis; improper treatment, or medical errors. Therefore, healthcare providers must establish processes for regularly updating patient records and ensuring that errors are promptly corrected. This requirement is also vital in research environments where accurate data is essential for generating valid clinical insights [28].

Protecting sensitive health information in healthcare is essential, especially considering the heightened risks of cyber-attacks and data breaches. Medical records, genetic information, and even anonymized datasets can become targets for malicious activities. The GDPR underscores the necessity for encrypted storage and transmission of patient data, particularly when it is shared between hospitals, researchers, or across borders. Healthcare institutions must demonstrate compliance with GDPR, which requires providers to maintain comprehensive records of data processing activities and implement effective privacy policies. Institutions should also conduct regular audits and assessments, such as Data Protection Impact Assessments (DPIAs), especially when adopting new technologies like AI. Furthermore, hospitals and research institutions must appoint a Data Protection Officer (DPO) if they process large volumes of sensitive health data. The DPO is responsible for overseeing compliance, advising on data protection obligations, and serving as the point of contact with regulatory authorities [29].

7.7.2.2 GDPR rights

Patients have the privilege of accessing data. This includes obtaining copies of their medical records, diagnostic data, and other personal health information collected during treatment. Healthcare organizations must provide this data in a readable format upon request within 30 days. This empowers patients to manage their health data actively and ensures transparency. For hospitals and clinics, it necessitates maintaining efficient systems for securely retrieving and sharing patient records. Under GDPR, patients can correct inaccuracies in their health records. Patients who discover their medical history is incorrect can request changes to ensure the data is accurate and current. For healthcare organizations, this means implementing mechanisms for patients to update their information quickly. This can be particularly important in AI systems, where accurate input data is critical to making valid predictions or recommendations.

Patients have the Claim to Erasure, which allows them to request the deletion of their data in certain circumstances. In healthcare, this can apply when the data is no longer needed for treatment, when a patient withdraws their permission for data handling, or when the data was unlawfully processed. However, this right is not absolute in healthcare. Medical data is often subject to legal retention requirements, meaning that hospitals cannot permanently delete a patient's records immediately. For example, healthcare providers may be required to retain medical records for a specific period to comply with national health regulations or in the context of ongoing treatment. Patients can request that their data be transferred from one healthcare provider to another. This right enables patients to switch providers more efficiently and ensures their medical history follows them. It is essential in cross-border healthcare services or when a patient seeks a second opinion at a different institution.

For healthcare organizations, this implies maintaining systems that can securely and efficiently transfer data to other providers while complying with GDPR's data protection requirements. Patients can object to processing their data in certain situations, such as when their data is being used for purposes beyond direct medical treatment (e.g., marketing or research). Healthcare organizations must respect these objections unless they can demonstrate overriding legitimate grounds for processing the data. In healthcare research, particularly in AI and federated learning initiatives, patients may object to using their anonymized data, raising challenges for researchers who must ensure that models do not rely on withdrawn data.

7.7.2.3 Challenges in complying with GDPR

GDPR encourages the anonymization or pseudonymization of personal data to protect patient privacy. Anonymization ensures that the data can no longer be linked back to an individual, while pseudonymization replaces identifying details with pseudonyms that require additional information to reverse. In healthcare, achieving proper anonymization can be difficult because of the richness and complexity of medical data. For example, MRI scans, genetic sequences, and clinical notes can often still be linked to individual patients, even after attempts to anonymize them. Effective data anonymization techniques are needed to comply with GDPR without compromising the utility of the data in research or diagnostics.

Healthcare [29] often involves cross-border collaborations, especially in research. GDPR imposes strict requirements on transferring personal data outside the EU to ensure it remains protected by GDPR standards. When data is shared with institutions in non-EU countries, such as for international clinical trials or federated learning initiatives, appropriate safeguards (e.g., Standard Contractual Clauses (SCCs)) must be in place. This challenges global healthcare projects that rely on sharing large datasets, as institutions must ensure compliance with GDPR while navigating differing national regulations [30].

While AI can improve healthcare outcomes, GDPR [31] places stringent requirements on such systems, particularly regarding transparency, explainability, and consent. AI systems must be able to explain how decisions are made, mainly when used in critical areas like diagnostics. Patients have the right to understand how their data is being used, and they can object if they feel their data is being used in ways they did not consent to. Therefore, healthcare providers and AI developers must design systems that comply with GDPR's transparency and consent requirements.

Key Differences between HIPAA and GDPR

- HIPAA is specific to the U.S. healthcare sector, while GDPR applies to all personal data processing across the EU and beyond.
- GDPR emphasizes explicit consent and provides broader individual rights compared to HIPAA.
- GDPR has a more stringent timeline for breach notification than HIPAA.
- Non-compliance penalties under GDPR can be significantly higher than those under HIPAA.
- GDPR has strict rules for international data transfers, while HIPAA does not explicitly address this issue.

These differences reflect the distinct cultural, legal, and regulatory environments in which HIPAA and GDPR were developed [32], with GDPR generally offering broader protections and rights related to personal data.

Table 7.4 Case studies

Year	*Country*	*Description*
2019	United States	A study focused on improving diagnostic algorithms for Alzheimer's disease using federated learning from multiple U.S. institutions, enhancing early detection accuracy while complying with HIPAA.
2020	Canada	A research initiative analyzed neuroimaging data for multiple sclerosis (MS) using federated learning across Canadian universities and hospitals, improving the identification of MS subtypes.
2021	United Kingdom	A project in the UK improved Parkinson's disease treatment by using federated learning to analyze clinical and genetic data, leading to tailored treatment options based on shared model insights.
2022	Germany	A federated learning project predicted outcomes for traumatic brain injury (TBI) patients, allowing hospitals to analyze patient data without compromising privacy and enhancing rehabilitation strategies.
2023	Australia	An initiative utilized federated learning to study autism spectrum disorder (ASD) across research centers, developing a predictive model that identified risk factors while protecting sensitive data.
2023	France	A collaborative project aimed at improving frontotemporal dementia (FTD) diagnosis through federated learning, analyzing clinical and neuroimaging data without transferring sensitive patient information.

7.8 CASE STUDIES

Here's a structured overview of case studies involving AI and FL that enhance cross-institutional research and treatment strategies for neural disorders, presented chronologically by year and country in Table 7.4.

The transformative role of AI and federated learning enhances cross-institutional research and treatment strategies for neural disorders. By enabling collaborative analysis of diverse datasets while ensuring patient privacy, federated learning represents a powerful approach to addressing the complexities of neurological disorders across various healthcare systems worldwide. Each project highlights advancements in predictive modeling, personalized treatment strategies, and the importance of collaborative efforts in the medical research landscape.

7.9 CONCLUSIONS AND FUTURE DIRECTIONS

AI and FL in the field of neural disorders have demonstrated significant potential in enhancing research and treatment strategies across institutions. By enabling collaborative analysis of decentralized data, federated learning has addressed critical challenges related to patient privacy and data security.

This approach has allowed researchers to develop robust predictive models and diagnostic tools without sharing sensitive health information, thereby fostering a more ethical framework for data utilization. The successful application of federated learning in various case studies demonstrates its effectiveness in enhancing diagnostic accuracy, personalizing treatment plans, and improving patient outcomes in neural disorders.

AI and federated learning in this domain are promising. As the healthcare landscape evolves, advancements in computational power, machine learning algorithms, and data interoperability will further bolster the capabilities of federated learning. Future initiatives could explore integrating multimodal data combining clinical, genomic, and imaging information to develop more comprehensive models that capture the complexities of neural disorders. Expanding federated learning networks to include more diverse healthcare institutions globally could enrich the datasets available for analysis, leading to models more representative of varied populations.

Continued collaboration among stakeholders such as healthcare providers, research institutions, and regulatory bodies will be essential in addressing the ethical, technical, and regulatory challenges associated with federated learning. Developing standardized protocols for data sharing, model training, and performance evaluation will enhance the reliability and validity of research findings. Furthermore, ongoing education and training for healthcare professionals in AI and data science will be critical to facilitate the adoption of these technologies in clinical settings. The application of AI and federated learning in enhancing cross-institutional research and treatment strategies for neural disorders has opened new avenues for innovation and collaboration. By leveraging the strengths of federated learning, the healthcare community can work together to advance our understanding of neural disorders, improve diagnostic and therapeutic approaches, and ultimately enhance the quality of care for patients worldwide. The potential for these technologies to revolutionize the field is immense, and ongoing efforts to refine and expand their application will be vital in addressing the pressing challenges faced by the healthcare sector.

REFERENCES

[1] R. Liu, Z. -A. Huang, Y. Hu, Z. Zhu, K. -C. Wong and K. C. Tan, "Spatial–Temporal Co-Attention Learning for Diagnosis of Mental Disorders From Resting-State fMRI Data," in IEEE Transactions on Neural Networks and Learning Systems, vol. 35, no. 8, pp. 10591–10605, Aug. 2024, doi: 10.1109/TNNLS.2023.3243000.

[2] R. Liu, Z. -A. Huang, Y. Hu, Z. Zhu, K. -C. Wong and K. C. Tan, "Attention-Like Multimodality Fusion With Data Augmentation for Diagnosis of Mental Disorders Using MRI," in IEEE Transactions on Neural Networks and Learning Systems, vol. 35, no. 6, pp. 7627–7641, June 2024, doi: 10.1109/TNNLS.2022.3219551.

[3] Z. -A. Huang, R. Liu, Z. Zhu and K. C. Tan, "Multitask Learning for Joint Diagnosis of Multiple Mental Disorders in Resting-State fMRI," in IEEE Transactions on Neural Networks and Learning Systems, vol. 35, no. 6, pp. 8161–8175, June 2024, doi: 10.1109/TNNLS.2022.3225179.
[4] T. Zhao and G. Zhang, "Enhancing Major Depressive Disorder Diagnosis With Dynamic-Static Fusion Graph Neural Networks," in IEEE Journal of Biomedical and Health Informatics, vol. 28, no. 8, pp. 4701–4710, Aug. 2024, doi: 10.1109/JBHI.2024.3395611.
[5] F. Noman, C. -M. Ting, H. Kang, R. C. -W. Phan and H. Ombao, "Graph Autoencoders for Embedding Learning in Brain Networks and Major Depressive Disorder Identification," in IEEE Journal of Biomedical and Health Informatics, vol. 28, no. 3, pp. 1644–1655, March 2024, doi: 10.1109/JBHI.2024.3351177.
[6] Y. Yang, C. Ye, X. Guo, T. Wu, Y. Xiang, and T. Ma, "Mapping Multi-Modal Brain Connectome for Brain Disorder Diagnosis via Cross-Modal Mutual Learning," in IEEE Transactions on Medical Imaging, vol. 43, no. 1, pp. 108–121, Jan. 2024, doi: 10.1109/TMI.2023.3294967.
[7] Z. Xia, T. Zhou, Z. Jiao and J. Lu, "Learnable Brain Connectivity Structures for Identifying Neurological Disorders," in IEEE Transactions on Neural Systems and Rehabilitation Engineering, vol. 32, pp. 3084–3094, 2024, doi: 10.1109/TNSRE.2024.3446588.
[8] D. -J. Lee et al., "Spectral Graph Neural Network-Based Multi-Atlas Brain Network Fusion for Major Depressive Disorder Diagnosis," in IEEE Journal of Biomedical and Health Informatics, vol. 28, no. 5, pp. 2967–2978, May 2024, doi: 10.1109/JBHI.2024.3366662.
[9] L. Liu et al., "H-Net: Heterogeneous Neural Network for Multi-Classification of Neuropsychiatric Disorders," in IEEE Journal of Biomedical and Health Informatics, vol. 28, no. 9, pp. 5509–5518, Sept. 2024, doi: 10.1109/JBHI.2024.3405941.
[10] J. Aina, O. Akinniyi, M. M. Rahman, V. Odero-Marah and F. Khalifa, "A Hybrid Learning-Architecture for Mental Disorder Detection Using Emotion Recognition," in IEEE Access, vol. 12, pp. 91410–91425, 2024, doi: 10.1109/ACCESS.2024.3421376.
[11] K. Sravani and P. Kuppusamy, "Optimized Deep Convolutional Neural Network for Autism Spectrum Disorder Detection Using Structural MRI and DTPSO," in IEEE Access, vol. 12, pp. 110035–110051, 2024, doi: 10.1109/ACCESS.2024.3441248.
[12] X. Sun, Y. Xu, Y. Zhao, X. Zheng, Y. Zheng and L. Cui, "Multi-Granularity Graph Convolution Network for Major Depressive Disorder Recognition," in IEEE Transactions on Neural Systems and Rehabilitation Engineering, vol. 32, pp. 559–569, 2024, doi: 10.1109/TNSRE.2023.3311458.
[13] J. -H. Oh et al., "Graph-Based Conditional Generative Adversarial Networks for Major Depressive Disorder Diagnosis With Synthetic Functional Brain Network Generation," in IEEE Journal of Biomedical and Health Informatics, vol. 28, no. 3, pp. 1504–1515, March 2024, doi: 10.1109/JBHI.2023.3340325.
[14] A. Ghimire, A. N. Asiri, B. Hildebrand and F. Amsaad, "Implementation of Secure and Privacy-aware AI Hardware using Distributed

Federated Learning," in 2023 IEEE 16th Dallas Circuits and Systems Conference (DCAS), Denton, TX, USA, 2023, pp. 1–6, doi: 10.1109/DCAS57389.2023.10130231.

[15] H. Kim, Y. Choi, J. Park, L. J. Mwasinga and H. Choo, "Federated Learning-Driven Edge AI for Enhanced Mobile Traffic Prediction," in NOMS 2024-2024 IEEE Network Operations and Management Symposium, Seoul, Korea, Republic of, 2024, pp. 1–4, doi: 10.1109/NOMS59830.2024.10575892.

[16] Z. A. El Houda, H. Moudoud, B. Brik and L. Khoukhi, "Securing Federated Learning through Blockchain and Explainable AI for Robust Intrusion Detection in IoT Networks," in IEEE INFOCOM 2023 – IEEE Conference on Computer Communications Workshops (INFOCOM WKSHPS), Hoboken, NJ, USA, 2023, pp. 1–6, doi: 10.1109/INFOCOMWKSHPS57453.2023.10225769.

[17] J. Moon, S. Kum, Y. Kim, V. Stankovski, U. Paščinski and P. Kochovski, "A Decentralized AI Data Management System In Federated Learning," in 2020 International Conference on Intelligent Systems and Computer Vision (ISCV), Fez, Morocco, 2020, pp. 1–4, doi: 10.1109/ISCV49265.2020.9204271.

[18] T. A. Khoa, D. -V. Nguyen, M. -S. Dao and K. Zettsu, "AOP: Towards Adaptive Offloading Point Approach in a Federated Learning Framework for Edge AI Applications," in 2023 IEEE 29th International Conference on Parallel and Distributed Systems (ICPADS), Ocean Flower Island, China, 2023, pp. 2846–2847, doi: 10.1109/ICPADS60453.2023.00403.

[19] Y. Rumesh, T. T. Senevirathna, P. Porambage, M. Liyanage and M. Ylianttila, Comprehensive Analysis Over Centralized and Federated Learning-Based Anomaly Detection in Networks with Explainable AI (XAI), ICC 2023 – IEEE International Conference on Communications, Rome, Italy, 2023, pp. 4853–4859, doi: 10.1109/ICC45041.2023.10278845.

[20] T. Patel, R. Murugan, G. Yenduri, R. H. Jhaveri, H. Snoussi and T. Gaber, "Demystifying Defects: Federated Learning and Explainable AI for Semiconductor Fault Detection," in IEEE Access, vol. 12, pp. 116987–117007, 2024, doi: 10.1109/ACCESS.2024.3425226.

[21] M. S. Nasir, M. S. Alam, F. I. Shahi, M. S. Kamal, K. Upreti and P. Vats, "Transformative Insights: Unveiling the Potential of Artificial Intelligence in the Treatment of Sleep Disorders – A Comprehensive Review," in 2023 International Conference on Emerging Trends in Networks and Computer Communications (ETNCC), Windhoek, Namibia, 2023, pp. 1–6, doi: 10.1109/ETNCC59188.2023.10284945.

[22] H. Cagnan, P. Brown, D. Bourget and T. Denison, "Inertial-based Control System Concepts for the Treatment of Movement Disorders," in 2015 Transducers – 2015 18th International Conference on Solid-State Sensors, Actuators and Microsystems (TRANSDUCERS), Anchorage, AK, USA, 2015, pp. 70–73, doi: 10.1109/TRANSDUCERS.2015.7180863.

[23] M. K. Sharma, M. N. Nachappa and R. Kumar, "Personalized Treatment Recommendations for Mental Health Disorders Using AI and Big Healthcare Data," in 2023 IEEE International Conference on ICT in

Business Industry & Government (ICTBIG), Indore, India, 2023, pp. 1–6, doi: 10.1109/ICTBIG59752.2023.10455991.

[24] Yi Lei, Han Qin, Xiaodan Li, Qing Wang, Lin Zang, Jun Tai, Jijiang Yang, "A Strategy for Aided Diagnosis of Obstructive Sleep Apnea in Children Based on Graph Neural Network," in 2023 IEEE 47th Annual Computers, Software, and Applications Conference (COMPSAC), Torino, Italy, 2023, pp. 1513–1518, doi: 10.1109/COMPSAC57700.2023.00233.

[25] C. M. Jayachandran and K. Shyamala, "Kohonen SOM Deployment in Android App-Based Cognitive Behavioral Therapy for Personality Disorders," in 2017 World Congress on Computing and Communication Technologies (WCCCT), Tiruchirappalli, India, 2017, pp. 255–257, doi: 10.1109/WCCCT.2016.69.

[26] A. Rahman, A., M.S. Hossain, G. Muhammad et al."Federated Learning-Based AI Approaches in Smart Healthcare: Concepts, Taxonomies, Challenges and Open Issues," in Cluster Computing, vol. 26, 2271–2311, 2023. https://doi.org/10.1007/s10586-022-03658-4.

[27] A. Nag, A. Das, R. Sil, A. Kar, D. Mandal and B. Das."Application of Artificial Intelligence in Mental Health," in Abraham, A., Pllana, S., Casalino, G., Ma, K., Bajaj, A. (eds) Intelligent Systems Design and Applications. ISDA 2022. Lecture Notes in Networks and Systems, vol. 646, 2023, Springer, Cham. https://doi.org/10.1007/978-3-031-27440-4_13

[28] A. Rahman, A. Nag and A. K. Bairagi, "A Hybrid Model for Recognizing Human Activity Using Extreme Learning," 2023 in 26th International Conference on Computer and Information Technology (ICCIT), Cox's Bazar, Bangladesh, 2023, pp. 1–6, doi: 10.1109/ICCIT60459.2023.10441574.

[29] Nag, A., Das, B., Sil, R., Hameed, A. A., Bhushan, B., & A. Jamil, "A Survey on Image-Based Cardiac Diagnosis Prediction Using Machine Learning and Deep Learning Techniques," in International Conference on Computing, Intelligence and Data Analytics (pp. 478-491), 2023, July. Cham: Springer Nature Switzerland.

[30] C. Kishor Kumar Reddy, C.H. Rupa and B. Vijaya Babu, "SPM: A Fast and Scalable Model for Predicting Snow/No-Snow", in World Applied Sciences Journal, vol. 32, no. 8, 1561–1570, 2014. ISSN 1818-4952, DOI: 10.5829/idosi.wasj.2014.32.08.1256

[31] A. Nag et al., "TumorGANet: A Transfer Learning and Generative Adversarial Network- Based Data Augmentation Model for Brain Tumor Classification," in IEEE Access, vol. 12, pp. 103060–103081, 2024, doi: 10.1109/ACCESS.2024.3429633

[32] A. Nag, B. Das, R. Sil, A.A. Hameed, B. Bhushan, and A. Jamil, "A Survey on Image-based Cardiac Diagnosis Prediction Using Machine Learning and Deep Learning Techniques," in García Márquez, F.P., Jamil, A., Ramirez, I.S., Eken, S., Hameed, A.A. (eds) Computing, Internet of Things and Data Analytics. ICCIDA 2023. Studies in Computational Intelligence, vol. 1145, 2024, Springer, Cham. https://doi.org/10.1007/978-3-031-53717-2_44

Chapter 8

Ensuring data privacy and security in federated learning for healthcare data

Chinna Ovu Reddi Umarani, Jahangeer Naskath, Nagarajan Karthikeyan, and Selvakumar Manickam

8.1 INTRODUCTION TO FEDERATED LEARNING IN NEURAL DISORDERS

Federated learning is a decentralized machine learning approach that permits multiple entities to collectively train models with no sharing of unprocessed data. In this technique, data remains stored locally, and only revised data is shared to maintain data integrity and privacy. The primary focus of federated learning is to safeguard sensitive patient health records. This method is particularly beneficial for predicting serious diseases such as Alzheimer's and Parkinson's at an early stage, enabling researchers to conduct studies without compromising data confidentiality. By enhancing overall accuracy and early-stage predictions, federated learning addresses significant concerns regarding data security, especially when dealing with real-world healthcare information. Various data-preserving methods and techniques are implemented in federated learning to ensure secure access. This approach paves the way for early diagnosis of patient conditions while upholding stringent security measures.

The main objective of this chapter is to develop a secure federated learning framework integrated with blockchain technology for the healthcare domain, focusing on protecting patient healthcare records. This objective is accomplished through the following tasks:

- Design a federated learning system that leverages blockchain to enhance data privacy, integrity, and decentralized management of patient data.
- Implement dual encryption techniques, combining both asymmetric and symmetric methods to ensure robust data protection during transmission.
- Analyze potential adversarial attacks on the federated learning model and propose preventive measures using blockchain and advanced encryption strategies.

DOI: 10.1201/9781003591085-8

- Evaluate the efficiency of the framework through edge computing integration, effective key management, and blockchain-based data transmission.
- Assess the real-world applicability and impact of the proposed system for predicting neural disorders and addressing challenges in secure data transfer.

The chapter is structured as follows: After this introduction and a brief state-of-the-art review, the integration of blockchain technology for reliable data transmission is discussed. Next, the two-factor encryption strategies are presented to ensure robust data security. The subsequent section addresses methods for mitigating adversarial attacks and associated risks in federated learning. The deployment framework for the proposed system is then described in detail. The final phase of the article provides real-world case studies, implementation insights, and a comparative analysis of encryption and decryption methods across various algorithms, highlighting the contributions and future directions of this research.

8.2 BLOCKCHAIN TECHNOLOGY FOR RELIABLE DATA TRANSMISSION

Blockchain is a rapidly emerging technology that facilitates data transmission across decentralized networks on a large scale. It is primarily utilized for secure and reliable data transfer through various advanced technological approaches.

8.2.1 Fundamentals of blockchain in healthcare

Blockchain is mainly used to secure and transfer the health record of patient data from diagnostic centers, hospitals, healthcare providers, and pharmacies. It's mainly used to predict the mistakes and in case of critical cases also can be accurately processed. In recent years, blockchain has become pivotal in ensuring secure data transmission globally. Its growing popularity and adaptation in congested network systems address significant challenges in data transfer techniques. Various parameters related to blockchain are represented in Table 8.1. Primarily focused on providing secure and reliable data transfer, overcoming issues faced in earlier methods where data was prone to modification and theft, and there was insufficient assurance of receiving original data. Utilize a three-dimensional approach with swarm intelligence in IoT-based methods to ensure secure data transmission [1]. Their method focuses on integrating physical hardware, software platforms, and communication links to achieve reliable data management. Focus on enhancing distributed data transfer by integrating blockchain with edge

Table 8.1 Parameters of Blockchain Techniques

Ref.	*Objective*	*Challenges*	*Results*	*Future Research*
[4]	Analyze risks of adversarial attacks on biometrics.	Focus on isolated modules.	Comprehensive risk assessment.	Incorporate attack execution time.
[5]	Unified malware classification framework.	Classifier aging.	Surveys classification methods.	Enhance classifier robustness.
[6]	Analyze double-spending attacks on blockchain.	Risks to blockchain reliability.	Develop a TR-DSA model.	Explore TR-DSA aspects.
[7]	Examine vulnerabilities in neural networks.	Poor transferability.	Increases transferability rates.	Enhance attack transferability.
[8,9]	Medical image classification with federated learning.	Centralized learning vulnerabilities.	Simulated collaborative training.	Explore advanced privacy techniques.

computing, with a primary emphasis on data security [2]. To verify reliable and secure information transfer in blockchain and IoT contexts, combine IPFS and PBF [3] to predict and trace data misuse. These combined methods are primarily used to provide comprehensive security throughout the data transmission process.

Integrate blockchain with machine learning to enhance secure data transmission and address data delivery issues using artificial neural networks (ANNs) [10]. This approach provides robust data privacy for secure transfer over extended periods and facilitates rapid data exchange. Figure 8.1 below illustrates the key components of blockchain technology fundamentals including data integrity and security, decentralization, interoperability, Cryptography, transparency, trust, and smart contracts. It highlights the essential elements involved in the technology's core principles.

8.2.1.1 Data integrity and security

Blockchain (BC) performs an essential role in securing records by enforcing data security and integrity. Once data is updated and recorded on the blockchain, it is not allowed to be modified or altered. Every block encompasses a cryptographic hash of the prior block, which maintains data consistency and accuracy, and prevents unauthorized modifications over time. Encryption techniques restrict unauthorized access, allowing only authorized users to view or modify the data.

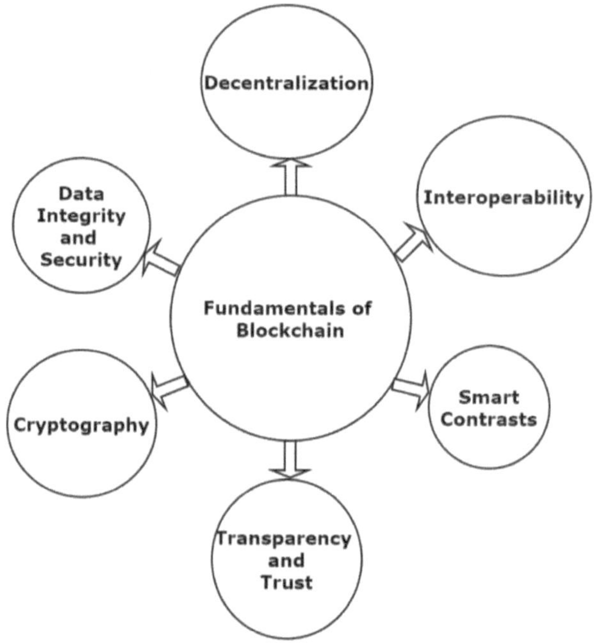

Figure 8.1 Fundamentals of Blockchain.

8.2.1.2 Decentralization

Blockchain does not rely on a centralized authority or network; instead, it operates across nodes in a decentralized network. Every blockchain ledger and transaction is replicated on each node, and transactions are authenticated by means of consensus protocol. This eliminates the chance of a single-spot failure, mitigates the threat of manipulation or centralized control, and enhances the system's resilience

8.2.1.3 Interoperability

It relates to the expertise of diverse BC frameworks and networks to perform simultaneously without any disturbance. It permits collaboration and transfer of information with various application frameworks, promoting effortless interactions and exchange between diverse systems and various innovation tools. It is very critical for working in this multi-chain location in order to get seamless solutions and facilitate different applications to work together.

8.2.1.4 Cryptography

It is a key principle of blockchain to uphold data protection and confidentiality. Various algorithms are employed to encrypt and decrypt data, ensuring proper storage and secure communication. A hash function is used by the blockchain to create a distinctive identifier for each block, along with digital signatures to authenticate the credentials of the contributors.

8.2.1.5 Transparency and trust

The details stored in the blockchain provide transparency for all transactions in an authenticated and immutable manner. Every transaction is observable by each participant in the network, facilitating trust among users. It supports real-time surveillance and assessment of transactions, ensuring the validity and authenticity of each transaction.

8.2.1.6 Smart contracts

Conventions are written directly into the code in the case of smart contracts, which are self-executing. They automatically enforce and impose the contract conditions once standardized specifications are met, eliminating the need for intermediaries. Smart contracts are primarily used for systematization, mitigating the risk of errors, enhancing efficiency by refining processes, and ensuring contract adherence without human intervention.

8.2.2 Application of blockchain in federated learning

Blockchain holds a vital role in addressing security and privacy challenges in decentralized ML. By enabling collaborative development, blockchain allows models to be trained across numerous decentralized devices or nodes without the need to share raw data, thereby preserving user confidentiality. Blockchain overcomes various issues and challenges, such as ensuring data safety and security and modifying conventional models. Its decentralized nature provides assurance and trust in the system. Integrating federated learning with BC enhances data confidentiality and integrity. The blockchain is of a decentralized nature to address single points of failure. It boosts trust in the system by eliminating the need for a core authority. Additionally, blockchain uses cryptographic methods to assure data updates, mitigate risks, prevent tampering, and verify each update. This approach is utilized across various sectors, including autonomous systems, healthcare, and finance.

In FL, before integrating BC, a central server serves as the trusted source of access for all users. However, blockchain eliminates the need for this

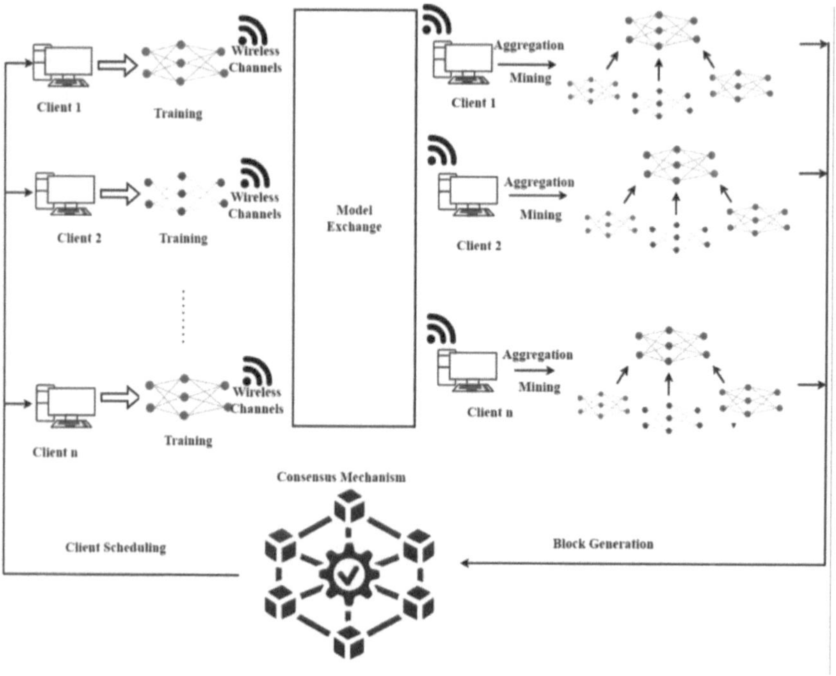

Figure 8.2 Working of Blockchain in Federated Learning Mechanism.

central authority by providing decentralized access to every user. This approach enables multiple participants to interact directly, removes entries from untrusted parties, and ensures the privacy of data. By combining these techniques, not only is privacy and security improved but the collaborative environment of machine learning is also enhanced, leading to increased trustworthiness. Figure 8.2 shows how a client or user shares their data in a federated learning environment using a blockchain consensus mechanism.

8.2.3 Advantages of decentralized, tamper-proof ledgers

Decentralized, tamper-proof ledgers offer significant advantages in blockchain technology. They enhance efficiency; and improve security, transparency, and data privacy, making them a powerful asset in various applications. By distributing data across a decentralized network and employing cryptographic techniques, these ledgers ensure the credibility and integrity of information, reducing the risk of manipulation or unauthorized access. The distributed characteristic of these ledgers confirms that no individual unit controls the entire system, which is a key benefit for enhanced security. This setup makes it challenging for any party to alter or modify data without the network's consensus. Additionally, cryptographic methods are employed to safeguard data entries, protecting them from unauthorized access and tampering, and thus maintaining the integrity of the information.

Decentralized ledgers significantly enhance trackability and transparency. Each transaction recorded in the ledger is permanent and immutable, creating a transparent and verifiable record of all activities. This improves reviewability, offering a clear and authentic record of changes and exchanges over time. As a result, it increases certainty and accountability among users. Additionally, these decentralized ledgers offer enhanced performance and superior information privacy. They systematize processes through the use of smart contracts, which streamline agreements and transactions when predefined criteria are met, eliminating the need for intermediaries. This accelerates transactions and reduces costs. Confidentiality is maintained through controlled access and selective disclosure. While ensuring transparency, sensitive data is protected. Moreover, seamless cooperation across geographical boundaries enhances collaboration by providing global accessibility, trustless interactions, and robust security.

8.3 TWO-FACTOR ENCRYPTION STRATEGIES

8.3.1 Overview of encryption methods

Encryption is a vital method for protecting data against unauthorized access. It transforms plaintext into ciphertext through the use of a cryptographic algorithm and a key. Figure 8.3 shows the basic encryption process. Below is a concise overview of common encryption techniques:

Symmetric Encryption: A unique key is used to perform the encryption and decryption processes together. This key must be kept confidential and shared only as required by the application. Algorithms such as DES and AES are commonly employed for this purpose. Figure 8.3 shows the basic symmetric encryption process.

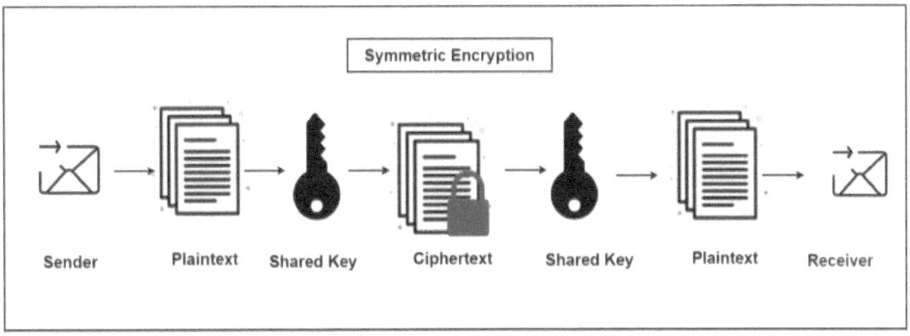

Figure 8.3 Symmetric Encryption.

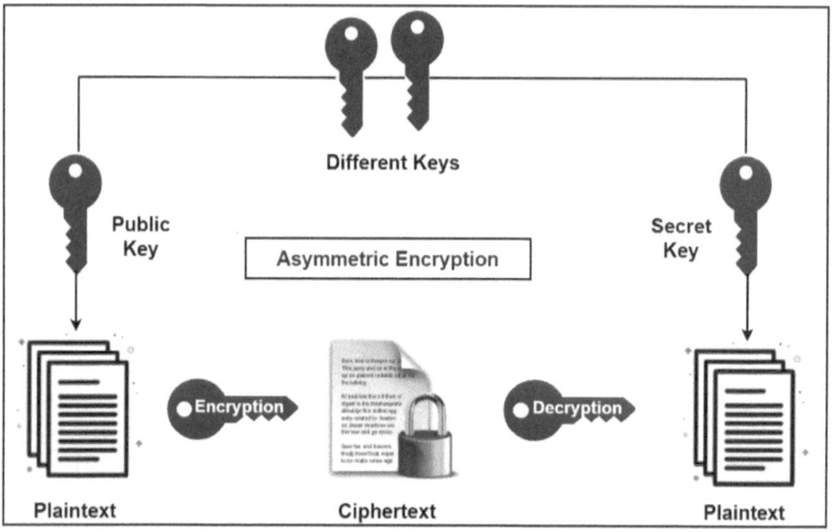

Figure 8.4 Asymmetric Encryption.

Asymmetric Encryption: Non-identical keys are used for the encryption and decryption processes, private key is used for decryption, while a public key is used for encryption. This method is generally considered more secure compared to symmetric encryption. Commonly used algorithms for this approach include ECC and RSA. Figure 8.4 shows the basic asymmetric encryption process.

For encryption, various techniques are aimed at enhancing data security across multiple applications. A 12-bit chaotic process using a 12x12 S-box is used for image encryption to improve speed and protection, especially in medical contexts [11]. Logistic maps, combined with reversible neural networks, provide secure key encryption and reconstruction [12], while homomorphic encryption enables secure data transfer by performing operations on encrypted data without decryption [13]. Studies highlight the need to address various attacks, such as brute force, during the encryption process [14, 15]. Fully homomorphic encryption with identity-based techniques allows for secure, multi-user encryption [16]. Additionally, encryption methods like combining multiple plaintexts [17], flexible encryption processes [18], and integrating linear and Latin square systems [19] contribute to more secure frameworks. Elliptic Curve Cryptography (ECC) further enhances encryption efficiency and security in high-performance systems [20].

Recent studies have focused on various techniques to enhance data security and decryption efficiency. Decryption methods leveraging block permutation have demonstrated lossless performance, ensuring that data integrity is maintained during the process [21]. The deployment of cloud setups has been shown to ensure the safe transmission of data [22], while strategies to combat eavesdropping attacks are crucial for protecting sensitive information [23]. The application of Paillier-type encryption provides robust security measures [24], complemented by quantized algorithms that ensure data integrity [25]. Efficient decryption is further achieved using the B-Plus Tree index method, which optimizes retrieval times, especially for resource-constrained devices [26]. Additionally, deep learning approaches, including backdoor attack algorithms, facilitate efficient and secure data access [27]. The outsourcing of decryption tasks has emerged as a viable method for effective data handling [28], and sliding methods have been employed to ensure safe access to sensitive information [29].

Hash Functions: Data integrity is maintained by using a fixed-size hash value derived from the given data. This hash value is non-reversible and ensures that operations are unique. Common hash functions include MD5 and SHA-256.

Hybrid Encryption: Combining both asymmetric and symmetric encryption is shown in Figure 8.5, it allows for leveraging the benefits of each technique. Asymmetric encryption plays a key role in securely exchanging data, while symmetric encryption is used to enhance efficiency.

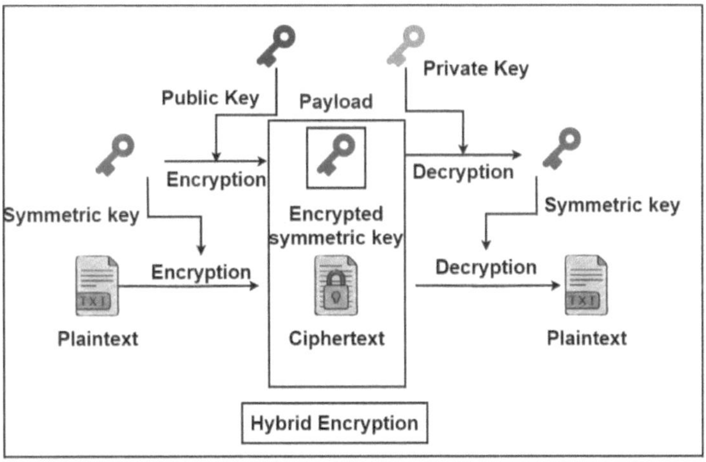

Figure 8.5 Hybrid Encryption.

8.3.2 Implementation of double encryption in federated learning

Double encryption, also known as layered encryption, involves applying encryption processes twice to enhance security. Several techniques are used in federated learning to implement this approach, as outlined in Figure 8.6:

Preliminary Encryption: Prior to data transmission, the data must be encrypted using symmetric key encryption. This technique ensures that the data transfer is conducted securely.

Subsequent Encryption: Encryption is performed twice; after the data is received at the server, it is encrypted again using an asymmetric key technique. This additional layer of encryption provides enhanced security, ensuring that data remains protected from unauthorized access even if the first layer fails.

Key Distribution: Managing the handling of keys is a complex process. An authorized key is required for each encryption layer, and it must be securely stored to prevent unauthorized access and ensure confidentiality.

Integration with FL: By integrating these elements, secure data transfer is ensured in FL. Training occurs on decentralized servers, while only the modified data is sent to a central server. Reliability and security are enhanced through the use of double encryption during data aggregation and transmission.

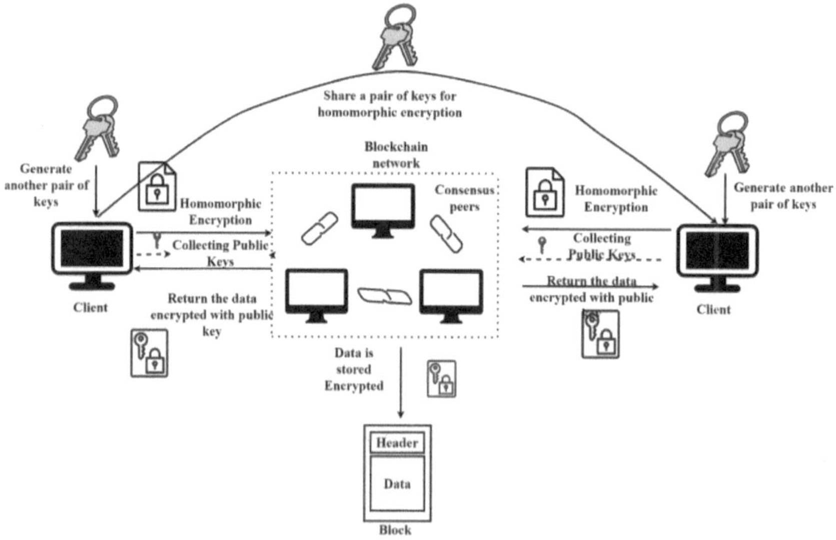

Figure 8.6 Dual Encryption Using Homomorphic Encryption Method.

Table 8.2 Encryption and Decryption Comparative Analysis, where ++ very high,+ high, – low, ⇧ – high, ⇔ – moderate, ⇩ – low, △ – fast, ⧗ – moderate, ▽ – slow

Algorithm	*Encryption Time*	*Decryption Time*	*Efficiency*	*Key Length (Bits)*	*Security Level*	*Rounds*	*Block Size (Bits)*
ECC	△	△	⇧	160, 256+	++	1	Variable
AES	△	△	⇔	128, 192, 256	+	10,12,14	18
AES with RSA	⧗	⧗	⇧	128 (AES) + 1024-4096 (RSA)	++	varies	varies
RSA	▽	▽	⇩	1024, 2048, 4096	+	1	Variable block size
DES	▽	▽	⇩	56	-	16	64

8.3.3 Enhancing data protection with dual-layer security

The dual encryption technique encompasses several processes, which are outlined in Table 8.2:

Stage 1 – Data Protection: This is the initial layer of data encryption, ensuring protection against unauthorized access. Its primary focus is to secure data during transmission.

Stage 2 – Authorization and Verification: Access to the encrypted data is granted only to authorized users to prevent unauthorized use. This stage involves the use of MFA, RBAC, and secure key transfer mechanisms.

Data Integrity: A key aspect of dual-layer security is verifying data integrity. This confirms that data remains unadjusted during transmission or repository. Verification is achieved through the use of digital signatures or hash functions.

8.4 MITIGATING ADVERSARIAL ATTACKS AND RISKS

8.4.1 Types of adversarial attacks in federated learning

Data privacy and security in FL are enhanced through decentralized machine learning algorithms. According to [30] FL is susceptible to various adversarial attacks depending on the specific type of federated learning being used. In HFL, attacks often exploit common samples and distinct features, while in VFL; adversaries may focus on distinct samples and common features.

For FLT, attacks are typically associated with distinct samples and features. Overall, the nature of the attacks varies with the approach to federated learning and the characteristics of the data involved.

Byzantine attacks: The performance of the unified model is compromised by corrupted data or inaccurate updates contributed by malicious users.

Data Poisoning: Incorrect predictions caused by the deliberate injection of false data during the training process.

Model Inversion: A malicious agent attempts to reconstruct confidential data by exploiting updates or model parameters.

Gradient Leakage: Sensitive data is extracted from the gradients during the training process.

8.4.2 Role of blockchain and encryption in mitigating risks

Blockchain plays a prominent part in secure and private data sharing [31]. This study emphasizes its importance across three aspects: transmission links, hardware, and platforms, leading to reduced risks in data transfer compared to traditional methods. There is a focus on transitioning from centralized to decentralized data transfer in smart cities, utilizing POS, ANN, and combined key encryption with blockchain for secure access in [32]. Highlighted in [33] is the reliable data transfer achieved through a three-tier architecture combining elliptic curve cryptography (EC) and blockchain. Study [34] explores various consensus algorithms for secure storage and access. Federated Learning (FL) with blockchain ensures immutable access, preventing record modifications and enhancing data traceability and transparency. Additionally, smart contracts automate model updates and data-sharing rules, further reducing risks.

8.4.3 Proactive defense mechanisms

To reduce the attacks and risks, it includes the following algorithms.

8.4.3.1 Robust aggregation algorithms

Algorithms are implemented to protect against unauthorized data access, using median or trimmed mean to safeguard the global model.

8.4.3.2 Median aggregation

To calculate the median for data aggregation in federated learning, follow these steps:

Sort the Values:
Sort the set of values Y in ascending order.

Calculate Median:
If m is (the number of values) odd, it is calculated as:

$$\text{Median}(Y) = \frac{y_{m+1}}{2}$$

For even, it is the average of two middle values,

$$\text{Median}(Y) = \frac{y_{\frac{m}{2}} + y_{\frac{m}{2}+1}}{2}$$

Trimmed mean aggregation
Before starting the trimmed mean aggregation, discard the least and largest values in the calculation. Let Y indicate the sorted data points, and t be the proportion of data to be trimmed from each end (e.g., 20% trimming indicates that 20% of the least and 20% of the largest values are discarded). The trimmed mean is calculated as follows:

```
Function Trimmed_Mean(Y,t)
a=length(Y)                              // Get the number of values
sort Y in ascending order                // Sort the values
trim_size=floor(t*a)                     // Calculate the number of
                                            values to trim
S_Start=trim_size+1                      // Start index for trimmed data
S_end=n-trim_size                        // End index for trimmed data
Trimmed_mean=sum(Y[S_Start:S_end])/      // Calculate trimmed mean
  (n-2*trim_size)
Return trimmed_mean
```

Abnormality Prediction: Using abnormality prediction methods to identify and eliminate improper patterns or variations in gradients and model updates.

Joint mitigation
Stimulating cooperation among users to share data regarding various vulnerabilities and associated risks enhances the overall security configuration.

Knowledge acquisition and development
Providing participants with training on security and risks related to federated learning helps mitigate the likelihood of successful attacks.

8.5 DEPLOYMENT FRAMEWORK

Various frameworks are involved in the process of federated learning model:

Versatile Framework: It ensures an interoperable architecture capable of handling all the loads from various healthcare IoT platforms.
Distributed Framework: It enhances the computation and storage of a system model without requiring a central server for data transfer.
Remote Computing: It implements cloud services for heavy computations, utilizing real-world data for processing and training local data on edge devices.
Packaging and Services: Utilize packaging services for easy and quick deployment, enabling scaling and maintenance for each individual system component.

8.5.1 Designing a secure federated learning system

To design a secure data transfer system for federated learning, several components must be considered. Figure 8.7 shows the process included in secure data transfer from various sources.

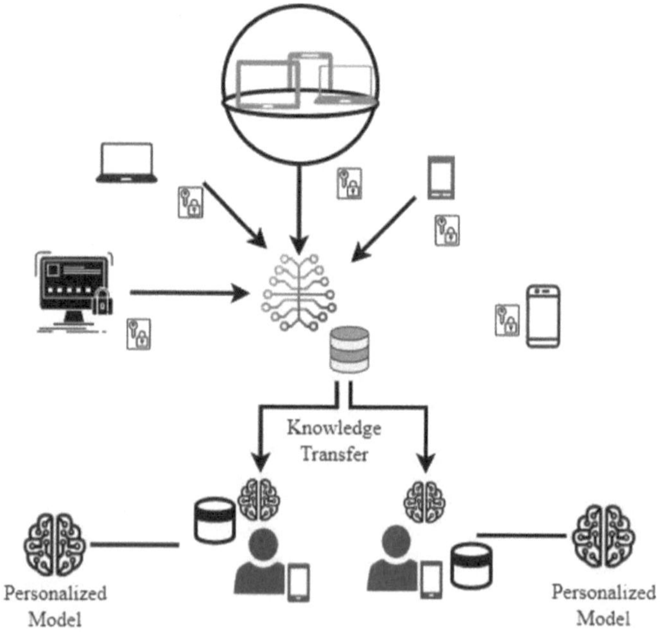

Figure 8.7 Secure Federated Learning.

Data Confidentiality: Edge nodes and local devices are crucial components for ensuring the secure storage of user data. Updates are performed for centralized access, with a focus on securing the private data of each user.

Model Consolidation: Global models are obtained by combining local models to achieve a secure, consolidated model, without disclosing individual updates separately.

Verification and Access Control: Implement a stringent authentication system for users and devices, ensuring that only authorized entities participate in this process.

Information Security: Encoded channels are utilized to update the model and ensure secure data transfer between the central server and devices.

8.5.2 Steps for integrating blockchain and encryption

To ensure data privacy, security, and integrity, integrating encryption techniques with blockchain is essential. This integration allows for the secure storage and access of confidential data, enabling decentralized access methods. Here are the steps for effective integration:

Phase 1: Determine BF Framework
Establish a framework to ensure privacy-preserving transactions by utilizing blockchain platforms such as Quorum and Hyperledger Fabric.

Phase 2: Deploy Exclusive Blockchain
Only trusted nodes can participate in the private, permissioned blockchain, ensuring a secure and exclusive environment.

Phase 3: Execute Digital Signatures
To verify transactions and ensure data integrity, utilize ECDSA (Elliptic Curve Digital Signature Algorithm) based on ECC (Elliptic Curve Cryptography).

Phase 4: Two-Layer Encryption
Before transmission, encrypt the data using the AES symmetric encryption technique, complemented by public key encryption methods such as ECC or RSA.

Phase 5: Execute Smart Contracts
Implement smart contracts to enforce rules, automate processes, and facilitate reward mechanisms for data sharing.

```
BEGIN
   // Step 1: Choose a Blockchain Configuration
   FUNCTION choose Blockchain_Configuration(platforms):
      SELECT framework FROM frameworks WHERE promotes Privacy enhancing
Transactions
      RETURN framework

// Step 2: Deploy a Private Blockchain
   FUNCTION deploy PrivateBlockchain(assured Nodes):
      CONFIGURE private Permissioned Network WITH assured Nodes
      RETURN private Network

// Step 3: Execute Digital Signatures
   FUNCTION execute DigitalSignatures(data, transaction):
      signature = ECC_ECDSA_SIGN(data)
      VERIFY integrity OF transaction USING signature
      RETURN signature

// Step 4: Deploy Dual Encryption
   FUNCTION deploy DualEncryption(data):
      encryptedData = AES_ENCRYPT(data)
      encryptionKey = FORMULATE_PUBLIC_KEY()
      secureKey = RSA_ECC_ENCRYPT(encryptionKey)
      RETURN encryptedData, secureKey

// Step 5: Smart Contract Establishment
   FUNCTION Establish SmartContracts(rules, rewards):
      CONTRACT smartContract FOR data SharingRules
      AUTOMATE rewards MECHANISM FOR federated Learning Participation
      RETURN smartContract

// Main Execution
   FUNCTION main():
      platforms = ["Hyperledger Fabric", "Quorum"]
      selected Platform = select BlockchainConfiguration(platforms)
         trusted Nodes = ["Node1", "Node2", "Node3"]
      private Network = deploy PrivateBlockchain(assuredNodes)
         data = "Sample data"
      transaction = "Sample transaction"
      signature = execute DigitalSignatures(data, transaction)
      encryptedData, secureKey = deploy DualEncryption(data)
      rules = "Data sharing rules"
      rewards = "Participation rewards"
      smartContract = establish SmartContracts(rules, rewards)
END
```

8.5.3 Technical considerations and best practices

The efficiency of a system is enhanced by minimizing latency through edge computing in real-time operations, ensuring minimal delay between model updates. Initially, data processed closer to the edge reduces the travel time between central servers and devices. This approach leads to improved efficiency and faster response times for real-time analysis applications. By leveraging edge computing, organizations can achieve quicker data processing and enhance overall system performance. Transactions can be verified more quickly, ensuring smooth operation and reduced computational load through the use of PoA (Proof of Authority) or PBFT (Practical Byzantine Fault Tolerance) algorithms. These consensus mechanisms are primarily focused on enhancing performance in financial and healthcare services, where efficiency and reliability are critical. By implementing these algorithms, organizations can streamline processes while maintaining robust security and transaction integrity. To maintain security and integrity, robust key management plays a crucial role. The regular rotation of key usage reduces the risk of unauthorized access, complicating access for hackers to compromise sensitive data. Cryptographic keys are securely stored in Hardware Security Modules (HSMs), which provide a safe environment for key management. Additionally, various design methodologies are incorporated to ensure secure system design, further enhancing the overall security framework and protecting against potential vulnerabilities.

8.6 REAL-WORLD CASES AND IMPLEMENTATION

8.6.1 Examples from neural disorder research

Numerous studies have explored neural disorders, and various real-world cases have contributed to advancements in technology. Machine learning has emerged as a promising approach for the early prediction and monitoring of diseases such as Parkinson's and Alzheimer's. Wearable devices have been introduced for continuous monitoring of patients' routines and behaviors, facilitating earlier diagnosis of diseases and enhancing patients' lifestyles. Table 8.3 compares prediction methodologies related to various diseases.

8.6.2 Future potential and ongoing challenges

Upcoming research in neural disorders encompasses neuroimaging technologies, machine learning (ML), and artificial intelligence (AI), paving the way for advancements in the medical system. The developed models can predict disorders such as Parkinson's and Alzheimer's before the onset of clinical symptoms. From the article GBD 2016, Table 8.4 shows various regional comparisons of these diseases. This creates new biomarkers [40]

Table 8.3 Techniques and Challenges in Neurodegenerative Disease Detection, AD – Alzheimer's Disease, PD – Parkinson's Disease

Author(s) & Year	*Prediction Technique*	*Challenges*	*Results*	*Disease Detection*
[35]	Enhances PD detection using speech signals.	Data collection is difficult; and requires large training data.	Best results from articulation features; modest improvements.	PD
[36]	Improves PD diagnosis via imaging genetics.	Data co-registration issues; overfitting due to small samples.	Detects biomarkers effectively; outperforms in feature selection.	AD
[37]	Video-based gait analysis for PD monitoring.	Non-portable equipment; low compliance with wearables.	Strong correlations in gait assessments; video outperforms others.	PD
[38]	Early AD diagnosis using machine learning.	No challenges mentioned.	Monitors AD progression; accuracy varies with noise.	AD
[39]	Machine learning for early AD diagnosis via radar.	Costly, time-consuming methods; low imaging resolution.	Improved accuracy with data augmentation.	AD

in the field of neurological disorders and enhances our understanding of disease mechanisms and therapies. To unlock these improvements, several changes must be addressed, primarily focusing on the confidentiality of data. The General Data Protection Regulation (GDPR) in Europe and the Health Insurance Portability and Accountability Act (HIPAA) in the U.S. enforce strict adherence [41] to the collection and analysis of sensitive patient data. Failure to adopt these regulations can lead to unauthorized access or illegal use of personal patient information, resulting in ethical and legal issues. Various methods used in blockchain and healthcare are shown in Figure 8.8. Advancing [42] encryption methods and developing secure data transfer models are crucial to ensuring patient trust in the widespread use of AI tools. Figure 8.8 shows the applications of blockchain in healthcare.

Collaboration between data scientists, bioengineers, neurologists, and machine learning experts is essential for advancing research in neurological disorders. However, each field has its terminologies, research focus, and methodologies, making integration challenging. Building strong interdisciplinary partnerships is crucial to the success of new technologies in this

Table 8.4 Compare Alzheimer's and Parkinson's Disease with Various Regions

Low	Low-mid	Mid	High
1	5	10	15

	Global	East Asia	Southern East Asia	Oceania	Central Asia	Central Europe	Eastern Europe	High-income Asia Pacific	Australia	Western Europe	SouthernLatin America	High income North America	Caribbean	Andean Latin America	Central Latin America	Tropical Latin America	North Africa and Middle East	South Asia	Central Sub-Saharan Africa	Eastern Sub-Saharan Africa	Southern Sub-Saharan Africa	Western Sub-Saharan Africa
Stroke	1	1	1	1	1	1	1	1	2	2	1	1	1	1	1	1	1	1	1	1	1	1
Migraine	2	3	3	3	2	2	2	2	1	1	2	2	2	2	2	3	2	2	4	3	3	3
Alzheimer's disease and other dementias	3	2	2	2	4	3	3	3	3	3	3	3	3	3	3	2	3	4	3	4	4	4
Meningitis	4	11	5	4	9	10	14	13	13	11	13	4	9	10	8	5	3	2	2	5	2	5
Epilepsy	5	5	4	5	3	8	6	7	6	5	6	5	4	4	4	4	4	6	5	5	2	5
Spinal cord injury	6	7	8	9	7	5	4	4	4	4	4	4	8	9	9	6	9	6	7	10	8	9
Traumatic brain injury	7	6	6	7	5	4	4	7	8	8	9	7	8	7	7	6	7	9	7	7	8	7
Brain and other CNS cancer	8	4	9	10	6	6	8	5	5	6	5	8	6	7	5	8	10	9	8	11	9	10
Tension-type headache	9	8	10	8	10	7	5	6	7	7	7	6	5	5	6	7	8	8	9	7	6	8
Encephalitis	10	9	7	6	8	11	11	14	14	12	14	11	10	11	12	10	5	10	10	11	8	10
Parkinson's disease	11	10	11	12	12	9	10	9	10	8	9	12	11	12	11	13	13	13	13	13	13	12
Other neurological disorders	12	12	12	11	11	12	9	10	9	10	10	10	10	12	8	10	11	12	12	12	8	12
Tetanus	13	15	13	14	15	15	15	15	15	15	15	15	13	15	15	15	14	11	11	6	14	11
Multiple sclerosis	14	14	15	15	13	13	11	13	12	11	13	11	15	14	14	14	15	14	14	14	15	15
Motor neuron diseases	15	13	14	13	14	14	14	12	11	12	11	14	13	13	13	15	15	15	15	15	14	14

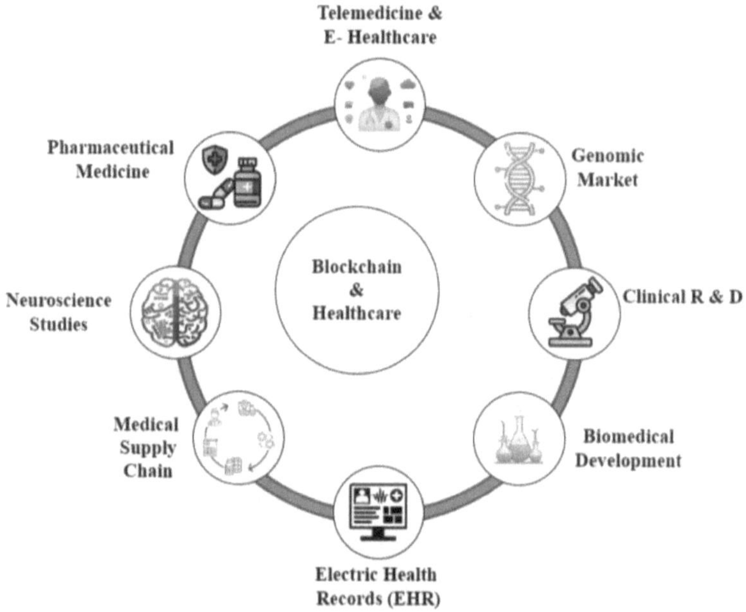

Figure 8.8 Various Applications of Healthcare with Blockchain.

area. While innovative therapeutic tools and cutting-edge technologies offer potential, obstacles remain primarily due to high costs and limited availability in research institutions that are typically well-funded by organizations or health centers located in urban areas. To improve access in underfunded regions and rural areas, it is vital to develop scalable, cost-effective solutions that can be deployed globally. Many researchers rely on datasets, but these are not always applicable to larger, diverse populations worldwide. AI and ML techniques offer a way to overcome these challenges by enabling early-stage diagnosis and treatment of neurological disorders, potentially helping millions across generations recover and manage their conditions.

8.7 COMPARISON CHART OF ENCRYPTION AND DECRYPTION METHODS ON VARIOUS ALGORITHMS

In federated learning, guaranteeing data security throughout the dissemination of framework updates among decentralized devices and the primary server is critical. AES is extremely efficient, operating with a wide range of key sizes: 128, 192, or 256 bits. It is particularly well-suited for instantaneous applications. Conversely, ECC provides a comparable level of security to RSA but primarily uses smaller key sizes, ensuring minimal power consumption in IoT devices and smartphones. This approach helps mitigate processing overhead, assuring rapid encryption and decryption to maintain security. For federated learning involving lightweight devices, this type of security process is often preferred. For higher security, blending algorithms such as AES-RSA or ECC-RSA are effective. RSA is employed for secure key exchange, while AES is mainly used for the encryption of the actual data. By collaborating with these methods, the system can efficiently handle large volumes of data while providing safe, secure, and speedy data transfer in federated learning [39].

Figure 8.9 presents an analysis of the encryption and decryption times for AES-128, AES-256, DES, ECC with AES, and RSA, as shown in another figure. It can be seen that AES 128 at 4.635 ms and DES at 5.746 ms, AES 256, ECC with AES and RSA have significantly higher combined encryption and decryption times at 7.328 ms, 8.188 ms, and 8.852 ms, respectively. A graphical comparison is given in Figure 8.9.

Figure 8.10, from [43] illustrates a comparison between the encryption time of the three files in the five cycles, which confirms that encryption takes longer with data of a larger size.

By comparing the decryption times of the three files in the five cycles, as in Figure 8.11, it is clear to us that decryption takes longer with data of a larger size [44].

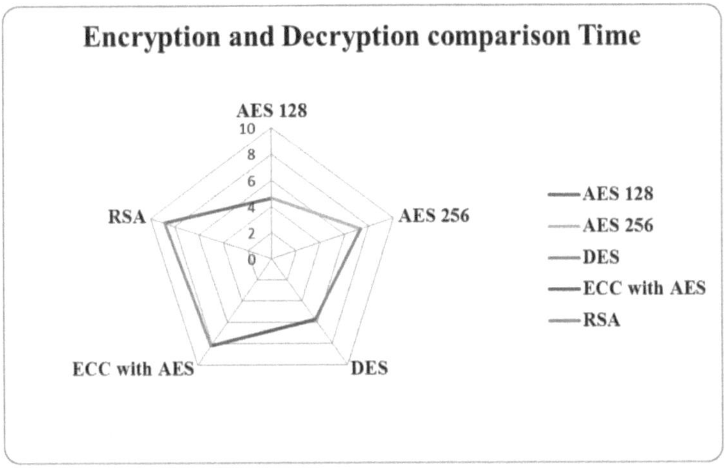

Figure 8.9 Encryption and Decryption Comparison Time.

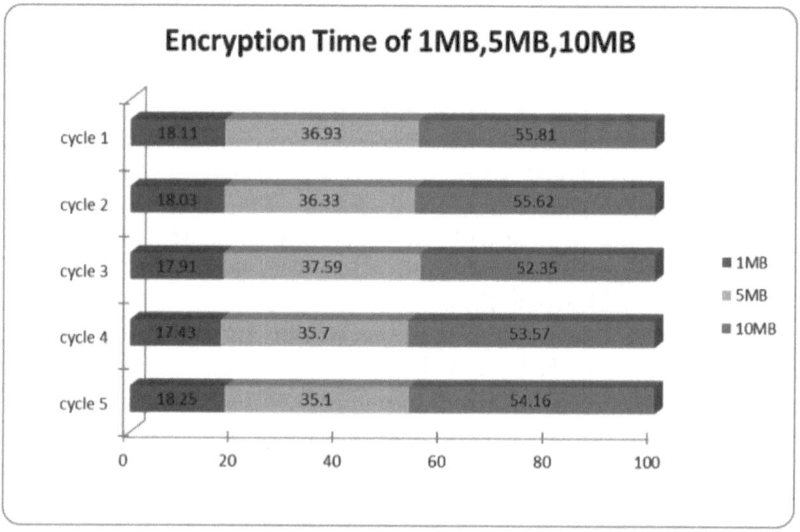

Figure 8.10 Encryption Time of 1 Mb, 5 Mb, 10 MB.

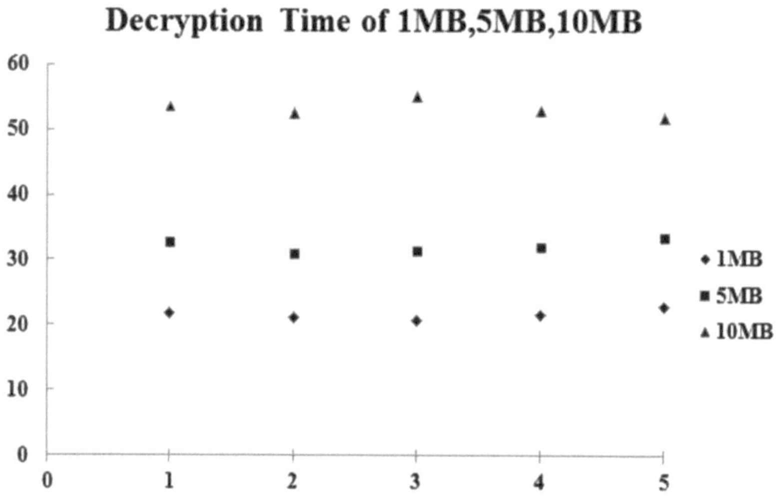

Figure 8.11 Decryption Time of 1 Mb, 5 Mb, 10 MB.

8.8 CONCLUSION

Federated learning plays a significant role in addressing neurological disorders by focusing on secure data processing. Ensuring that data transfer methods utilize secure communication channels is crucial to prevent misinformation and facilitate accurate diagnoses under optimal conditions. Various techniques, such as multi-layer encryption and blockchain technology, are employed to maintain data integrity and security, ensuring safe access to information throughout the analysis process. This approach enhances research in the medical field by fostering secure collaboration among various institutions. To predict and diagnose patient conditions at an early stage, it is essential to enable secure data transfer among institutions for effective treatment analysis, thereby overcoming the cost barriers associated with diagnosis. Moreover, utilizing AI detection systems can help identify diseases at earlier stages, allowing patients to receive timely treatment. By integrating these technologies with secure data transfer, both underfunded and well-funded institutions can contribute to improving patients' quality of life throughout their healthcare journey.

REFERENCES

1. Y. Jiao and C. Wang, "A Blockchain-Based Trusted Upload Scheme for the Internet of Things Nodes," in International Journal of Crowd Science, vol. 6, no. 2, pp. 92–97, June 2022, DOI: 10.26599/IJCS.2022.9100010.
2. L. Li, D. Jin, T. Zhang, and N. Li, "A Secure, Reliable and Low-Cost Distributed Storage Scheme Based on Blockchain and IPFS for Firefighting IoT Data," in IEEE Access, vol. 11, pp. 97318–97330, 2023, DOI: 10.1109/ACCESS.2023.3311712.
3. M. Shi, Z. Zhang, Q. Lv, Miao, and C.-M. Pun, "Universal Object-Level Adversarial Attack in Hyperspectral Image Classification," in IEEE Transactions on Geoscience and Remote Sensing, vol. 61, pp. 1–14, 2023, Art no. 5532714, DOI: 10.1109/TGRS.2023.3336734.
4. Z. Chen, J. Du, X. Hou, K. Yu, J. Wang, and Z. Han, "Channel Adaptive and Sparsity Personalized Federated Learning for Privacy Protection in Smart Healthcare Systems," in IEEE Journal of Biomedical and Health Informatics, vol. 28, no. 6, pp. 3248–3257, June 2024, DOI: 10.1109/JBHI.2024.3353791.
5. M. Kim, I. Oh, K. Yim, M. Sahlabadi, and Z. Shukur, "Security of 6G-Enabled Vehicle-to-Everything Communication in Emerging Federated Learning and Blockchain Technologies," in IEEE Access, vol. 12, pp. 33972–34001, 2024, DOI: 10.1109/ACCESS.2023.3348409.
6. Y. Jiang and J. Zhang, "Profitability Analysis of Time-Restricted Double-Spending Attack on PoW-Based Large Scale Blockchain With the Aid of Multiple Types of Attacks," in IEEE Transactions on Information Forensics and Security, vol. 19, pp. 8155–8171, 2024, DOI: 10.1109/TIFS.2024.3449224.

7. S. Yan, J. Ren, W. Wang, L. Sun, W. Zhang, and Q. Yu, "A Survey of Adversarial Attack and Defense Methods for Malware Classification in Cyber Security," in IEEE Communications Surveys & Tutorials, vol. 25, no. 1, pp. 467–496, First Quarter 2023, DOI: 10.1109/COMST.2022.3225137.
8. S. H. Park, S. -H. Lee, M. Y. Lim, P. M. Hong, and Y. K. Lee, "A Comprehensive Risk Analysis Method for Adversarial Attacks on Biometric Authentication Systems," in IEEE Access, vol. 12, pp. 116693–116710, 2024, DOI: 10.1109/ACCESS.2024.3439741.
9. P. Zhang, X. Pang, N. Kumar, G. S. Aujla, and H. Cao, "A Reliable Data-Transmission Mechanism Using Blockchain in Edge Computing Scenarios," in IEEE Internet of Things Journal, vol. 9, no. 16, pp. 14228–14236, Aug. 15, 2022, DOI: 10.1109/JIOT.2020.3021457.
10. A. Khan et al., "Secure Remote Sensing Data With Blockchain Distributed Ledger Technology: A Solution for Smart Cities," in IEEE Access, vol. 12, pp. 69383–69396, 2024, DOI: 10.1109/ACCESS.2024.3401591.
11. A. Khan et al., "Secure Remote Sensing Data With Blockchain Distributed Ledger Technology: A Solution for Smart Cities," in IEEE Access, vol. 12, pp. 69383–69396, 2024, DOI: 10.1109/ACCESS.2024.3401591.
12. S. Fugkeaw, L. Hak and T. Theeramunkong, "Achieving Secure, Verifiable, and Efficient Boolean Keyword Searchable Encryption for Cloud Data Warehouse," in IEEE Access, vol. 12, pp. 49848–49864, 2024, DOI: 10.1109/ACCESS.2024.3383320.
13. Y. Hualong and G. Daidou, "Research on Double Encryption of Ghost Imaging by SegNet Deep Neural Network," in IEEE Photonics Technology Letters, vol. 36, no. 10, pp. 669–672, 15 May, 2024, DOI: 10.1109/LPT.2024.3379554.
14. T. R. Ningthoukhongjam, S. Devi Heisnam and M. Singh Khumanthem, "Medical Image Encryption Through Chaotic Asymmetric Cryptosystem," in IEEE Access, vol. 12, pp. 73879–73888, 2024, DOI: 10.1109/ACCESS.2024.3404088.
15. G. Tu, W. Liu, T. Zhou, X. Yang and F. Zhang, "Concise and Efficient Multi-Identity Fully Homomorphic Encryption Scheme," in IEEE Access, vol. 12, pp. 49640–49652, 2024, DOI: 10.1109/ACCESS.2024.3384247.
16. G. Zu, Y. Lu, and J. Li, "Comment on an Attribute-Based Searchable Encryption Scheme With Receiver Anonymity," in IEEE Transactions on Services Computing, vol. 17, no. 4, pp. 1875–1876, July-Aug. 2024, DOI: 10.1109/TSC.2023.3332864.
17. S. Ahmad, S. Rass and P. Schartner, "False-Bottom Encryption: Deniable Encryption From Secret Sharing," in IEEE Access, vol. 11, pp. 62549–62564, 2023, DOI: 10.1109/ACCESS.2023.3288285.
18. Y. Zhang, W. Zhou, R. Zhao, X. Zhang and X. Cao, "F-TPE: Flexible Thumbnail-Preserving Encryption Based on Multi-Pixel Sum-Preserving Encryption," in IEEE Transactions on Multimedia, vol. 25, pp. 5877–5891, 2023, DOI: 10.1109/TMM.2022.3200310.
19. G. Cao, Y. Tao, X. Liu and T. Zhang, "Image Encryption Based on a Coined Chaotic System and High-Intensity Encryption Primitives," in IEEE Access, vol. 12, pp. 92043–92061, 2024, DOI: 10.1109/ACCESS.2024.3423691.

20. Y. Yuan, H. He, H. Amirpour, L. Qu, C. Timmerer and F. Chen, "IoT Privacy Protection: JPEG-TPE With Lower File Size Expansion and Lossless Decryption," in IEEE Internet of Things Journal, vol. 11, no. 13, pp. 23485–23496, 1 July, 2024, DOI: 10.1109/JIOT.2024.3385268.
21. N. H. Sultan, M. Laurent and V. Varadharajan, "Securing Organization's Data: A Role-Based Authorized Keyword Search Scheme With Efficient Decryption," in IEEE Transactions on Cloud Computing, vol. 11, no. 1, pp. 25–43, 1 Jan.–March, 2023, DOI: 10.1109/TCC.2021.3071304.
22. H. Yang, H. Yan, Y. Li, P. Wen and F. Yang, "Secure Zonotopic Set-Membership State Estimation for Multirate Complex Networks Under Encryption–Decryption Mechanism," in IEEE Transactions on Automatic Control, vol. 69, no. 8, pp. 5109–5124, Aug. 2024, DOI: 10.1109/TAC.2023.3347599.
23. B. Qu, Z. Wang, B. Shen, H. Dong and X. Zhang, "Secure Particle Filtering With Paillier Encryption–Decryption Scheme: Application to Multi-Machine Power Grids," in IEEE Transactions on Smart Grid, vol. 15, no. 1, pp. 863–873, Jan. 2024, DOI: 10.1109/TSG.2023.3271949.
24. W. Chen, Z. Wang, Q. Ge, H. Dong and G.-P. Liu, "Quantized Distributed Economic Dispatch for Microgrids: Paillier Encryption–Decryption Scheme," in IEEE Transactions on Industrial Informatics, vol. 20, no. 4, pp. 6552–6562, April 2024, DOI: 10.1109/TII.2023.3348816.
25. N. Gao, K. Fan, H. Wang, K. Zhang, H. Li and Y. Yang, "Public-Key Inverted-Index Keyword Search With Designated Tester and Multiuser Key Decryption in IoT," in IEEE Internet of Things Journal, vol. 11, no. 1, pp. 1065–1079, Jan. 1, 2024, DOI: 10.1109/JIOT.2023.3288119.
26. Y. Ding et al., "Backdoor Attack on Deep Learning-Based Medical Image Encryption and Decryption Network," in IEEE Transactions on Information Forensics and Security, vol. 19, pp. 280–292, 2024, DOI: 10.1109/TIFS.2023.3322315.
27. C. Ge, Z. Liu, W. Susilo, L. Fang and H. Wang, "Attribute-Based Encryption With Reliable Outsourced Decryption in Cloud Computing Using Smart Contract," in IEEE Transactions on Dependable and Secure Computing, vol. 21, no. 2, pp. 937–948, March–April 2024, DOI: 10.1109/TDSC.2023.3265932.
28. C. -Y. Lin, S. -C. Wu, P. -H. Kuo, M. -J. Huang, S. -W. Hong and H. -T. Yau, "Application of Chaotic Encryption and Decryption in Wireless Transmission From Sensory Tool Holders on Machine Tools," in IEEE Sensors Journal, vol. 23, no. 11, pp. 11453–11468, June 1, 2023, DOI: 10.1109/JSEN.2023.3265777.
29. K. N. Kumar, C. K. Mohan and L. R. Cenkeramaddi, "The Impact of Adversarial Attacks on Federated Learning: A Survey," in IEEE Transactions on Pattern Analysis and Machine Intelligence, vol. 46, no. 5, pp. 2672–2691, May 2024, DOI: 10.1109/TPAMI.2023.3322785.
30. Barnawi, P. Chhikara, R. Tekchandani, N. Kumar and B. Alzahrani, "A Differentially Privacy Assisted Federated Learning Scheme to Preserve Data Privacy for IoMT Applications," in IEEE Transactions on Network

and Service Management, vol. 21, no. 4, pp. 4686–4700, Aug. 2024, DOI: 10.1109/TNSM.2024.3393969.

31. R. Ullah, Y. Dong, T. Arslan and S. Chandran, "A Machine Learning-Based Classification Method for Monitoring Alzheimer's Disease Using Electromagnetic Radar Data," in IEEE Transactions on Microwave Theory and Techniques, vol. 71, no. 9, pp. 4012–4026, Sept. 2023, DOI: 10.1109/TMTT.2023.3245665.
32. S. Xu, X. Han, G. Xu, J. Ning, X. Huang and R. H. Deng, "An Adaptive Secure and Practical Data Sharing System with Verifiable Outsourced Decryption," in IEEE Transactions on Services Computing, vol. 17, no. 3, pp. 776–788, May–June 2024, DOI: 10.1109/TSC.2023.3321314.
33. GBD 2016 Neurology Collaborators. "Global, Regional, and National Burden of Neurological Disorders, 1990–2016: A Systematic Analysis for the Global Burden of Disease Study 2016," Lancet Neurology, 2019 May, vol. 18, no. 5, pp. 459–480. DOI: 10.1016/S1474-4422(18)30499-X. Epub 2019 Mar 14. PMID: 30879893; PMCID: PMC6459001.
34. S. Xu, X. Han, G. Xu, J. Ning, X. Huang and R. H. Deng, "An Adaptive Secure and Practical Data Sharing System With Verifiable Outsourced Decryption," in IEEE Transactions on Services Computing, vol. 17, no. 3, pp. 776–788, May–June 2024, DOI: 10.1109/TSC.2023.3321314.
35. N. P. Narendra, B. Schuller and P. Alku, "The Detection of Parkinson's Disease From Speech Using Voice Source Information," in IEEE/ACM Transactions on Audio, Speech, and Language Processing, vol. 29, pp. 1925–1936, 2021, DOI: 10.1109/TASLP.2021.3078364.
36. M. Kim, J. H. Won, J. Youn and H. Park, "Joint-Connectivity-Based Sparse Canonical Correlation Analysis of Imaging Genetics for Detecting Biomarkers of Parkinson's Disease," in IEEE Transactions on Medical Imaging, vol. 39, no. 1, pp. 23–34, Jan. 2020, DOI: 10.1109/TMI.2019.2918839.
37. C.G. Sabo, A. Fasano, A. Iaboni, and B. Taati, "Concurrent Validity of Zeno Instrumented Walkway and Video-Based Gait Features in Adults with Parkinson's Disease," in IEEE Journal of Translational Engineering in Health and Medicine, vol. 10, pp. 1–11, 2022, Art no. 2100511, DOI: 10.1109/JTEHM.2022.3180231.
38. D. Pan et al., "Adaptive 3DCNN-Based Interpretable Ensemble Model for Early Diagnosis of Alzheimer's Disease," in IEEE Transactions on Computational Social Systems, vol. 11, no. 1, pp. 247–266, Feb. 2024, DOI: 10.1109/TCSS.2022.3223999.
39. Z. Bassfar, A. Sayeed, P. Bala, A. Alshehri, A. Alanazi, A. Abdulaziz and S. Zubair, "Toward Secure and Resilient Networks: A Zero-Trust Security Framework with Quantum Fingerprinting for Devices Accessing Network," Mathematics. vol. 11, 2023, p. 2653. DOI: 10.3390/math11122653
40. G. Sreelatha, C. Kishor Kumar Reddy, M. Mohd Hanafiah and R. MadanaMohana. "Hybrid Electro Search Beetle Optimization Based Task Scheduling and Game Theory SOA Based Resource Allocation in Multi Cloud Computing." Wiley Journal of Software: Practice and Experience, September 2024. DOI: https://doi.org/10.1002/spe.3370

41. C. Kishor Kumar Reddy, A. Daduvy, R. Madana Mohana, B. Assiri, M. Shauib, S. Alam and A. Sheneamer, "Enhancing Precision Agriculture and Land Cover Classification: A Self-Attention 3D Convolutional Neural Network Approach for Hyperspectral Image Analysis," IEEE Access, 2024. DOI: 10.1109/ACCESS.2024.3420089
42. C. Kishor Kumar Reddy, P. Anaghaa Reddy, H. Janapati, B. Assiri, M. Shauib, S. Alam and A. Sheneamer, "A Fine Tuned Vision Transformer (FTVT) Based Enhanced Multi-Class Brain Tumor Classification using MRI Scan Imagery." Frontiers in Oncology Cancer Imaging and Image-directed Interventions, August 2024. DOI: 10.3389/fonc.2024.1400341
43. S. Khaldi, M. AlZain and M. Masud, "SCES Proposed a Model for Data Protection in Cloud Educational Systems in Saudi Arabia," International Journal of Health Sciences, 2022. DOI: 10.53730/ijhs.v6nS3.7018
44. C. Kishor Kumar Reddy, A. Rangarajan, D. Rangarajan, M. Shuaib, F. Jeribi and S. Alam, "A Transfer Learning Approach: Early Prediction of Alzheimer's Disease on US Healthy Aging Dataset," MDPI Mathematics, July 2024, 2204. DOI: 10.3390/math12142204.

Chapter 9

Federated learning and personalized medicine

Tailoring neural disorder therapies in healthcare 6.0

Lingala Thirupathi, Gundekari Anusha, Thejoramnaresh Reddy Boya, and Hari Chandra Prasad Cheerla

9.1 INTRODUCTION

Federated learning (FL) represents a transformative approach to machine learning, particularly in the context of Healthcare 6.0, which emphasizes personalized and patient-centered care. This innovative method enables multiple healthcare institutions to collaboratively train machine learning models without the need to share sensitive patient data. Instead, the models learn directly from local datasets, which helps preserve patient privacy and adhere to regulatory standards like HIPAA. Table 9.1 depicts the main features of FL in healthcare.

9.1.1 Importance of Personalized Medicine

Precision medicine, another name for personalized medicine, is a practice that customizes medical care to each patient's unique needs. This methodology stands in stark contrast to the conventional "one-size-fits-all" approach, especially in complicated domains such as brain illnesses where treatment response varies greatly among patients. Neural disorders, such as Alzheimer's, Parkinson's, and multiple sclerosis, exhibit a wide range of symptoms and progression rates. Each patient may experience unique combinations of these symptoms, necessitating highly individualized treatment plans to achieve optimal outcomes. The genetic makeup of individuals plays a critical role in how they respond to therapies. Personalized medicine considers genetic variations that can influence drug metabolism, efficacy, and the likelihood of adverse effects, ensuring that patients receive treatments that align with their biological profiles.

Environmental factors, such as lifestyle, diet, and socio-economic status, also impact the development and progression of neural disorders. Personalized medicine incorporates these elements to develop more comprehensive and effective treatment strategies. Advancements in technology, including genomic sequencing and bioinformatics, enable healthcare providers to gather

 DOI: 10.1201/9781003591085-9

Table 9.1 Key Features of FL in Healthcare

Feature	*Description*
Data Privacy and Security	By giving healthcare providers autonomy over their data, FL lowers the dangers of illegal access and data breaches.
Collaborative Model Development	Institutions can contribute to a shared model, improving its accuracy and robustness by leveraging diverse datasets while ensuring that sensitive information remains local.
Personalized Treatment	By utilizing data from various demographics and patient backgrounds, FL facilitates the development of tailored therapeutic interventions that better meet individual patient needs.
Addressing Data Heterogeneity	FL is designed to handle the variability in patient data across different healthcare settings, making it well-suited for the complexities of real-world healthcare scenarios.
Algorithmic Fairness	The decentralized nature of FL helps to mitigate biases in AI models, ensuring that the resulting algorithms are more inclusive and representative of the patient population.
Integration with Clinical Workflows	FL can be seamlessly integrated into existing healthcare processes, enhancing decision-making without disrupting routine practices.
Accelerating Research and Innovation	By facilitating collaborative research, FL can speed up the development of new treatments and interventions, contributing to advancements in precision medicine.

and analyze vast amounts of data. This wealth of information supports the customization of treatment plans based on detailed patient profiles. Federated learning enhances the capabilities of personalized medicine by allowing healthcare institutions to collaboratively develop machine learning models without sharing sensitive patient data. This decentralized approach fosters innovation while maintaining data privacy. By tailoring therapies to the specific needs of patients, personalized medicine has the potential to significantly improve treatment efficacy. Customization ensures that patients receive the most effective interventions for their unique conditions.

Personalized approaches can reduce the incidence of adverse drug reactions. By considering individual patient factors, healthcare providers can select treatments that are less likely to cause harmful side effects, enhancing patient safety. When patients understand that their treatment plans are tailored specifically for them, they are more likely to engage actively in their care. This improved engagement can lead to better adherence to treatment protocols and overall health outcomes. Personalized medicine can accelerate drug development processes by identifying patient subgroups that are more likely to respond to specific therapies. This targeted approach can streamline clinical trials, making them more efficient and effective. Figure 9.1 explores the different FL frameworks.

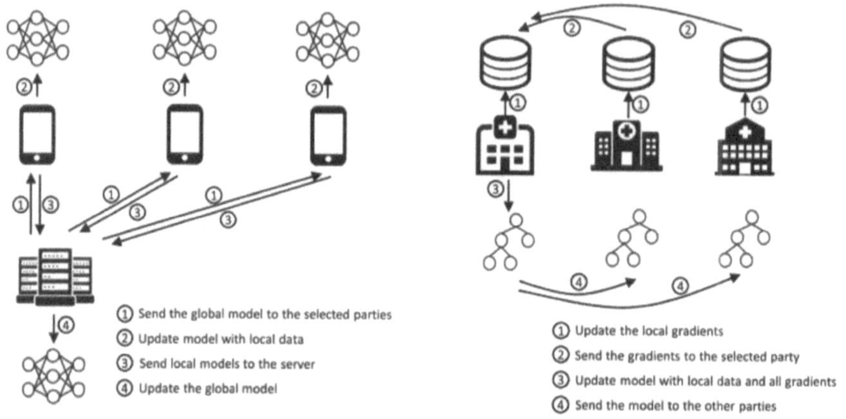

(a) FedAvg (b) SimFL

Figure 9.1 FL frameworks.

Artificial intelligence (AI) is being used in customized medicine to analyze large, complicated datasets and find patterns and insights that human analysts would miss. AI-powered algorithms can help medical professionals make data-driven decisions for specific patients. By ensuring that therapies are successful for a variety of populations, personalized medicine can reduce health inequities. By including varied demographic data, FL can help develop inclusive models that account for different responses to therapies. Personalized medicine provides healthcare professionals with valuable decision-support tools. These tools can analyze patient data in real time, offering insights that guide treatment choices and improve outcomes for neural disorders.

Despite its benefits, personalized medicine faces challenges in implementation, such as the need for robust data-sharing frameworks and overcoming regulatory hurdles. However, FL offers a promising solution by enabling collaborative data use while safeguarding patient privacy. The paradigm shift towards personalized medicine encourages collaboration among various stakeholders, including researchers, clinicians, and patients. This collaborative spirit is essential for advancing the field of neural disorder therapies. Personalized medicine raises important ethical questions regarding data ownership and consent. Healthcare providers must navigate these complexities to ensure that patient rights are respected while leveraging data for improved outcomes. As personalized medicine continues to evolve; it is poised to revolutionize therapeutic interventions for neural disorders. Future treatments may include gene therapies and targeted biologics that are specifically designed for individual patients.

Personalized medicine emphasizes long-term follow-up and outcomes tracking, allowing healthcare providers to adjust treatment plans based on patient responses over time. This adaptability is crucial for managing chronic conditions like neural disorders. The shift toward personalized medicine aligns with the broader movement toward patient-centered care. This model prioritizes patient preferences and values, ensuring that treatment decisions reflect the unique needs and goals of individuals. The importance of personalized medicine in tailoring therapies for neural disorders in Healthcare 6.0 cannot be overstated. By leveraging technology, addressing individual patient factors, and fostering collaboration, personalized medicine is set to enhance treatment efficacy, safety, and overall patient satisfaction, ultimately paving the way for a more effective and equitable healthcare landscape.

9.1.2 Focus on Neural Disorders

A wide range of illnesses are classified as neural disorders, such as autism spectrum disorders, multiple sclerosis, Parkinson's disease, and Alzheimer's disease. Every one of these illnesses poses different difficulties for diagnosis, management, and therapy, frequently mandating individualized strategies to maximize care. The integration of FL and personalized medicine offers promising avenues to address these challenges, enhancing patient outcomes and driving advancements in therapeutic strategies. Neural disorders are characterized by significant variability in symptoms, progression rates, and treatment responses among patients. Because of this intricacy, individualized treatment plans that take into account each patient's unique genetic, environmental, and lifestyle characteristics are required. By enabling healthcare professionals to work together on model development without violating patient privacy, FL makes this personalization easier. Federated learning has several benefits when it comes to brain illnesses, one of which is its capacity to leverage a variety of datasets from various healthcare organizations. Federated learning makes sure that machine learning models are more inclusive and representative by training them on data from different groups. This inclusivity is crucial for developing personalized interventions that consider the wide range of demographic and clinical variables present in neural disorder patients.

Federated learning can significantly improve the accuracy of diagnostic tools used in identifying neural disorders. By aggregating insights from numerous datasets, FL-based models can learn to identify subtle patterns that may be indicative of specific conditions. This enhanced diagnostic capability allows for earlier and more accurate identification of disorders, enabling timely and effective intervention. Personalized medicine emphasizes the customization of treatment plans based on individual patient characteristics. With FL, clinicians can access models that reflect the best practices derived from a diverse pool of patient data. This enables them to tailor interventions more effectively, ensuring that treatments align with the specific needs and responses of each patient.

Many patients with neural disorders experience resistance to standard treatments. Federated learning can help identify patient subgroups that may benefit from alternative therapies by analyzing diverse treatment outcomes. This insight allows for the development of more effective, targeted therapies that cater to these resistant populations. Federated learning supports a continuous learning environment where models can be updated with new patient data over time. This adaptability is particularly beneficial for chronic neural disorders, where treatment needs may evolve. Clinicians can refine treatment plans based on real-time feedback from ongoing patient responses, ensuring that interventions remain relevant and effective. Figure 9.2 shows personalized medicine in sleep and cancer.

The use of FL addresses critical ethical concerns surrounding data privacy in healthcare. By keeping patient data local while still contributing to a collaborative model, FL mitigates risks associated with data breaches. This is especially important in the context of neural disorders, where sensitive information is often involved. Personalized medicine fosters patient

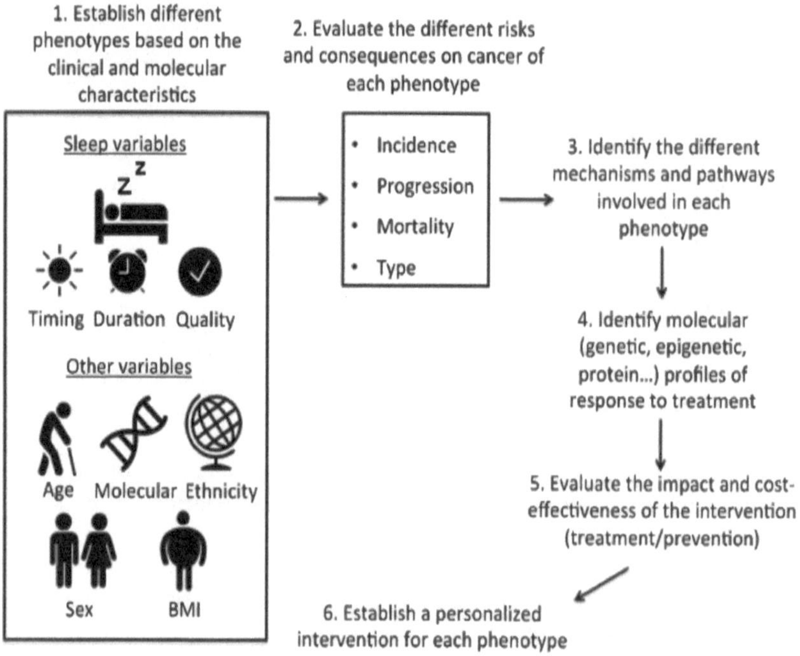

Figure 9.2 Personalized medicine in sleep and cancer. (Original.)

engagement by involving individuals in their treatment decisions. Federated learning can enhance this process by providing clinicians with robust data-driven insights, allowing them to explain treatment options in a way that resonates with patients. This empowerment can lead to improved adherence and better health outcomes.

Federated learning promotes collaboration among researchers and clinicians, breaking down silos that often exist in healthcare. By pooling knowledge and data without compromising privacy, FL accelerates the development of innovative treatment strategies and clinical trials tailored to neural disorders. The combination of FL and personalized medicine holds great promise for the future of neural disorder therapies. Ongoing advancements in AI and machine learning will likely lead to even more sophisticated models that can predict patient responses with high accuracy, ultimately transforming the landscape of treatment for neural disorders. The focus on neural disorders within the context of FL and personalized medicine underscores a critical shift towards more individualized, data-driven healthcare. By leveraging the strengths of FL to enhance data privacy, diversity, and collaboration, healthcare providers can develop more effective, tailored interventions that address the unique challenges presented by neural disorders.

The main contribution of this chapter is to highlight the FL role in personalized medicine for neural disorders, enabling collaborative model development while preserving privacy. It emphasizes inclusivity in AI models, accelerates precision medicine by tackling data heterogeneity and algorithmic fairness, and discusses integration into clinical workflows, ultimately paving the way for more effective treatments.

This chapter is organized into different sections, starting with the literature survey, next FL: A paradigm shift in Healthcare, then after applications of FL in neural disorders, privacy preservation, and data security, addressing data heterogeneity, algorithmic fairness in FL, integration within clinical workflows, conclusions, finally the references.

9.2 LITERATURE SURVEY

To integrate IoT, big data, machine learning, 6G, and cloud computing with digital twin implementation in aircraft lifecycle management, a comprehensive framework is presented in study [1]. The system addresses major industry difficulties by enabling accurate, real-time representations of aircraft. To improve efficiency and safety, it examines lifecycle stages, models, and tools for making decisions. Additionally, it highlights a knowledge-driven approach for deeper insights. Despite challenges like data quality and security, future research directions include advanced analytics and emerging technologies, positioning digital twins as vital for the aviation industry's evolution.

Strategy [2] enhances adversarial defense in FL under non-IID scenarios using a server-side model-contrastive correction framework and a client-side adaptive correction module. It effectively mitigates adversarial training instability, particularly in intelligent driving systems, while requiring further research for broader applications beyond image data and improving algorithm robustness across diverse client environments. The study tackled the complexity of electricity consumption prediction in educational institutions using cooperative ensemble learning, SHAP-based feature selection, and hyperparameter optimization. The GA–LSTM model outperformed traditional methods, achieving the lowest error metrics. Insights from SHAP values highlighted key predictors, emphasizing the importance of temporal variables over climatic factors [3].

Study [4] introduced a reputation-based interpretable distributed semi-supervised fusion mechanism for intelligent labeling systems, improving accuracy and reducing overhead. While effective, it faces challenges such as increased computational demands, scalability issues, and vulnerability to malicious nodes. Article [5] presented a distributed infrastructure for federated learning, addressing performance and stability challenges in heterogeneous systems. It discusses implementation details, privacy implications through differential privacy, and the use of Kubernetes for managing diverse architectures like Intel and ARM, potentially accelerating federated learning application development across various devices.

The PolyFLAM and PolyFLAP frameworks [6] enhance federated learning security using polymorphic encryption, with unique keys for each server-client message to mitigate risks from key compromise. They balance security and efficiency but incur additional computational costs. Synergizing with established methods can improve scalability and learning efficiency while addressing these challenges. Introduced in [7], SoFLis a clustered federated learning algorithm designed to tackle non-IID data challenges. Experiments show that SoFL improves accuracy by 13–18% over FedAvg and converges faster. Suitable for various fields, it forms multiple federated models by clustering clients with shared optimization goals, although it may increase server computation costs.

Paper [8] presented an efficient and secure federated learning framework for underwater wireless IoT networks, utilizing IoT edge device scheduling and a voting mechanism for enhanced security. While the UCB-SC and UCB-SCP policies improve efficiency and security, their effectiveness depends on data quality and stable communication conditions, which can vary underwater. Explores federated learning as a promising technique for enhancing machine learning adoption while emphasizing privacy and security. It highlights that while existing aggregation algorithms perform well in security and robustness, they struggle with privacy and inference attacks. Techniques like homomorphic and polymorphic encryption can significantly improve these aspects [9].

Paper [10] presented FBLearn, a blockchain-based federated learning platform enhancing data security and model accuracy. It addresses challenges like data quality and adversarial attacks through innovative global model aggregation strategies, adaptive weight calculations, and ensemble techniques. The platform's flexibility supports various algorithms, enabling efficient private data utilization across different sectors. Paper [11] introduced a new caching strategy for federated NDN learning in smart city IoT, optimizing energy efficiency and content retrieval. The proposed approach outperforms benchmarks in cache hit ratio, reduces content access delays, and minimizes energy consumption, contributing to sustainable development and enhancing network resilience for smart city applications.

Paper [12] presented a Byzantine-robust multimodal federated learning framework for intelligent connected vehicles (ICVs), addressing data privacy, security, and adversarial robustness. By integrating diverse sensor data, it enhances object detection accuracy. Evaluations on benchmark datasets demonstrate high performance and low communication overhead, paving the way for future secure distributed machine learning research. Study [13] presented a methodology for accurately detecting gas leaks using intelligent multimodal data in pipelines, comparing gas detector readings and infrared thermal imaging. Employing CNN and LSTM models, the findings show improved accuracy with multimodal data. The approach supports privacy-preserving federated learning for effective gas leak monitoring in Industry 5.0.

To pick clients with better local model performance for global aggregation, the Fed-RHLP algorithm [14] uses a roulette wheel technique, which encourages participation fairness. It solves the Non-IID problem by allowing clients with lesser performance to align with the global model, consistently achieving faster convergence and greater accuracy compared to FedAvg and Power-of-Choice. Study [15] demonstrated the effectiveness of federated learning (FL) in enhancing IoT security by detecting routing vulnerabilities through various ML algorithms. SVM and KNN achieved approximately 95% accuracy, highlighting FL's advantages in data confidentiality and scalability. The FL-DSFA model showed improved detection efficiency, with future research aimed at extending its capabilities.

Paper [16] presented a novel technique that combines group signatures (GSs) with secure aggregation (SA) to enhance privacy in federated learning. By sharing secret keys between the admin and clients, the method reduces computational and communication costs. Simulation results demonstrate superior privacy preservation and resilience against various security attacks compared to existing algorithms. The greedy hierarchical FL model [17] achieved an accuracy of 86.72%, only 3.217% lower than the original model, demonstrating its effectiveness with similar data distributions. While requiring more communication rounds, it optimizes memory allocation in trusted execution environments, highlighting its practicality and potential for further optimization in scenarios with significant data bias.

The proposed FL approach [18] using the Inception-V3 model achieved remarkable accuracy in classifying lung and colon histopathological images, with an overall accuracy of 99.720%. It achieved 100% accuracy in colon cancer classification and 99.867% for lung cancer, demonstrating effective compliance with patient data regulations and precise cancer cell categorization. The research in study [19] presented the Embedded Federated Learning-Driven LSTM (EFL-LSTM) model, enhancing cybersecurity in IoHT environments. By integrating feature selection techniques with federated learning, it achieved accuracies of 97.16% and 99.78% in detecting cyberattacks. Future work aims to refine detection for specific threats and expand FL applications in healthcare.

Review [20] explored machine learning methods for medical imaging analysis, highlighting challenges like dataset accessibility and privacy preservation. It discusses non-IID data handling and privacy-enhancing strategies, emphasizing that while federated learning is promising, its effectiveness depends on various factors including dataset quality, algorithm efficiency, and computational resources. While it does not lessen pain, combining regular physical treatment with neural mobilization greatly increases mobility in patients with cervical radiculopathy and chronic neck pain [21]. This review adds important new information to the clinical management of nerve-related neck discomfort by highlighting the usefulness of neural mobilization as a practical strategy for improving functionality.

The first RCT [22] of Acoustic CR® Neuro modulation found no significant therapeutic benefit over a placebo. The device is unlikely to surpass other sound-based tinnitus treatments or psychological interventions. Further trials are needed for FDA approval, suggesting alternative study designs for more informative comparisons and enhancing patient choice in tinnitus management. Study [23] reveals that children with functional neurological disorders (FND) often experience illness-promoting psychological processes influenced by daily challenges and their environment. Cumulative adverse childhood experiences (ACEs) activate stress responses, potentially amplifying future reactions to stress and contributing to ongoing distress if not effectively addressed.

A large body of research [24] has demonstrated the therapeutic advantages of invasive and non-invasive neuromodulator treatments for eating disorders. To clarify contradictory results and improve knowledge of the network alterations connected to the onset and treatment of various illnesses, more research is necessary. Through ADMSC transplantation and exosomes produced from the cells, advancements in ADMSC-related therapy [25] for CNS diseases show promise in improving immune control and brain regeneration. Though preliminary research has yielded encouraging results, additional studies are needed to validate safety and effectiveness in clinical contexts. Additionally, better dose and delivery techniques are needed to improve therapeutic precision.

Nanomedicine [26] is transforming neuro-protection and treatment of CNS disorders through drug delivery and therapies like immunotherapy and gene therapy. Key challenges include assessing long-term effects, biosafety, and standardization. Continued interdisciplinary collaboration and innovation are essential for optimizing nanomaterials and unlocking their potential for improving patient outcomes in neurological care. The analysis in [27] highlights the positive impact of personalized medicine (PM) strategies on oncology care, particularly in mNSCLC and TNBC. By integrating PM into treatment workflows, institutions enhance effectiveness and options for patients. The findings support policy changes and investments, aiming to reduce barriers and improve access to quality cancer care.

Bioprinting [28] enables the creation of 3D tissue-like constructs using living cells and biocompatible materials, with techniques like inkjet and extrusion printing. While promising for personalized tissue regeneration and drug development, challenges remain, such as improving resolution and understanding immune responses. Advances could transform personalized medicine and regulatory practices. The ICPerMed document [29] outlines a roadmap for integrating personalized medicine (PM) into healthcare, providing strategies to overcome barriers and enhance health outcomes. Successful implementation relies on collaboration, ethical commitment, and sustainable investments. Engaging all stakeholders can transform PM into a cornerstone of modern, equitable, and patient-centered healthcare.

Study [30] looked at how professionals, users, and healthy people felt about Personal Health Data Spaces (PHDS) and genetic medicine. Interest in genetic data worries about data ownership, and the significance of autonomy and trust were among the major themes. Although there were several implementation challenges identified, participants thought that PHDS was helpful for decision-making. Technological developments in 3D printing [31] healthcare promise more accurate medications and quicker organ and tissue creation, improving quality of life and individualized medicine. In addition to offering more trustworthy data for medication research and perhaps replacing animal testing, bioprinting can enhance medical education and drastically lower healthcare expenditures.

Advancements in genomics enhance patient care but face challenges like therapy resistance [32]. Incorporating comprehensive genomic profiling, novel immune subtypes, and breakthroughs in transcriptomics can improve personalized medicine and the TNM staging system. Collaborative efforts among healthcare providers, researchers, and policymakers are essential for better managing colorectal cancer and optimizing treatment options.

9.3 FEDERATED LEARNING: A PARADIGM SHIFT IN HEALTHCARE

Federated learning is a decentralized machine learning technique that allows several organizations to work together to jointly train models using locally relevant data. By training models on local datasets and then sharing just the model updates with a central server, FL allows each participating site to maintain control over its own data, as opposed to pooling sensitive data in a single location. This creative framework is especially helpful in the healthcare industry, where patient confidentiality and data security are critical.

9.3.1 Federated learning principles

Data Security and Privacy: Protecting personal information is one of FL's core tenets. By storing patient data locally on servers or devices, FL reduces the possibility of illegal access and data breaches. This is particularly important in the healthcare industry because of how sensitive data is.

Decentralization: FL functions in a decentralized fashion, in contrast to conventional machine learning techniques that depend on centralized data repositories. By allowing each participant to contribute to the model training process without having to divulge their raw data, institutional boundaries are respected and a collaborative environment is fostered.

Model Aggregation: Using its own data, each participating institution in FL trains a local model. A central server receives the resulting model changes (such as gradients), which it then aggregates to produce a global model. By combining knowledge from several datasets, this combined model is more effective and generalizable.

Federated learning follows cycles of iterative learning. The global model is returned to the participants for additional training using their local data once it has been updated. This procedure keeps on until the model performs at a level that is satisfactory, enabling ongoing improvement and modification.

Handling Data Heterogeneity: FL is designed to address the inherent heterogeneity of healthcare data, where patient populations, treatment protocols, and data collection methods can vary significantly across institutions. By accommodating these differences, FL helps create models that are more representative and effective across diverse settings.

Scalability: The decentralized nature of FL allows for easy scaling. As more institutions join the collaborative effort, they can contribute their data insights without overburdening a central database. This scalability is crucial in healthcare, where a wide range of data sources can enhance model training.

Regulation Compliance: FL complies well with laws like HIPAA, which regulates how patient data is used in the healthcare industry. Federated learning assists in ensuring compliance with privacy rules by letting institutions keep control over their data while yet promoting communal learning.

The implementation of FL represents a paradigm change in the healthcare industry, moving away from the conventional centralized data processes and toward a more private-focused, collaborative strategy. This change is especially significant in the context of personalized medicine, since creating individualized treatment plans requires the capacity to use a variety of data sources while maintaining patient privacy. Healthcare practitioners can leverage FL's collective intelligence capabilities without violating patient privacy. This builds confidence between patients and healthcare institutions while also improving the resilience of machine learning models. Federated learning is poised to transform healthcare data utilization and open up opportunities for more efficient, inclusive, and customized medical solutions as it continues to gain popularity.

9.3.2 Collaborative Model Development in Healthcare

Collaborative model development in healthcare involves the collective effort of multiple institutions to create machine learning models that can better analyze and predict patient outcomes. Traditionally, this process required aggregating large datasets in a centralized location, raising significant concerns around data privacy and security. On the other hand, FL presents a novel strategy that permits organizations to work together on model development without exchanging private patient information. Due to FL's ability to provide local model training on each participating institution's dataset, the collaborative model creation process is radically transformed. Each site changes its model based on local patient data rather than providing raw data to a central server; only the model parameters, or gradients, are shared with a central server thereafter. This strategy guarantees that the models benefit from the diversity of data across various healthcare settings while simultaneously protecting patient privacy. The benefits of collaborative model creation are displayed in Table 9.2.

While the benefits of collaborative model development through FL are significant, several challenges must be addressed. Those are, firstly, technical complexity, implementing FL requires sophisticated technical infrastructure and expertise. Healthcare organizations need to invest in the necessary tools and training to effectively participate in collaborative learning. Secondly, data heterogeneity, variations in data formats, collection methods, and patient populations across institutions can complicate model development.

Table 9.2 Advantages of Collaborative Model Development

Advantage	*Description*
Enhanced Data Diversity	Collaborative model development through FL enables the incorporation of diverse patient populations, treatment protocols, and clinical practices from various institutions. This richness of data helps create more robust and generalizable models, ultimately improving their predictive accuracy and effectiveness in real-world scenarios.
Data Privacy and Compliance	FL mitigates privacy concerns associated with centralized data sharing. By keeping sensitive patient information local, healthcare organizations can comply with regulations such as HIPAA while still contributing valuable insights to the collaborative effort. This fosters trust between patients and providers, encouraging participation in research and model development.
Accelerated Innovation	Collaborative efforts facilitated by FL can speed up the development of new predictive models and treatment strategies. By pooling knowledge and insights without compromising data privacy, institutions can share best practices and accelerate research, leading to faster advancements in healthcare solutions.
Reduced Costs	Traditional centralized approaches often require significant investment in data infrastructure and storage. FL reduces these costs by enabling institutions to leverage existing infrastructure while still contributing to collective learning. This makes it more feasible for smaller healthcare organizations to participate in cutting-edge research.
Improved Clinical Decision-Making	Models developed through collaborative efforts in FL can provide healthcare providers with more comprehensive insights into patient care. By analyzing data from multiple sources, these models can help identify trends and outcomes that may not be apparent when examining data from a single institution.

Addressing these differences is crucial to ensure that the resulting models are valid and applicable across diverse settings. Thirdly, regulatory frameworks, although FL helps address privacy concerns, navigating the regulatory landscape remains a challenge. Clear guidelines and frameworks are needed to support the ethical use of federated approaches in healthcare. The paradigm shift brought about by FL is likely to redefine collaborative model development in healthcare. As more institutions recognize the value of shared insights while preserving data privacy, the potential for innovation and improvement in patient care will expand. Future advancements may include the integration of advanced AI techniques, enabling even more sophisticated models that can address complex healthcare challenges.

9.4 APPLICATIONS OF FEDERATED LEARNING IN NEURAL DISORDERS

In 2021, the United States took significant strides in the application of federated learning (FL) within healthcare, particularly concerning neural disorders. Researchers at Stanford University embarked on a groundbreaking study aimed at early detection of Alzheimer's disease. This study utilized FL to analyze MRI data sourced from multiple healthcare institutions. By allowing each hospital to train models on their local data without sharing sensitive patient information, the researchers demonstrated that FL could enhance diagnostic accuracy while ensuring compliance with stringent data privacy regulations like HIPAA. This approach not only improved the model's performance but also set a vital precedent for future research, showcasing how collaborative learning could effectively tackle complex neurological conditions while maintaining patient confidentiality.

Germany emerged as a key player in the realm of FL applications for neural disorders in 2020, particularly with a focus on Parkinson's disease. A collaborative initiative led by the University of Freiburg involved several hospitals that contributed mobility data collected from wearable devices. This data was crucial for understanding the progression of Parkinson's disease. By employing FL, the researchers developed predictive models that could analyze this data collaboratively, thereby optimizing treatment plans for patients. The study highlighted the power of real-time data integration and underscored FL's potential in providing personalized healthcare solutions. It showcased how data from diverse patient populations could lead to a more comprehensive understanding of disease progression, ultimately improving clinical decision-making.

In 2019, Canada made significant contributions to the application of FL in the study of multiple sclerosis (MS). A team at the University of Toronto spearheaded a research project that leveraged federated approaches to analyze imaging data across multiple clinical sites. This study not only focused on the technical aspects of model training but also emphasized the clinical implications of utilizing FL in a real-world healthcare setting. By enabling healthcare providers to draw insights from distributed datasets while preserving the confidentiality of patient information, this research laid the groundwork for more personalized treatment strategies in MS. It demonstrated that collaborative efforts in research could yield better diagnostic tools and treatment options, ultimately leading to enhanced patient outcomes.

Australia's contribution in 2018 focused on advancing FL applications for epilepsy diagnosis and management. Researchers at the University of Sydney implemented a federated framework to analyze electroencephalogram (EEG) data collected from various hospitals across the country. This innovative study allowed clinicians to develop more accurate seizure classification models while ensuring that sensitive EEG recordings remained within the local institutions. By facilitating real-time analysis of patient data, the research aimed to improve the precision of diagnoses and tailor treatment approaches for individuals with epilepsy. This case illustrated the potential of FL to enhance clinical workflows and provide timely interventions, ultimately improving quality of life for patients.

The United Kingdom made noteworthy advancements in FL applications for neural disorders in 2017, particularly in the context of autism spectrum disorder (ASD). A collaborative project among several universities explored the potential of FL to analyze behavioral data collected from children diagnosed with ASD. By employing a federated approach, researchers were able to develop predictive models based on distributed datasets, enriching the understanding of ASD and informing intervention strategies. This initiative emphasized the importance of multi-institutional collaboration in advancing research while protecting patient data. By enabling a richer analysis of diverse behavioral patterns, FL paved the way for more effective and personalized interventions in managing ASD, demonstrating the broader implications of collaborative healthcare research.

The application of FL in neural disorders has evolved significantly over the past several years, with a wealth of contributions from various countries illustrating its transformative potential in healthcare. The case studies from the United States, Germany, Canada, Australia, and the United Kingdom collectively demonstrate how FL enables healthcare institutions to collaborate effectively while preserving patient privacy. From improving diagnostic accuracy and optimizing treatment plans to facilitating real-time data analysis and enhancing clinical decision-making, the benefits of FL are profound. As researchers and healthcare providers continue to explore the capabilities of FL, the resulting innovations are likely to lead to more personalized, efficient, and effective healthcare solutions for individuals suffering from neural disorders.

Customizing treatment plans for neurological illnesses is a challenging task that greatly benefits from the FL collaborative environment. Federated learning makes it easier to create customized therapies that cater to each patient's particular needs by utilizing dispersed data from several healthcare facilities. Patients with neural illnesses, such as those with Parkinson's, Alzheimer's, and multiple sclerosis, vary greatly in terms of their symptoms, course of the disease, and reaction to therapy. A thorough comprehension of this heterogeneity is necessary for these efforts. With the use of FL, researchers can examine data from various patient populations in various healthcare environments, capturing a wide range of patient attributes like as socioeconomic status, environmental impacts, and genetic makeup. This thorough understanding is essential for creating individualized treatment programs that meet the unique requirements of every patient.

Federated learning enables the aggregation of insights from multiple datasets while maintaining patient privacy. For example, institutions can contribute their local models trained on proprietary data, which can then be aggregated to create a more robust global model. This global model, enriched with information from various sources, can provide valuable data-driven insights that inform treatment strategies. By identifying trends and patterns that emerge from a broader dataset, healthcare providers can better predict how individual patients might respond to specific interventions. Federated learning aligns seamlessly with the principles of precision medicine, which aims to tailor treatments based on individual patient profiles. In the context of neural disorders, this could mean developing specific pharmacological interventions that consider a patient's genetic makeup, disease stage, and co-morbidities. For instance, researchers can use FL to analyze the effectiveness of different medications across various demographics, identifying which treatments work best for specific patient subgroups. This information can guide clinicians in selecting the most appropriate therapies, enhancing the likelihood of successful outcomes.

One of the significant advantages of FL is its ability to support continuous learning. As new patient data is generated whether from ongoing clinical trials or real-world treatment FL allows models to be updated iteratively without compromising data privacy. This adaptability is particularly important for chronic neural disorders, where treatment responses can change over time. Clinicians can use these updated models to adjust treatment strategies in real time, ensuring that interventions remain effective as patient needs evolve. Federated learning can enhance clinical decision support systems (CDSS) by providing access to robust, real-time predictive models that incorporate insights from diverse patient populations. For example, an FL model trained on data from multiple hospitals could help clinicians assess the risk factors for complications in patients with Parkinson's disease. By analyzing data from a broader demographic, the CDSS can generate personalized recommendations that help clinicians make informed decisions about treatment options and patient management strategies.

The collaborative nature of FL fosters innovation in treatment strategies. By enabling multiple institutions to share insights without compromising patient data, researchers can work together to develop and validate new therapeutic approaches. For instance, a consortium of hospitals could focus on a specific neural disorder, pooling their findings to identify novel biomarkers or treatment pathways that would not be apparent in isolated studies. This collaborative environment accelerates the pace of research and enhances the quality of treatment strategies developed. Customizing treatment strategies in healthcare raises ethical considerations regarding data use and patient consent. Federated learning addresses these concerns by enabling institutions to maintain control over their patient data while still contributing to collective learning. This respect for patient privacy fosters trust and encourages participation in research, ultimately leading to more comprehensive and effective treatment strategies.

The integration of FL into clinical practice can transform how healthcare providers approach the customization of treatment strategies. Training and equipping clinicians with the tools to leverage FL insights will empower them to make data-informed decisions tailored to each patient. This could lead to improved patient adherence to treatment plans, as individuals are more likely to engage with interventions that are specifically designed for their unique circumstances. By harnessing the collective intelligence derived from diverse patient data while safeguarding privacy, FL enables the development of tailored interventions that improve patient outcomes. This collaborative approach not only enhances the understanding of neural disorders but also empowers healthcare providers to make informed, personalized treatment decisions. As FL continues to evolve, its applications in customizing treatment strategies are poised to play a pivotal role in advancing precision medicine and improving the quality of care for individuals affected by neural disorders.

9.5 PRIVACY PRESERVATION AND DATA SECURITY

The integration of FL in personalized medicine, particularly for tailoring therapies for neural disorders, hinges on the effective protection of patient data. As healthcare increasingly adopts data-driven approaches, safeguarding sensitive patient information while enabling collaborative research is paramount. Key mechanisms that FL employs to protect patient data are shown in Table 9.3.

Protecting patient data in the context of federated learning and personalized medicine is multifaceted, involving a combination of data locality, model updates, advanced cryptographic techniques, and robust access controls. As healthcare continues to evolve toward more data-driven approaches, these mechanisms are essential for ensuring that patient privacy is maintained while enabling the collaborative development of tailored therapies for neural disorders.

9.5.1 Ethical Considerations in FL

As FL becomes increasingly integrated into personalized medicine, particularly for neural disorders, several ethical considerations emerge. These considerations are essential to ensure that the deployment of FL respects patient rights, promotes equity, and adheres to legal standards. Key ethical dimensions associated with FL are shown in Table 9.4.

Ethical considerations in FL are vital for fostering a responsible approach to the integration of advanced technologies in personalized medicine. By addressing issues such as patient privacy, informed consent, equity, bias, accountability, data ownership, and the impact on clinical practice, stakeholders can ensure that FL serves the best interests of patients and contributes positively to the healthcare landscape. As FL continues to evolve, ongoing dialogue about these ethical dimensions will be crucial for maintaining trust and integrity in the pursuit of tailored therapies for neural disorders.

Table 9.3 Mechanisms for Protecting Patient Data

Mechanism	*Description*
Data Locality	Instead of centralizing patient data in a single repository, FL allows each healthcare institution to retain control of its data. Local models are trained on-site, meaning that sensitive information never leaves the institution's secure environment.
Model Updates Instead of Raw Data	Only model updates such as gradients or weights are shared with a central server, rather than the raw patient data itself. This mechanism minimizes the exposure of sensitive information, as the updates do not contain identifiable patient details. The aggregation of these updates from multiple institutions creates a robust global model without compromising individual patient privacy.
Differential Privacy	It involves altering the model updates by adding noise before sharing them. Differential privacy ensures that each patient's data contribution gets hidden within the broader dataset, offering a mathematical assurance that individual data points cannot be re-identified. This method is critical to the healthcare industry since patient trust and regulatory compliance depend on maintaining confidentiality.
Secure Multi-Party Computation (SMPC)	It permits the joint computation of a function over the inputs of many people while maintaining the privacy of those inputs. This implies that institutions can work together to create models in the framework of FL without ever disclosing their raw data to one another. Throughout the collaborative learning process, sensitive information is protected by utilizing cryptographic techniques.
Homomorphic Encryption	Makes it possible to compute on encrypted data, thus model training and evaluation can take place without the need to first decrypt the data. Without the right decryption keys, data stays safe and unreadable even if it is intercepted during transit. This approach guarantees confidentiality at all times and is especially helpful for securing patient data when it is in transit.
Access Control and Authentication	Updates to the models and sensitive data should only be accessible by authorized staff. Ensuring that only authorized individuals can interact with the data and participate in the model training process is made possible by the implementation of robust authentication procedures. It also improves the collaborative research effort's overall integrity.
Auditing and Compliance	Regular auditing of data access and usage is essential to ensure compliance with regulations such as HIPAA. By maintaining detailed logs of who accessed data, what actions were taken, and when, healthcare institutions can monitor for unauthorized access and ensure that patient data is being handled responsibly. These auditing mechanisms foster accountability and help institutions maintain compliance with legal and ethical standards.
Transparency and Patient Consent	Engaging patients in the process is crucial for building trust. Clear communication about how their data will be used, the measures in place to protect their privacy, and the benefits of participating in FL initiatives can enhance patient willingness to share data for research purposes. Obtaining informed consent ensures that patients are aware of the data protection mechanisms in place, fostering a collaborative relationship between healthcare providers and patients.

Table 9.4 Ethical Considerations in FL

Parameter	*Description*
Patient Privacy & Confidentiality	It is imperative to guarantee that the shared model parameters do not allow for the re-identification of specific patient information. To maintain ethical standards in data management, researchers and institutions need to have strong privacy protections in place, like secure multi-party computation and differential privacy.
Informed Consent	Patients must be fully aware of how their data will be used, the implications of participating in FL initiatives, and the potential benefits and risks involved. Clear communication about the processes involved in FL, including how data will be protected and utilized, is essential to foster trust and ensure ethical participation.
Equity & Access	There is a risk that some institutions, particularly those with fewer resources, may be left out of collaborative FL efforts, potentially exacerbating existing healthcare disparities. Ensuring that all healthcare providers have the opportunity to participate in FL initiatives can help create a more equitable healthcare landscape, where diverse patient populations are represented in the development of personalized therapies.
Bias & Fairness	Data bias can significantly impact the outcomes of machine learning models. If the data used to train FL models is not representative of the broader population, it can lead to biased treatment recommendations, particularly for underrepresented groups. Ethical FL practices must include strategies for identifying and mitigating bias, ensuring that models are fair and equitable across different demographics, including age, gender, ethnicity, and socioeconomic status.
Accountability & Transparency	Researchers and healthcare institutions must be transparent about the methodologies used, the sources of data, and the algorithms implemented in the training of models. Establishing clear lines of accountability ensures that stakeholders can be held responsible for any adverse outcomes resulting from the use of FL, reinforcing trust in the system.
Data Ownership and Control	Institutions and patients must have clarity regarding who owns the data and the models generated from that data. Ethical guidelines should address how data can be used and shared, ensuring that patient rights are respected. Patients should retain the right to withdraw their consent at any time, and there must be mechanisms in place to honor such requests.
Impact on Clinical Practice	Healthcare providers should be trained to interpret and contextualize the outputs of FL models, ensuring that they supplement rather than replace clinical judgment.
Long-Term Consequences	As FL models evolve and are integrated into clinical practice, ongoing evaluations of their impact on patient outcomes and healthcare systems will be necessary. Researchers and institutions must remain vigilant about the potential unintended consequences of deploying FL, continuously assessing whether the benefits outweigh any ethical concerns that arise.

9.6 ADDRESSING DATA HETEROGENEITY

Table 9.5 explores the different challenges in heterogeneous datasets in the context of addressing data heterogeneity.

Successfully addressing data heterogeneity in diverse datasets is critical for the effective tailoring of neural disorder therapies. Collaborative approaches, robust privacy safeguards, and continuous engagement with clinical stakeholders are essential to overcoming these challenges and improving patient outcomes. Integrating varied data sources to address data heterogeneity in tailoring neural disorder therapies involves several

Table 9.5 Challenges in Diverse Datasets

Challenge	*Description*
Variability in Data Sources	Data collected from various hospitals and clinics may follow different protocols, leading to inconsistencies in measurements, imaging techniques, and diagnostic criteria. Variations in demographics, genetic backgrounds across patient populations can affect treatment responses and complicate model training.
Non-IID Data Distribution	Since patient data is frequently not identically distributed or independent (non-IID), creating a generalized model that works effectively for all patient groups is challenging. Dataset outliers have the potential to change model predictions and affect how well-customized treatments work.
Model Personalization	Tailoring therapies requires models that can adapt to individual patient characteristics, necessitating complex algorithms that can handle this variability without overfitting. Finding the right balance between personalized models and those that generalize well across populations is a significant challenge.
Privacy & Security	Requiring robust mechanisms to protect patient information during model training. Ensuring compliance with healthcare regulations (e.g., HIPAA) while leveraging diverse datasets adds complexity to data handling and model deployment.
Communication and Computational Constraints	Healthcare institutions may have varying levels of computational resources and internet connectivity, impacting the feasibility of centralized data sharing or federated learning. Delays in communication for model updates can hinder timely interventions, which are crucial in treating neural disorders.
Interpretability and Trust	The complexity of neural networks can lead to difficulties in interpreting model decisions, making it hard for clinicians to trust AI-driven recommendations. Ensuring that model outputs are clinically relevant and understandable is essential for acceptance in practice.
Evaluation & Validation	Developing standardized evaluation metrics that account for diverse patient populations and clinical outcomes is challenging. Addressing potential biases in training datasets is crucial to ensure that tailored therapies are equitable and effective for all patient groups.

strategic approaches. First, establishing common data models (e.g., FHIR, OMOP) ensures consistency across healthcare systems, while data harmonization aligns terminologies and measurement units. Utilizing FL allows decentralized model training without centralizing sensitive data, ensuring privacy through secure aggregation techniques.

Implementing robust data integration methods, such as data fusion and multimodal learning, enhances predictive accuracy by combining diverse datasets. Addressing non-IID challenges with adaptive learning algorithms and transfer learning facilitates better generalization across populations. Ensuring data quality through rigorous cleaning and quality assurance is essential, alongside fostering collaborative data-sharing frameworks and ethical guidelines for data governance. Training stakeholders on these practices and maintaining continuous feedback loops for model updates further enhance the integration process. Collectively, these strategies improve the effectiveness of personalized therapies in healthcare, ultimately leading to better patient outcomes.

9.7 ALGORITHMIC FAIRNESS IN FL

9.7.1 Importance of inclusivity in AI models

Inclusivity in AI models is crucial for ensuring algorithmic fairness, particularly in the context of federated learning. As FL involves collaboration across diverse datasets from multiple institutions, incorporating inclusivity helps address several key issues. Inclusive AI models are designed to account for the diverse characteristics of different population groups. By incorporating a wide range of data sources, federated learning can mitigate biases that arise from underrepresented groups, leading to fairer outcomes. Models trained on inclusive datasets are better equipped to generalize across various demographics. This is particularly important in healthcare, where patient characteristics can significantly affect treatment responses. Ensuring that models learn from diverse data enhances their applicability in real-world scenarios.

Incorporating inclusivity fosters trust among stakeholders, including patients and healthcare providers. When AI systems are perceived as fair and representative, there is greater confidence in their recommendations and outcomes, facilitating broader acceptance and usage. Inclusivity aligns with ethical guidelines and regulatory requirements regarding fairness and non-discrimination. By proactively addressing potential disparities, organizations can avoid legal pitfalls and uphold ethical standards in AI development. AI models that reflect diverse populations are more likely to identify effective treatments for various groups, ultimately leading to improved health outcomes. Inclusivity ensures that all patients receive personalized care tailored to their unique characteristics. Incorporating inclusivity in AI models within federated learning frameworks is vital for achieving algorithmic fairness. It helps reduce bias, enhances model generalization, builds trust, ensures compliance with ethical standards, and improves patient outcomes, paving the way for more equitable AI applications in healthcare and beyond.

The different types of inclusive AI models in the context of FL are shown below. Fairness-aware models in FL focus on mitigating biases that arise from imbalanced datasets across participating nodes. By employing techniques such as reweighting or adjusting loss functions to emphasize underrepresented groups, these models aim to ensure that all demographic segments are treated equitably. In the healthcare context, this could mean adjusting the model to account for variations in disease prevalence or treatment responses among different ethnic or socioeconomic groups, thereby promoting equitable healthcare outcomes. Federated transfer learning models leverage knowledge gained from one dataset to improve performance on another, especially in scenarios where some nodes have limited data. By transferring learned features from well-represented groups to those with fewer samples, these models enhance inclusivity. In healthcare, this approach can be particularly beneficial when training models on data from diverse populations, allowing insights from larger datasets to inform better predictions for minority groups, thus enhancing personalized treatment strategies.

Multi-task learning models in federated learning allow simultaneous training on multiple related tasks across different institutions, facilitating the sharing of knowledge while maintaining data privacy. This approach is beneficial in healthcare, where related outcomes (such as various health conditions) can be predicted collaboratively. By training on multiple tasks, these models can capture diverse patient profiles and interactions among diseases, leading to more holistic and inclusive healthcare solutions. Diverse ensemble models combine predictions from multiple individual models trained on different subsets of data, thereby leveraging the strengths of each. In the federated learning context, each node can contribute a unique perspective based on its local dataset, resulting in a more comprehensive model. This approach increases inclusivity by ensuring that diverse patient experiences and responses are considered, ultimately improving the model's robustness and fairness across varied populations.

Privacy-preserving inclusive models prioritize patient confidentiality while ensuring diverse representation in training. Techniques like differential privacy or homomorphic encryption allow models to learn from varied datasets without exposing sensitive information. In healthcare, this enables institutions to collaborate on AI models that benefit from inclusivity while adhering to stringent privacy regulations, ensuring that all patient demographics can contribute to and benefit from the model's insights. Each of these inclusive AI models plays a vital role in enhancing fairness and representation in federated learning, particularly in healthcare, where diversity in patient data is critical for effective treatment and outcomes. By addressing biases and promoting equitable solutions, these models help ensure that AI applications are just and effective for all population segments.

9.7.2 Techniques for Ensuring Fair Outcomes

Ensuring fair outcomes in the context of algorithmic fairness in FL involves several key techniques designed to mitigate biases and enhance equity across diverse datasets. Here are some of the most effective techniques. Data preprocessing techniques focus on addressing imbalances before model training. This may involve re-sampling methods like under-sampling majority classes or over-sampling minority classes to create a more balanced dataset. Additionally, techniques like data augmentation can help generate synthetic data for underrepresented groups, ensuring that the model learns adequately from all demographics.

Incorporating fairness-aware loss functions during training allows models to explicitly account for fairness metrics. These loss functions can penalize models for making biased predictions against certain groups, effectively guiding the learning process to produce fairer outcomes. For instance, a loss function might be adjusted to prioritize minimizing error rates equally across different demographic groups, rather than just focusing on overall accuracy. Bias mitigation algorithms are designed to identify and correct for biases during the model training process. Techniques such as adversarial debiasing, where an adversarial model is trained to detect and reduce bias in predictions, can be employed. In FL, these algorithms can help ensure that the model's predictions are equitable across various participating nodes, making adjustments based on the demographic makeup of the data.

Regularization techniques can help promote generalization while reducing the risk of overfitting to biased data. By applying constraints that encourage the model to perform uniformly well across different groups, these techniques help mitigate the impact of data imbalance. For example, group fairness regularization can ensure that the model's performance is similar for all demographic groups, thereby fostering equitable outcomes. Utilizing specific evaluation metrics to assess fairness is crucial for understanding and improving model performance across different groups. Metrics such as demographic parity, equal opportunity, and disparate impact can be applied to evaluate how well the model treats various demographic segments. Regularly monitoring these metrics during the model development process allows practitioners to make informed adjustments to enhance fairness.

Ensemble methods combine predictions from multiple models trained on different subsets of data, allowing for a more comprehensive understanding of diverse patient profiles. By aggregating outputs from various models, ensemble approaches can balance biases that individual models might have.

This technique can lead to more robust and fair predictions by ensuring that diverse perspectives are included in the final decision-making process. In FL, implementing collaborative model updates allows different nodes to contribute to a shared model while maintaining local data privacy. Techniques such as secure aggregation ensure that model updates are shared in a way that reflects the performance across diverse datasets. This collaborative approach can help identify and rectify biases, leading to more equitable outcomes.

Establishing mechanisms for continuous monitoring of model performance and fairness after deployment is essential. Gathering feedback from stakeholders and using real-world performance data can help identify potential biases that were not evident during training. Regular audits and updates based on this feedback ensure that the model remains fair and effective over time. By employing these techniques, FL can significantly enhance algorithmic fairness, ensuring that AI models produce equitable outcomes across diverse populations. This commitment to fairness is particularly important in sensitive domains like healthcare, where biased predictions can have profound implications for patient care and outcomes.

9.8 INTEGRATION WITHIN CLINICAL WORKFLOWS

Federated learning has shown promise as a means of improving healthcare, especially in the area of treating neurological disorders. Federated learning's ability to train machine learning models on decentralized data without requiring the centralization of sensitive patient data is one of its main features. This quality is especially important in the healthcare industry, where regulatory compliance and privacy concerns are top priorities. Federated learning may enhance the efficacy of therapeutic interventions and predictive models by permitting institutions to cooperate on training models while maintaining the localization of patient data, all while guaranteeing data security.

In the context of neural disorder therapies, FL can facilitate the development of personalized treatment plans. For instance, hospitals can share insights on patient outcomes and treatment responses without disclosing individual patient data. By aggregating knowledge across diverse datasets from various demographics and clinical settings FL can help create more robust models that account for variability in response to therapies. This approach is especially crucial in treating neural disorders, where patient responses can be highly individualized. For example, models developed through FL can identify specific biomarkers or genetic markers associated with treatment efficacy, leading to tailored therapies that optimize outcomes for different patient populations.

The field of remote patient monitoring and rehabilitation for individuals with neurological diseases is one area where FL is being used practically in healthcare settings. Real-time data on patients' neurological status can be gathered using wearable technology and mobile health apps, facilitating ongoing evaluation and prompt actions. Federated learning enables these devices to learn from the data generated across multiple patients, enhancing the algorithms that drive the monitoring systems. As these systems improve, healthcare providers can better understand how different therapies impact patient progress, leading to more informed clinical decisions and improved rehabilitation protocols. Federated learning can support research and clinical trials by providing access to a broader range of patient data without compromising privacy.

Collaborative research initiatives can utilize FL to analyze data from multiple institutions, increasing the statistical power of studies and enabling the discovery of new insights into neural disorders. This collaborative approach can accelerate the development of innovative therapies and enhance the overall understanding of neural disorders, fostering a more effective and responsive healthcare system. By leveraging decentralized data, improving personalized treatment strategies, enhancing remote monitoring, and facilitating collaborative research, FL can contribute to more effective and secure healthcare solutions. As technology and regulatory frameworks continue to evolve, the integration of FL into healthcare practices may well redefine how we approach the treatment of complex neural disorders.

The integration of FL into clinical decision-making, particularly in the context of personalized medicine for neural disorder therapies, represents a transformative shift in how healthcare providers approach treatment strategies. By leveraging decentralized data from multiple institutions, FL enhances the ability to tailor interventions to individual patient needs, ultimately leading to improved clinical outcomes. One of the most significant impacts of FL on clinical decision-making is the enhancement of predictive models used in diagnosing and treating neural disorders. Traditional models often rely on centralized datasets, which may not capture the full spectrum of patient variability. In contrast, FL enables the aggregation of diverse patient data while maintaining privacy, leading to the development of more generalized models that account for variations in genetics, demographics, and disease progression. This ability to create robust, data-informed models allows clinicians to make better-informed decisions, optimizing therapy selection and timing for each patient.

Federated learning promotes continuous learning from real-world patient outcomes. By allowing healthcare providers to contribute insights from their own clinical experiences without compromising patient confidentiality, FL facilitates the dynamic refinement of treatment algorithms. Clinicians can access updated models that reflect the latest trends in patient responses, which is particularly crucial for neural disorders that can vary widely in manifestation and treatment effectiveness. This continuous feedback loop enhances the agility of clinical decision-making, enabling practitioners to adjust therapies based on the most current evidence and patient experiences. The personalized approach fostered by FL also empowers patients to become active participants in their care. With access to tailored treatment recommendations and ongoing monitoring, patients can engage more meaningfully in their health management.

Federated learning can facilitate collaborative decision-making among multidisciplinary teams in healthcare settings. By sharing insights derived from aggregated data across various specialties neurology, psychiatry, and rehabilitation clinicians can develop holistic treatment plans that consider the multifaceted nature of neural disorders. This collaborative approach can lead to more comprehensive care strategies that address not just the clinical symptoms but also the psychosocial aspects of patient well-being. The impact of FL on clinical decision-making in the context of personalized medicine for neural disorder therapies is profound. By enhancing the accuracy of predictive models, promoting continuous learning from diverse patient data, empowering patient engagement, and fostering collaborative care, FL paves the way for more tailored, effective, and responsive healthcare solutions. As these technologies continue to evolve, they hold the potential to significantly improve outcomes for individuals affected by neural disorders, marking a new era in personalized medicine.

Federated learning is poised to revolutionize precision medicine, particularly in the field of neural disorder therapies. By enabling the secure and efficient use of decentralized data from diverse healthcare institutions, FL facilitates the development of highly personalized treatment strategies. This approach allows researchers and clinicians to build robust models that reflect a wide array of patient experiences and genetic backgrounds, significantly enhancing the precision of diagnoses and treatment plans. As a result, FL [31] accelerates the shift from a one-size-fits-all model to tailored therapies that consider individual patient characteristics, ultimately improving patient outcomes in neural disorders.

The implementation of FL has demonstrated notable improvements in treatment efficacy. By aggregating data from multiple sources, while maintaining patient confidentiality, FL enables the training of algorithms that can identify which treatments are most effective for specific subgroups of patients. For example, in neural disorders such as depression or epilepsy, FL can help identify biomarkers that predict responses to various therapies, allowing clinicians to personalize interventions more accurately. This enhanced [32] understanding not only improves the likelihood of successful treatment but also minimizes adverse effects and ineffective interventions, thereby optimizing resource utilization in healthcare.

Looking ahead, several future directions for FL in the context of personalized medicine are emerging. One promising avenue is the integration of multimodal data sources, such as genetic, imaging, and behavioral data, to develop more comprehensive models of neural disorders. Additionally, as wearable technology and remote monitoring systems proliferate, FL can facilitate real-time data collection and analysis, enabling clinicians to adjust treatments dynamically based on ongoing patient feedback. Another important direction is the establishment of regulatory frameworks that support the widespread adoption of FL in clinical practice.

The future of FL in precision medicine is ripe with potential developments that can further enhance its impact on neural disorder therapies. For instance, advancements in federated optimization techniques could lead to faster convergence of models, reducing the time required to translate research findings into clinical applications. Moreover, integrating artificial intelligence with FL could provide even more sophisticated analytical tools, enabling deeper learning from complex datasets and enhancing the precision of treatment recommendations. In addition, fostering patient engagement through digital platforms that allow individuals to contribute their data securely could create a more participatory model of care. This not only empowers patients but also enriches the data pool available for FL, leading to more nuanced insights into treatment efficacy across diverse populations. Federated learning holds tremendous promise for accelerating precision medicine and tailoring neural disorder therapies. By enhancing treatment efficacy, exploring future directions, and embracing potential developments, FL can significantly transform the landscape of healthcare, offering more effective, personalized solutions that cater to the unique needs of each patient.

9.9 CONCLUSIONS

Federated learning [33] marks a pivotal advancement in the pursuit of personalized medicine, especially within the realm of neural disorders. By facilitating collaborative model development across diverse datasets while prioritizing patient privacy, FL enables healthcare providers to tailor therapeutic interventions to individual needs. This decentralized approach not only enhances the effectiveness of treatments but also ensures that AI models reflect a broad spectrum of patient demographics, thereby mitigating biases that can affect clinical outcomes. Furthermore, FL accelerates the evolution of precision medicine by addressing critical challenges such as data heterogeneity, algorithmic fairness, and seamless integration into clinical workflows. Federated learning has the potential to advance tailored medicines as it continues to transform healthcare procedures, which would eventually improve patient outcomes and provide a more welcoming healthcare atmosphere. Federated learning is establishing [34] the way for a future when individualized, successful therapies become the norm, greatly improving the management of brain illnesses and supporting the larger objectives of Healthcare 6.0 by utilizing the combined knowledge of multiple institutions. With further innovation and cooperation, FL is positioned to significantly alter the personalized medicine scene.

With FL, customized medicine has enormous [35] promise to improve patient outcomes and change the way healthcare is delivered, especially when it comes to neurological illnesses. Federated learning can result in more robust and comprehensive models that more accurately reflect the varied needs of patient populations since it makes it possible for data to be shared securely and effectively across numerous healthcare organizations. The capacity of FL to combine data from multiple sources, including real-time health monitoring equipment, genetic data, and electronic health records, without compromising patient privacy, is one of its most promising features. By giving medical professionals a more comprehensive understanding of each patient, this integration can help them create extremely individualized treatment programs that are based on a patient's unique genetic, environmental, and lifestyle characteristics.

Federated learning can enhance the speed and accuracy of clinical decision-making. By continuously learning from real-world data and patient outcomes, FL-enabled systems can adapt and refine therapeutic strategies, ensuring that treatments remain relevant and effective. This dynamic learning process is crucial in managing complex neural disorders, where treatment responses can vary widely among individuals. Federated learning promotes collaboration among researchers and clinicians, facilitating the sharing of insights and best practices across institutions. This collaborative approach can accelerate the discovery of new biomarkers and treatment modalities, fostering innovation in therapeutic strategies. As FL technology advances, we can also expect improvements in algorithmic fairness and inclusivity. By aggregating data from diverse populations, FL helps ensure that AI models are not only accurate but also representative, minimizing health disparities and improving access to personalized care.

In summary, the future of personalized medicine with FL is bright, characterized by more tailored, effective, and equitable healthcare solutions. As the integration of FL into clinical practice continues to evolve, it will likely play a central role in shaping the next generation of personalized therapies, making healthcare more responsive to the unique needs of each patient.

REFERENCES

[1] Kabashkin, I. Digital Twin Framework for Aircraft Lifecycle Management Based on Data-Driven Models. *Mathematics* 2024, *12*, 2979. https://doi.org/10.3390/math12192979

[2] Zhang, Y.; Shi, Y.; Zhao, X. Bidirectional Corrective Model-Contrastive Federated Adversarial Training. *Electronics* 2024, *13*, 3745. https://doi.org/10.3390/electronics13183745

[3] Alba, E.L.; Oliveira, G.A.; Ribeiro, M.H.D.M.; Rodrigues, É.O. Electricity Consumption Forecasting: An Approach Using Cooperative Ensemble Learning with SHapley Additive exPlanations. *Forecasting* 2024, *6*, 839–863. https://doi.org/10.3390/forecast6030042

[4] Sheng, X.; Yu, C.; Zhou, Y.; Cui, X. Reputation-Driven Asynchronous Federated Learning for Optimizing Communication Efficiency in Big Data Labeling Systems. *Mathematics* 2024, *12*, 2932. https://doi.org/10.3390/math12182932

[5] Liberti, F.; Berardi, D.; Martini, B. Federated Learning in Dynamic and Heterogeneous Environments: Advantages, Performances, and Privacy Problems. *Applied Sciences* 2024, *14*, 8490. https://doi.org/10.3390/app14188490

[6] Moshawrab, M.; Adda, M.; Bouzouane, A.; Ibrahim, H.; Raad, A. A Maneuver in the Trade-Off Space of Federated Learning Aggregation Frameworks Secured with Polymorphic Encryption: PolyFLAM and PolyFLAP Frameworks. *Electronics* 2024, *13*, 3716. https://doi.org/10.3390/electronics13183716

[7] Zhang, J.; Qiao, Z. SoFL: Clustered Federated Learning Based on Dual Clustering for Heterogeneous Data. *Electronics* 2024, *13*, 3682. https://doi.org/10.3390/electronics13183682

[8] Yan, L.; Wang, L.; Li, G.; Shao, J.; Xia, Z. Secure Dynamic Scheduling for Federated Learning in Underwater Wireless IoT Networks. *Journal of Marine Science and Engineering* 2024, *12*, 1656. https://doi.org/10.3390/jmse12091656

[9] Moshawrab, M.; Adda, M.; Bouzouane, A.; Ibrahim, H.; Raad, A. Securing Federated Learning: Approaches, Mechanisms and Opportunities. *Electronics* 2024, *13*, 3675. https://doi.org/10.3390/electronics13183675

[10] Djolev, D.; Lazarova, M.; Nakov, O. FBLearn: Decentralized Platform for Federated Learning on Blockchain. *Electronics* 2024, *13*, 3672. https://doi.org/10.3390/electronics13183672

[11] Naeem, M.A.; Meng, Y.; Chaudhary, S. The Impact of Federated Learning on Improving the IoT-Based Network in a Sustainable Smart Cities. *Electronics* 2024, *13*, 3653. https://doi.org/10.3390/electronics13183653

[12] Wu, N.; Lin, X.; Lu, J.; Zhang, F.; Chen, W.; Tang, J.; Xiao, J. Byzantine-Robust Multimodal Federated Learning Framework for Intelligent Connected Vehicle. *Electronics* 2024, *13*, 3635. https://doi.org/10.3390/electronics13183635

[13] Sharma, A.; Khullar, V.; Kansal, I.; Chhabra, G.; Arora, P.; Popli, R.; Kumar, R. Gas Detection and Classification Using Multimodal Data Based on Federated Learning. *Sensors* 2024, *24*, 5904. https://doi.org/10.3390/s24185904

[14] Sittijuk, P.; Tamee, K. Fed-RHLP: Enhancing Federated Learning with Random High-Local Performance Client Selection for Improved Convergence and Accuracy. *Symmetry* 2024, *16*, 1181. https://doi.org/10.3390/sym16091181

[15] Khan, R.; Tariq, N.; Ashraf, M.; Khan, F.A.; Shafi, S.; Ali, A. FL-DSFA: Securing RPL-Based IoT Networks against Selective Forwarding

Attacks Using Federated Learning. *Sensors* 2024, *24*, 5834. https://doi.org/10.3390/s24175834
[16] Kanchan, S.; Jang, J.W.; Yoon, J.Y.; Choi, B.J. GSFedSec: Group Signature-Based Secure Aggregation for Privacy Preservation in Federated Learning. *Appl. Sci.* 2024, *14*, 7993. https://doi.org/10.3390/app14177993
[17] Yan, J.; Li, Y.; Yin, S.; Kang, X.; Wang, J.; Zhang, H.; Hu, B. An Efficient Greedy Hierarchical Federated Learning Training Method Based on Trusted Execution Environments. *Electronics* 2024, *13*, 3548. https://doi.org/10.3390/electronics13173548
[18] Hossain, M.M.; Islam, M.R.; Ahamed, M.F.; Ahsan, M.; Haider, J. A Collaborative Federated Learning Framework for Lung and Colon Cancer Classifications. *Technologies* 2024, *12*, 151. https://doi.org/10.3390/technologies12090151
[19] Kumar, M.; Kim, S. Securing the Internet of Health Things: Embedded Federated Learning-Driven Long Short-Term Memory for Cyberattack Detection. *Electronics* 2024, *13*, 3461. https://doi.org/10.3390/electronics13173461
[20] Hernandez-Cruz, N.; Saha, P.; Sarker, M.M.K.; Noble, J.A. Review of Federated Learning and Machine Learning-Based Methods for Medical Image Analysis. *Big Data and Cognitive Computing* 2024, *8*, 99. https://doi.org/10.3390/bdcc8090099
[21] López-Pardo, M.J.; Calvache-Mateo, A.; Martín-Núñez, J.; Heredia-Ciuró, A.; López-López, L.; Valenza, M.C.; Cabrera-Martos, I. Routine Physical Therapy with and without Neural Mobilization in Chronic Musculoskeletal Neck Disorders with Nerve-Related Symptoms: Systematic Review and Meta-Analysis. *Healthcare* 2024, *12*, 1225. https://doi.org/10.3390/healthcare12121225
[22] Nag, A., Das, A., Sil, R., Kar, A., Mandal, D., Das, B. Application of Artificial Intelligence in Mental Health. In: Abraham, A., Pllana, S., Casalino, G., Ma, K., Bajaj, A. (eds) *Intelligent Systems Design and Applications. ISDA 2022*. Lecture Notes in Networks and Systems, vol. 646, 2023. Springer, Cham. https://doi.org/10.1007/978-3-031-27440-4_13
[23] Kozlowska, K.; Schollar-Root, O.; Savage, B.; Hawkes, C.; Chudleigh, C.; Raghunandan, J.; Scher, S.; Helgeland, H. Illness-Promoting Psychological Processes in Children and Adolescents with Functional Neurological Disorder. *Children* 2023, *10*, 1724. https://doi.org/10.3390/children10111724
[24] Wu, K.; Lo, Y.T.; Cavaleri, J.; Bergosh, M.; Ipe, J.; Briggs, R.G.; Jann, K.B.; Murray, S.B.; Mason, X.L.; Liu, C.Y.; et al. Neuromodulation of Eating Disorders: A Review of Underlying Neural Network Activity and Neuromodulatory Treatments. *Brain Science* 2024, *14*, 200. https://doi.org/10.3390/brainsci14030200
[25] Wu, H.; Fan, Y.; Zhang, M. Advanced Progress in the Role of Adipose-Derived Mesenchymal Stromal/Stem Cells in the Application of Central Nervous System Disorders. *Pharmaceutics* 2023, *15*, 2637. https://doi.org/10.3390/pharmaceutics15112637
[26] Krsek, A.; Jagodic, A.; Baticic, L. Nanomedicine in Neuroprotection, Neuroregeneration, and Blood–Brain Barrier Modulation: A Narrative

Review. *Medicina* 2024, *60*, 1384. https://doi.org/10.3390/medicina60091384

[27] Agarwal, A.; Pritchard, D.; Winzeler, A.; Mohammed, H.; Brown, T.D.; Gustavsen, G.G. Improvements in Clinical Cancer Care Associated with Integration of Personalized Medicine. *Journal of Personalized Medicine* 2024, *14*, 997. https://doi.org/10.3390/jpm14090997

[28] Lam, E.H.Y.; Yu, F.; Zhu, S.; Wang, Z. 3D Bioprinting for Next-Generation Personalized Medicine. *International Journal of Molecular Sciences* 2023, *24*, 6357. https://doi.org/10.3390/ijms24076357

[29] Cinti, C.; Trivella, M.G.; Joulie, M.; Ayoub, H.; Frenzel, M. On behalf of the International Consortium for Personalised Medicine and Working Group 'Personalised Medicine in Healthcare' (WG2). The Roadmap toward Personalized Medicine: Challenges and Opportunities. Journal of Personalized Medicine 2024, *14*, 546. https://doi.org/10.3390/jpm14060546

[30] Tommel, J.; Kenis, D.; Lambrechts, N.; Brohet, R.M.; Swysen, J.; Mollen, L.; Hoefmans, M.-J.F.; Pusparum, M.; Evers, A.W.M.; Ertaylan, G.; et al. Personal Genomes in Practice: Exploring Citizen and Healthcare Professionals' Perspectives on Personalized Genomic Medicine and Personal Health Data Spaces Using a Mixed-Methods Design. *Genes* 2023, *14*, 786. https://doi.org/10.3390/genes14040786

[31] Shopova, D.; Yaneva, A.; Bakova, D.; Mihaylova, A.; Kasnakova, P.; Hristozova, M.; Sbirkov, Y.; Sarafian, V.; Semerdzhieva, M. (Bio) printing in Personalized Medicine—Opportunities and Potential Benefits. *Bioengineering* 2023, *10*, 287. https://doi.org/10.3390/bioengineering10030287

[32] Kishor Kumar Reddy, C.; Badam, R.; Ahmed, S. IoT Driven Accessibility:A Refreshable OCR-Braille Solution for Visually Impaired and Deaf-Blind Users Through WSN. *JETECH Elsevier*, April 2024, https://doi.org/10.1016/j.ject.2024.04.007

[33] Kishor Kumar Reddy, C;, Kaza, V.S.; Anisha, P.R.; Khurbani, M.M.; Shauib, M.; Alam, S. Optimizing Barrier Placement for Intrusion Detection and Prevention in WSNs. *PLOS ONE*, February 2024. https://doi.org/10.1371/journal.pone.0299334

[34] P R Anisha, C Kishor Kumar Reddy, Marlia Mohd Hanafiah, B V Ramana Murthy, R Madana Mohana Y V S S Pragathi, An Intelligent Deep Feature Based Feature Based Metabolism Syndrome Prediction System for Sleep Disorder Diseases. *Multimedia Tools and Applications*, Springer, November 2023. https://doi.org/10.1007/s11042-023-17296-4

[35] Ahluwalia, P.; Ballur, K.; Leeman, T.; Vashisht, A.; Singh, H.; Omar, N.; Mondal, A.K.; Vaibhav, K.; Baban, B.; Kolhe, R. Incorporating Novel Technologies in Precision Oncology for Colorectal Cancer: Advancing Personalized Medicine. *Cancers* 2024, *16*, 480. https://doi.org/10.3390/cancers16030480

Chapter 10

Federated machine learning and augmented reality (AR)/virtual reality (VR)-based framework for schizophrenia diagnosis and therapy

Vijayakumar Ponnusamy, Nandini Manickam, Emilija Kisic, and Nemanja Zdravković

10.1 INTRODUCTION

The medical field requires constant updates of technologies, advancements in medical equipment, therapeutic interventions, medication, and drugs. There is a huge requirement for a proper healthcare management system to maintain patient records, medical history, and treatments undergone to track the patient's health conditions and predict treatment plans after every visit to the healthcare center. These advancements in technologies assist physicians and healthcare providers in effectively diagnosing diseases. The healthcare sector has incorporated various emerging technologies to provide an efficient and reliable way of handling data between patients and healthcare providers. The main drawbacks in safeguarding sensitive information are data privacy and security as well as managing massive volumes of data. Federated learning (FL) provides a solution for the above concerns through a decentralized network where multiple devices are connected to a central server. Initially, all the connected devices receive a model from the central server. These devices train the models using local data and then transmit the revised models to a central server. This prevents the user data from getting shared. Integrating the model updates received from multiple devices, the central server updates the central training model based on the weighted training outcomes. A new version, the global model is then released to get deployed in the edge devices using their data. Thus, FL works by training a centralized model through decentralized devices. Each edge device trains the model locally and shares only the model updates. This prevents data privacy and helps to protect sensitive information through secure encryption and decryption processes.

Schizophrenia is a severe mental disorder that disturbs cognitive functions like thoughts, processing, attention, problem-solving, and memory which disconnects them from the real world. The World Health Organization

DOI: 10.1201/9781003591085-10

(WHO) reports that worldwide nearly 24 million people (0.32%) suffer from schizophrenia. This rate shows that about 1 in 222 people are adults. At least one-third of people experience schizophrenia with a complete decrease in symptoms. Some people show drastic worsening conditions and slowly decrease over time, and other people show gradual worsening of symptoms over time. Schizophrenia is often identified with distress and disruptions in personal, family, social, emotional, professional, and other areas of life. This disorder is mostly affected during the age of late adolescence and twenties and is most likely found among men than women. Individuals who are affected generally face extreme stress, fear, easy breakdown, less motivation, and negligence in taking care of themselves. This leads to physical illness, cardiovascular, and infectious diseases. Comparing the degree of severity of disorders between the general population and the affected individuals, schizophrenia patients have a two-to-three-times higher risk of dying at a young age than the general population. Hence, diagnosing this disorder early is crucial to improving the quality of life. Federated learning helps in training the models by extracting the features of schizophrenia and classifying them using machine learning algorithms.

After the stage of diagnosis, the affected individuals are given therapy through game-based activities to measure their motor activities, cognitive impairments, and emotional behaviors like happiness, fear, and sadness. Virtual Reality (VR)/ Augmented Reality (AR) is a therapeutic tool designed to enhance the learning and training experience through immersive, interactive environments that simulate real-time scenarios. Fears and phobias are the basis for game-based activities, which expose people to their anxieties and traumas in a virtual environment. Based on their performance in the game, a score will be generated. This score is used to analyze the severity of traumas which can further be monitored through a feedback session or by making them perform the same activity and comparing the newly generated score with the previous one. This will show the effectiveness of the therapy given.

This paper mainly focuses on providing a privacy-secured framework for the diagnosis of schizophrenia and an effective therapeutic tool using AR/VR technology. The previous work has contributed to the diagnosis of schizophrenia through machine learning (ML) and employing several convolutional neural network (CNN) architectures for designing deep learning (DL) models. Though the performance metrics showed better accuracy in the diagnosis, they still faced data privacy and security issues. To resolve this, the proposed federated learning (FL) framework is designed to provide a decentralized network with multiple edge devices connected without sharing its data. This improves the efficiency and performance in diagnosing the presence of schizophrenia. Similarly, VR and AR technologies are used as a therapeutic tool for affected individuals. Game-based activities that trigger emotional behaviors like fear, and anger, and improve motor activities like the movement of limbs are developed in the virtual environment. Scores are generated and the effectiveness of therapy is measured by comparing their performances in the activities on every visit. This technology has proved to be an effective tool in improving cognitive skills.

This chapter is comprised of the following sections. The first section starts with a comparison between ML and FL. To have a better understanding, first, we learn about machine learning (ML) and its importance. Then, study deep learning (DL) and its importance. Finally, study the importance of federated learning (FL). This helps in distinguishing the characteristics of ML, DL, and FL. The next section deals with the features, characteristics, and workflow of augmented reality (AR) and virtual reality (VR) in the therapy process. The next section deals with the advantages of FL, AR, and VR and thereby illustrates the advantages of integrating these technologies. The next section depicts the need to integrate these technologies into the medical field. The next section gives an overview of schizophrenia, its types, and signs and symptoms. The disadvantages of the existing ML technologies are mentioned in the next section followed by the design of the FL framework in the diagnosis of schizophrenia. The next section describes the role of VR/AR in the therapy of schizophrenia followed by the challenges in FL, AR, and VR in the diagnosis and therapy of schizophrenia. The final section of the chapter is concluded with a conclusion.

10.1.1 Machine learning (ML) versus federated machine learning (FL)

The two key methods used to train the models over a huge dataset are federated learning (FL) and machine learning (ML). These technologies have revolutionized data processing for large-scale applications in recent decades. The conventional ML trains the model using a centralized server. The data is gathered here and the training process is executed. There is a requirement for enhancements in classical data training models to improve data privacy. Federated learning (FL) has gained attention over distributed data training. Here multiple users are allowed to cooperatively use their data to train the model, then only share the trained model with the central cloud server, keeping sensitive data private. This improves data privacy and secures patients' sensitive information. In the following section, let us understand ML and FL in detail.

10.1.1.1 Machine learning (ML) and its importance

The field of Artificial Intelligence (AI) includes ML, which is the process of creating algorithms that can learn from data and forecast future events. By employing machine learning algorithms to learn from tremendous amounts of data and develop predictions on previously unseen fresh data, models are trained. Hence, it is a process of learning from large data, identifying patterns, and deciding based on the patterns that were found. The three main subcategories of ML are listed below:

- **Supervised learning:** In this case, the known data is used to train the algorithm. It learns to map input features to output with the aid of the labeled training data. The capacity to extrapolate from the data and predict data that hasn't been observed is gained. There are mainly two types: regression, in which the system learns to anticipate continuous values based on features, and classification when the algorithm gains the ability to group input data into certain categories according to certain attributes. frequently employed in the prognosis of illnesses
- **Unsupervised learning:** Here the algorithm is trained on unknown information. Investigating the data's distribution is the primary goal. commonly used in medical imaging where the models are trained on clusters of data. There are mostly two kinds of primarily dimensionality reduction, which lowers the amount of input variables in the dataset, and clustering, which clusters related data points according to their shared properties. This helps in retaining the original information for future use.
- **Reinforcement learning:** This is about an agent's interaction with an environment in aiming at maximizing the reward signal. Action and rewards or costs are based on actions. Commonly used in personalized therapy, treatment plans that monitor patients' outcomes. There are two types: mainly model-based and model-free reinforcement learning.

Machine learning algorithms are implemented by learning patterns and relationships from the available data to make predictions. The following stages represent the working of ML algorithms.

- Data collection: features that are important for the task.
- Data preprocessing: cleaning the data, normalizing and splitting the dataset.
- Choosing a model: A suitable ML model is chosen based on the task.
- Training: Training data is utilized to train the selected model. This involves modifying the parameters of the model to reduce the discrepancy between the actual outputs and those that are expected.
- Evaluating: After training, the model is trained using test data, and its performance is evaluated.

- Fine-tuning: Adjusting hyperparameters tuning parameters like learning rate or amount of a neural network's hidden layers that are not explicitly learned during training. This improves the performance.
- Prediction: The trained models are used to make decisions on unseen data. learned patterns are applied to new inputs to generate outputs like classification in regression tasks.
- Deployment: After training and tuning the model, it is deployed in the environment to make predictions for new data by integrating the model into an existing software system and the created new system.
- Monitoring and maintenance: monitor the system's performance in the deployed environment and perform maintenance whenever required. This involves retraining the model and updating the model according to newly available data.

10.1.1.2 Deep learning (DL) and its importance

A subfield of AI called deep learning (DL) uses artificial neural networks (ANNs) to teach machines new skills. Deep learning is a type of ML and AI that trains the model from large datasets and simulates cognitive processes. Deep learning models are used to learn classification tasks and identify patterns in sources like photos, text, images, and other types of data. Deep learning is also used for automating tasks that require the assistance of human intelligence. Deep learning features consist of neural networks interconnected by multiple layers of nodes. Nodes present in each layer are connected to adjacent layers. More the layers, the deeper the network. In ANN, signals propagate between nodes, and weights are assigned to them. The adjacent layer of nodes will be more affected by a weight node with a larger size. The weighted inputs are added up in the last layer to create the output. A sizable collection of labeled data and architectures are used to train the models. To train these models, DL models often consist of three or more layers—often hundreds or thousands of layers. With the use of unsupervised learning, this model can accurately predict outcomes from unstructured and raw data by extracting features, traits, and associations. Neural networks are composed of weights, biases, and data inputs. Together, these components enable precise item identification, classification, and description within the data. Deep learning has become a critical component of advanced technologies.

Deep learning algorithms are quite complicated, and depending on the properties of the datasets, there are several kinds of neural networks. Each type has its advantages and disadvantages which are overcome by other types of neural networks. Some of them are:

- **Convolutional Neural Networks (CNN):** Mostly utilized in image classification and computer vision. They are able to identify patterns and characteristics in pictures and movies. They can perform object identification, image recognition, pattern recognition, and face recognition from the images and videos. Uses matrix multiplication and linear algebraic concepts to identify the patterns. One or more hidden layers, an input layer, and an output layer make up this. CNN is composed of three layers: convolutional, pooling, and fully connected.

- **Recurrent Neural Networks (RNN):** Employed in language process and speech recognition. Identifies itself through feedback loops and operates with sequential or time series data. They gather information from past inputs that influence the current input and output. Uses an approach known as backpropagation through time (BPTT) to find the gradients that differ from the conventional backpropagation. RNN can produce one-to-many, many-to-one, or many-to-many outputs.
- **Autoencoders and variational autoencoders:** Produce voice and visuals that are authentic utilization of sophisticated generative modeling. Data that has not been labeled is encoded into a compressed format and then decoded back into its original form. Using simple autoencoders, one may reconstruct corrupted images and variational autoencoders not only reconstruct the data but also output variations on the original data.
- **Generative Adversarial Networks (GANs):** used both in and out of AI. Data that resembles the initial training set is generated as a result. consists of a discriminator that compares the generated picture to the original images in the dataset, and a generator whose output is based on the input and the generative model's training efficiency of the layers.

10.1.1.3 Federated learning (FL) and its importance

One of the most significant advancements in data science and AI is federated learning (FL). Federated learning or collaborative learning is an ML method that eliminates the need to transfer or store raw data on a central server and enables a collection of distributed edge devices or systems to train ML models. Federated learning applications use an iterative training procedure that can take place on numerous edge devices or servers multiple times. A base model is generated by a central server and transmitted to the edge devices that are linked. The pre-trained models are sent to each connected device, which then uses its own local data to train them. After training, the devices send the locally trained models back to the central server, protecting their privacy by not disclosing the raw data. After that, the server combines the local model based on weights to produce a shared global model. By updating the more recent model and contrasting it with the current model, it will be possible to evaluate the correctness and monitor the performance of the updated global model. Until the model achieves a predefined number of iterations or a suitable degree of accuracy, the shared model procedure is repeated for every iteration. Federated learning methods are deployed in various environments in different industries. The benefit of this framework is that it keeps personal sensitive data safe and secure. This FL framework generally finds application in the medical field for predicting and diagnosing diseases.

Federated learning comes in three varieties: federated transfer learning, vertical FL, and horizontal FL. In horizontal FL, sampled data are distributed among the connected devices, and the model is trained collaboratively. Features are split between the devices and models are trained that focus on the complementary features in vertical FL. Federated transfer learning deals with pre-trained models that are adapted to decentralized data for performing specific tasks in such a way it reduces the need for external local data. Similarly, there are three approaches to FL. First is the centralized FL approach where the devices are connected to a central server. This approach selects the required device and collects the model updates from those devices during the training. Here the communication happens between the central server and individual devices. Though they can generate accurate models, network failures can stop the process which is a major drawback of this approach. Second is the decentralized FL where the system does not require any central server to carry out the training process. Here the model updates are shared only among the connected edge devices. The most recent global model update is dispersed to the connected edge devices by aggregating local updates from those devices. This approach reduces the single point of failure but still, the performance depends upon the network topology. The third approach is the heterogeneous FL where the devices connected can be either mobile, computers, or IoT which may differ in terms of hardware, software, and computation. HeteroFL generates a single global model that communicates between varied local models.

Various FL algorithms are used for the prediction and classification of diseases accurately. The process known as federated stochastic gradient descent (FedSGD) divides the central global model among the linked devices, with each device calculating the gradient using its own local data. Based on the number of samples present in each device, the gradients are aggregated in a proportion that measures the gradient descent step which is fed to the central server. Federated averaging (FedAvg) is another algorithm that is an extension of FedSGD. Here instead of sharing the gradients with the central server weights or model parameters on the local models are aggregated.

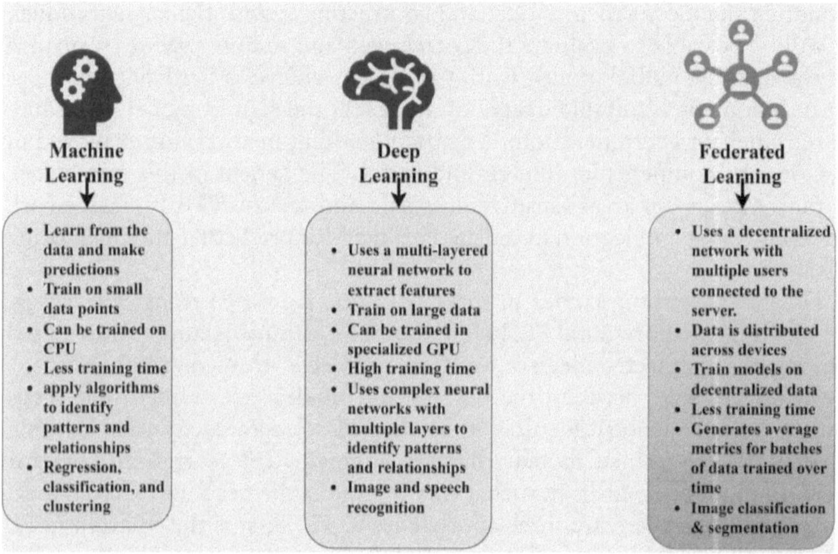

Figure 10.1 Comparison between Machine Learning (ML), Deep Learning (DL), and Federated Learning (FL).

The averaging of gradients is equal to the averaging of weights. There is a chance for tuning parameters before sending them to the central server for averaging. Federated learning with dynamic regularization (FedDyn) is an algorithm mainly used for minimizing the local losses that occur due to the heterogeneity of users thereby regularizing the global losses from the central server. This also helps in reducing the computational cost. Figure 10.1 distinguishes ML, DL, and FL in terms of complexity, training, algorithms, and applications.

10.1.2 Comparison of ML, DL and FL

Machine learning, DL, and FL are promising technologies that play a significant role in data processing for large-scale applications. From the importance, types, and advantages of these techniques that were mentioned above, this section performs a convergence comparison between ML, DL, and FL. Table 10.1 elaborates on the characteristics, features, advantages, challenges, and applications in enhancing the performance of the system.

Table 10.1 Characteristics of ML, DL, and FL

Parameter	*Machine Learning (ML)*	*Deep Learning (DL)*	*Federated Learning (FL)*
Definition	Without the need for explicit programming, this subset of AI can learn from data and generate predictions	Multi-layered neural networks are used in this area of machine learning to assess different data aspects	The kind of machine learning used to train models on decentralized data that is spread across several devices
Data points	Train on small data points	Needs a lot of data to train	Requires sufficient amount of data to get the right prediction accuracy
Hardware for training	Models can be trained on CPU	Models can be trained on a specialized GPU	It requires large amounts of devices
Training time	Requires less training time because of its smaller size	Requires high training time due to a higher volume of data	As the data is not huge, training time will be less
Output	Generates numerical values as output	Generates anything from numerical values to free-from elements as output	Generates average metrics over all batches of data trained across all clients
Analysis complexity	Uses training algorithm to identify patterns and relationships of data	Uses complex neural networks with multiple layers to analyze patterns and relationships	Image classification and segmentation tasks from medical images
Algorithm complexity	ML algorithms can range from simple linear models to more complex models	DL algorithms are based on ANN that consists of multiple layers and nodes	The central server chooses a stratified model to be trained
Applications	Used in a wide range of applications such as regression, classification, and clustering	Mostly used for complex tasks such as image and speech recognition, natural language processing, and autonomous systems	Mostly used in data-driven insights in healthcare analytics, and predictive analysis

10.2 INTRODUCTION TO AUGMENTED REALITY (AR) AND VIRTUAL REALITY (VR)

Future developments in gaming, marketing, e-commerce, education, healthcare, and other applications are greatly foreseen by the use of virtual reality (VR) and augmented reality (AR). There are several key distinctions between the two technologies though they can be easily misunderstood. VR replaces the entire real world with a virtual one to completely immerse the user whereas AR adds items to the real world that still exists in the real world. The following section explores VR and AR in detail.

10.2.1 Introduction to augmented reality (AR)

The immersive experience of the real world is known as augmented reality (AR). Perceptual data produced by computers, which often encompasses a variety of experiences including visual, auditory, haptic, somatosensory, and olfactory enhances realism. From music to video, graphics to GPS overlays, and more, designers enhance the physical world with computer-generated input that adjusts in real-time to changes in the user's surroundings and activity. Because AR is accessible to everyone with a smartphone, it is a more potential tool for gaming and branding. Clear lenses or a pass-through camera are commonly used in AR systems to let users see their surroundings in real time while virtual components are seen on the camera output or projected onto the lenses. AR is only as good as virtual content visualization and internal data processing. Users don't notice any delays because they occur concurrently. This guarantees that the AR program may be used in real time. There are abundant options available in AR for visual presentations. Either a display on headgear that doesn't obstruct the user's field of vision or an opaque device that shows the viewing image as though the user isn't wearing any equipment at all—like smart glasses—must allow the user to still see their surroundings. There are a few AR headsets available, such as the Magic Leap and the Microsoft Hololens. This can also be implemented without a headset.

10.2.2 Introduction to virtual reality (VR)

A computer-generated environment known as virtual reality (VR) immerses users in their surroundings with objects and images that look realistic. VR applications can mimic reality or completely deviate from it. People can see this world with the use of a virtual reality headset or helmet. We may get completely immersed in video games and experience the characters' emotions through virtual reality. Virtual reality has uses in commercial, entertainment, medical, and educational fields. People can learn how to do cardiac surgery, participate in space projects and military simulations, and enhance the caliber of their sports training to maximize performance. VR systems usually use headgear and a variety of sensors to track the user's movement and communicate the necessary pictures or input, giving the impression that the user is interacting with the virtual world. Replaces the entire real world with a virtual one to completely immerse the user. Virtual reality involves wearing a headset with a screen of some kind that shows a virtual environment to fully submerge the user in it. Additionally, these headsets make use of head-tracking technology, which lets the user physically move their head to look around the scene. They will be able to see the virtual world in all directions as the display moves with them. There are two major types of headsets. The first type has a screen built into the headset. These gadgets are computer-connected and need a reasonably strong system to function properly. They work well and have excellent visuals, but they are expensive. The Oculus Rift, Vive, and PlayStation VR which are compatible with the PlayStation 4 gaming system are a few well-known examples. To make the experience more engaging, several of these gadgets also include handheld controls that follow the movements of your hands. The other kind of headgear stores your phone inside and shows content from its screen. These operate entirely off apps on your smartphone and don't need a PC. These headsets tend to be significantly less expensive than those with built-in screens, but their performance and graphics aren't quite as impressive. The Gear VR and Google Cardboard are two well-known examples.

10.2.3 Advantages of AR and VR

The AR and VR applications have created endless opportunities for many professional fields. VR and AR enhance users' satisfaction of apps, games, and movies in the entertainment industry. In the medical industry, virtual reality can help students gain a better understanding of the human body, and it can allow surgeons to safely perform risky treatments. VR has applications in education, military training, and space exploration. Scientists can conduct experiments in a synthetic environment by utilizing virtual reality technology. Augmented reality can be used by the business sector to create product designs and by the construction industry to locate and correct architectural defects in buildings. Figure 10.2 represents the workflow of VR in healthcare.

10.2.4 Recent applications of AR and VR

AR and VR find tremendous applications in various fields. To enhance education, learning, and understanding of various concepts by creating a virtual environment. VR and AR are used in healthcare as a therapeutic tool. Some of the applications of AR are:

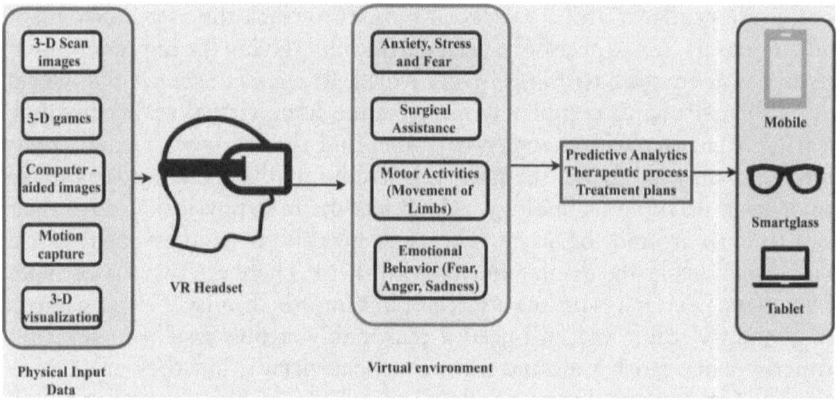

Figure 10.2 Workflow of VR in Healthcare.

- Food and beverages AR-integrated menus
- Makeup virtual try-ons
- Medical imaging
- Education in language learning
- Warehouse management

Many industries have seen a lot of benefits from VR technology. This technology offers an innovative and safe way to simulate real-life scenarios. Some of the applications of VR are:

- Specialized military training
- Surgery simulation
- Theme parks
- Virtual walkthroughs
- Digital marketing

10.3 BENEFITS OF FEDERATED LEARNING (FL), VIRTUAL REALITY (VR), AND AUGMENTED REALITY (AR)

- The outcome of this chapter is that every participant will receive an effective diagnosis and therapeutic analysis of schizophrenia.
- Headsets and wristbands collect the EEG and HRV data. stores the values in the system.
- Effective diagnosis of schizophrenia is predicted by determining the correlation between physiological data and the questionnaire scale.

- Federated learning framework is a decentralized network where models are trained by multiple devices without sharing the data preserving the patients' information.
- Therapy treatment is given through task-based activities designed in VR/AR to evaluate the characteristics of stress and anxiety, and to measure the severity.
- The effectiveness of therapy is measured through repeated processes and comparing the scores from the previous activity-based tasks taken.

10.4 NEED FOR FL, AR, AND VR IN THE MEDICAL FIELD

Federated learning has become crucial in healthcare in recent years because it offers the benefits of data security and transparency in ML models. Federated learning is a decentralized network that allows multiple devices to connect through a central cloud server. Here multiple devices are used to train the models in their local data. So, the model is distributed among various edge devices and is trained. This reduces the amount of data in training the model since the size is small. This technology also reduces the need for large-scale data transfers between multiple clients and servers. The benefit of this design is that since the models are trained in the devices' local data only the model is shared without sharing the data keeping the sensitive data secure.

AR can transform healthcare by providing a more interactive and realistic experience for both patients and healthcare professionals. This assists the surgeons with the surgery and educates the students and patients through physical therapy. With the help of AR, patients can connect with doctors to check their symptoms and receive personalized healthcare. Doctors can check the medical reports for accuracy and suggest treatment plans.

VR in healthcare uses immersive technology that enhances medical treatments, training, and therapy. This medical service is done with the help of VR headsets to create a virtual environment that allows the patients to interact. This immersive technology is mainly designed to evaluate the degree of mental health through game-based activities. Several studies have proved that VR provides an effective solution for anxiety, post-traumatic stress disorder (PTSD), and phobias.

10.5 INTRODUCTION TO SCHIZOPHRENIA

On April 24, 1908, during a convention of the German Psychiatric Association in Berlin, Prof. Bhauler coined the term schizophrenia. He emphasized that the division of psychological functioning is the main feature of schizophrenia. The National Institute of Health (NIH) reports that in

India, the prevalence of schizophrenia spectrum disorder was 1.41% during lifetime and 0.41% currently. Of the 149 people who underwent screening, 149 had schizophrenia, and 55 of them tested positive for a co-occurring mental illness. In this group, the prevalence of depression was 9.4%, anxiety was 8.1%, alcohol use disorder was 10.7%, and tobacco use disorder was 27.5%. When the severity of the disease was evaluated over the past month, the individuals at work accounted for 53.4% of the handicap, the social life for 59.5%, and the home life for 59.5%. Phrenia: split mind, schizo: split mind. It investigates the impact on people's thoughts and behavior. Signs and symptoms of schizophrenia are portrayed in Figure 10.3.

Schizophrenia is a complex mental condition that involves multiple components, including genetic, physiological, environmental, and psychological aspects. Research indicates that an individual's risk of acquiring schizophrenia is increased if they have a close relative with the illness, like a parent or sibling. Numerous genes have been connected to an elevated risk through genetic research, including genome-wide association studies (GWAS), yet no single gene is entirely to blame. Rather, a mix of genetic mutations and variations determines susceptibility. There is a link between abnormal brain development and function and schizophrenia. According to the neurodevelopmental hypothesis, schizophrenia may arise from abnormalities in the prenatal or early postnatal stages of brain development. Possible causes include delivery issues that affect the brain's oxygen supply, malnutrition, and exposure to viruses during pregnancy. Moreover, aberrant neurotransmitters have a major effect. For a long time, the dopamine hypothesis was in charge, contending that dysregulation of dopamine is a significant factor.

The development of schizophrenia is significantly influenced by the environment as well. Risk factors include prenatal infections, malnourishment,

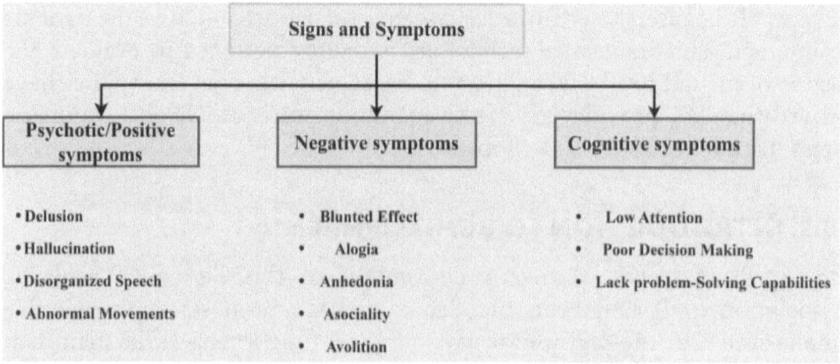

Figure 10.3 Signs and Symptoms of Schizophrenia.

difficult births, and maternal stress. Psychological elements also play a significant part in the sickness. Exposure to severe life stressors such as abuse and childhood trauma may heighten one's susceptibility. There is a list of environmental risk factors, such as social isolation, urban upbringing, migration, and social adversity. Schizophrenia has a psychological component to both its genesis and progression. Information processing issues and cognitive impairments are common in people with schizophrenia. These cognitive issues can affect the course of the condition and frequently appear before clinical signs. Problems with executive function, memory, and attention are commonly observed. In summary, there is a complex interplay between genetic predispositions and environmental exposures that contribute to the development of schizophrenia. change the way the brain develops and functions. The goal of ongoing research is to better understand these intricate networks in order to improve treatment, diagnosis, and preventive approaches.

10.5.1 Disadvantages of existing ML

Despite the advantages of applying ML in the medical field, there are still open issues that data scientists and professionals face when they are trying to use ML algorithms for medical diagnosis. Some of the challenges are:

- Lack of professionals
- Bias in the ML model that affects the performance
- Lack of quality data
- Data annotation must be done accurately
- Need for hyperparameter tuning

10.6 FRAMEWORK OF FL IN THE DIAGNOSIS OF SCHIZOPHRENIA

The diagnosis model of schizophrenia disease is developed based on aperiodic neural activity that has a connection with the balance between excitation and inhibition as well as brain neural spikes [1]. The connection between the First Episode's anomalies of Schizophrenia Spectrum Psychosis (FESSP) and severity is analyzed through a questionnaire and resting-state electroencephalography (EEG). The symptoms were assessed using the Brief Psychiatric Rating Scale (BPRS), the Scale for Assessment of Negative Symptoms (SANS), and the Scale for Assessment of Positive Symptoms (SAPS). A 10-10 international system 60-channel cap was used to collect EEG data. Power spectral density was measured for every electrode for each individual. The correlation between the exponent and the aperiodic offset was $p<0.001$ and $r=0.89$.

The growth of the Internet of Medical Things (IoMT) in physiological signal processing meets dynamic distribution changes in signals and data privacy issues. Meta continual learning method (MetaCL) is used for preserving patient data by incorporating a horizontal federated learning mechanism [2]. This method consists of a blockchain module, a knowledge base, a micro classifier, and a feature extractor. Using the INCART and MIT-BIH-AR datasets, experiments were carried out to assess MetaCL's scalability, task increment, time increment, domain increment, and institute increment. MetaCL demonstrated an accuracy of 98.57% on MIT-BIH-AR while INCART demonstrated an accuracy of 95.49%. similarly, INCART on MIT-BIH-AR showed an accuracy of 96.15%, and INCART with an accuracy of 98.24% after the completion of INCART training when processed through the horizontal mechanism.

Natural Language Processing (NLP) and Automatic Speech Recognition (ASR) are the emerging tools used in the classification of schizophrenia [3]. The ASR data are estimated quantitatively through Word Error Rate (WER) and the nature of speech is analyzed qualitatively through its error type and position. Word similarity measures also help in enhancing the accuracy of classification. Two random forest classifiers were implemented in order to compare the similarity measures between automatic and manual transcripts and evaluate their performance. Automatic transcriptions showed an accuracy of 76.7% and manual transcriptions showed an accuracy of 79.8%. integration of NLP and ASR achieves accuracy in the classification of schizophrenia.

An automatic EEG recognition system is developed using a vision transformer for early diagnosis of schizophrenia [4]. ID EEG sequence data are mapped into 3D images using electrode positioning of 10–20 international systems of 19 channels. This preserves the temporal and spatial features of EEG data. Ten-fold cross-validation and leave-one-subject-out cross-validation techniques are used to assess the model's performance. This was evaluated for subject-dependent and subject-independent categories. On average, the model's accuracy was 98.99%. for the subject-independent category and 85.04% for the subject-dependent category. This assists the physicians in early diagnosis and treatment.

Electroencephalogram (EEG) waveforms are extracted to detect hidden patterns using AI models for the classification of schizophrenia [5]. EEG waveforms consist of healthy control and schizophrenia patients' data. In order to classify the presence of schizophrenia, a convolutional neural network (CNN) model is created to extract features and compare data from patients and healthy individuals. The CNN model achieves a test accuracy of 60%, specificity of 55.55%, and precision of 55.55%. these models are cost-effective and improve the diagnosis of schizophrenia.

Automatic diagnosis of schizophrenia with minimal input data can be achieved using an optimized system that contains single-channel EEG [6].

This EEG data is extracted creating a model through transfer learning and knowledge distillation. This strategy contributes to the system's increased efficiency. Additionally, Continuous Wavelet Transform (CWT) is used to convert EEG signals into pictures in order to efficiently use pre-trained models. This change improves the automatic diagnosis of schizophrenia and raises the pre-trained models in the picture domain. When self-distillation and VGG16 are combined for the P4 channel, 97.81% accuracy is obtained.

CALSczNet is a new deep learning-based technique that extracts the temporal and spatial patterns from EEG using temporal and spatial convolution to improve detection performance [7]. This technique uses Long Short-Term Memory (LSTM), Temporal Attention (TA), and Local Attention (LA) to deal with the discriminative characteristics of non-stationarity in EEG signals. The publicly accessible Kaggle dataset for simple sensory tasks with ten-fold cross-validation for assessing the model's performance. The model detects schizophrenia early with an accuracy of 98.6%, sensitivity of 98.65%, specificity of 98.72%, and F1-score of 98.65%.

Wearable Internet of Medical Things (IoMT) devices have become promising technology in the real-time monitoring of health through wrist-worn/body-worn sensors [8]. Actigraph devices are used to collect the position, sleep/wake cycle, and motion activities of an individual for early diagnosis of schizophrenia. Motor activity data are analyzed using a deep CNN using an attention mechanism. The characteristics of motor activities are analyzed. The missing values from the dataset are dealt with through the imputation method, and imbalance in class is dealt with through Synthetic Minority Over-sampling Technique (SMOTE) techniques. Actigraph device data are extracted from the 'Psykose' dataset. Using 24-hour actigraphy data, the model achieves an accuracy of 94% and provides non-invasive and real-time mental health services.

For early diagnosis of schizophrenia, resting-state functional magnetic resonance imaging (rs-fMRI) is increasingly being used to examine the brain's functional connectivity (FC) network [9]. Node-level features are extracted using the Graph Attention Network (GAT) in order to quantify the correlation of brain connectivity data. The bilinear convolution (BC) neural network architecture combined with the multi-graph attention network (MGAT) facilitates the estimation of functional connectivity. MGAT-BC model uses grid search and nested cross-validation for performance evaluation. This model achieves an accuracy of 92% in capturing topological features that improve the diagnosis of schizophrenia.

Mental health disorders (MHD) have become more common and have diversified into many forms of severities of symptoms that make it difficult to differentiate between a particular disorder with others [10]. A support system with deep learning is developed which receives data from wearable devices and helps the physicians to make differential diagnoses and early treatments. Publicly available datasets namely, 'Psykose' and 'Depresjon' are used to analyze motor activity signals from wearables that differentiate schizophrenia from mood disorders patients. This study is deployed in Long Short-Term Memory (LSTM) and Gated Recurrent Unit (GRU) and trained on an attention-selected mechanism. The LSTM model's performance yielded an F-score of 0.88, correlation coefficient of 0.77, accuracy of 0.88, and sensitivity of 0.93.

Data-driven diagnosis through the identification of brain connectivity biomarkers using EEG data provides a solution for the overlapping of symptoms of schizophrenia from other disorders [11]. A novel feature interaction-based explainability technique for multimodal explanations is developed by extracting the EEG spectral power data. The effects of schizophrenia are studied on the alpha, beta, and theta frequency bands from the explainable machine learning models in order to identify the neuropsychiatric disorder biomarkers. The evaluation of the model was measured using mean and standard deviation relevance across each fold. This model's accuracy was 0.73, its F1-score for mean and accuracy was 0.70, and its F1-score for standard deviation was 0.13.

Identification of psychotic episodes has become a challenge due to their nature and varied symptoms among individuals [12]. Extracting information from electronic health records (EHR) may also sometimes fail to provide essential information. In order to diagnose psychosis, NLP algorithms are utilized to extract admission notes, analyze them using a rule-based algorithm, and train models using keywords. Two models were developed, and their performance of extracting keywords efficiently was measured. With an F1-score of 0.8881, the first model was created using an XGBoost classifier that extracted features from notes using expert-curated keywords utilizing Term Frequency-Inverse Document Frequency (TF-IDF). Another model was developed using BlueBERT that showed an F1-score of 0.8841 on extracting the same notes.

Psykose is a publicly available dataset that contains motor activity signals extracted from body sensors [13]. Actigraph devices are used to monitor the movement, position, and sleep/wake patterns of an individual. The dataset consists of 22 schizophrenia patients and 32 healthy control subjects' data. Sensor data set for 24-h for a particular period is monitored. This also contains demographic and medical assessments for each subject during the observed period. This model's performance is assessed using either leave-one-patient-out cross-validation or N-fold cross-validation. Random forest showed a better performance of 0.183 false-positive, precision of 0.836, recall of 0.837, F1-score of 0.836, and MCC of 0.662 compared to other classifiers.

P300 is used to study the instability of brain abnormalities, processing, and stimulus-based responses [14]. When examining the locations of the brain during the cognitive process, trial-to-trail variability (TTV) attracts more attention. TTV is examined in a time-varying EEG network that spans the beta1, beta2, alpha, theta, and delta bands of schizophrenia. According to performance evaluation, a cross-band time-varying network can effectively extract the characteristics of schizophrenia with 83.39% accuracy, 89.22% sensitivity, and 74.55% specificity.

An optimized federated learning model is developed for the detection of schizophrenia through functional magnetic resonance imaging (fMRI) and structural magnetic resonance imaging (sMRI) [15]. EEG data and deep learning are analyzed and the EEG data are converted into images using time series data conversion algorithms [16]. These images were fed into a convolutional neural network (CNN) to train models based on VGGNet. An accuracy and loss of 0.963 and 0.184 were obtained in predicting schizophrenia. Application of 3D CNN on T1-weighted MRI scans and processing is done through deep learning models to predict patients with schizophrenia [17]. The proposed model outperformed benchmarks achieving an accuracy of 90.7% in classifying schizophrenia through structural MRI data. Diagnosis of schizophrenia is explored through deep learning-based methods for automated analysis of EEG signals [18]. CNN-LSTM models showed 99.25% accuracy in the prediction of schizophrenia.

The current developments in the prognosis of schizophrenia using machine learning and deep learning are explored [19]. This combines physiological data with genetic information for early diagnosis of schizophrenia. The impact of different parts of the brain and their regional data in schizophrenia diagnosis are studied [20]. This uses empirical wavelet transform and empirical mode decomposition for extracting features and applied to the convolutional neural network (CNN) achieving an accuracy of 99.93% and 94.13%. The system is applied to a light gradient boosting machine (light GBM) algorithm for the prediction of schizophrenia using EEG signals [21]. The accuracy of this model was 98%. The application of dimensionality reduction in the EEG signals when fed into deep learning is studied [22]. For analyzing multichannel EEG signals, the crossover-boosted Archimedes optimization algorithm detected schizophrenia. This achieved an accuracy of 96.34%. Table 10.2 depicts the role of FL in the diagnosis of schizophrenia.

10.6.1 Role of AR/VR in therapy of schizophrenia

The efficacy of Immersive VR (IVR) is evaluated by implementing positive reinforcement components in motor coordination [23]. 18 participants who had motor impairment in the upper limb (UL) were exposed to IVR and physical therapy (PT) sessions. Treatment effects on motor recovery were analyzed based on the virtual image of UL and measuring the speed of movements. VR is used in creating an environment based on fear of falling (FOF) using physiological data as input [24]. Evaluation is done on movement scenarios such as walking, turning, reaching, sitting to standing,

Table 10.2 Role of FL in the Diagnosis of Schizophrenia

Ref	*Purpose*	*Method*	*Results*
[1]	Aperiodic neural activity with inhibition and excitation balance	Questionnaire, resting-state EEG	Correlation coefficient of r=0.89 and p<0.001
[2]	IoMT in physiological signal processing	Meta Continual learning methods (MetaCL) and horizontal FL	MIT-BIH-AR showed an accuracy of 98.57% and INCART with an accuracy of 95.49%
[3]	Classification of schizophrenia through speech recognition	NLP and ASR	Automatic transcription accuracy=76.7% and Manual transcription accuracy=79.8%
[4]	Automatic EEG recognition system	Vision transformer	Subject-dependent accuracy=85.04% and subject independent accuracy=98.99%
[5]	Detect hidden patterns of EEG data	CNN model	Test accuracy=60%, specificity=55.55%, precision=55.55%
[6]	CalSczNet for the detection of schizophrenia	Temporal and spatial convolution and LSTM	Accuracy=98.6%, sensitivity=98.65%, specificity=98.72% and F1=98.65%

and crossing an obstacle. Individuals with and without Parkinson's disease [25] are considered targets for the study. Feasibility, acceptability, usability, and safety are measured based on the score. Cognitive impairments in elder people are assessed using a non-invasive instrument that includes video images captured from frontal cameras [26]. A new multimodal database that consists of 191 elderly subjects that analyze cognitive impairments through handwriting tasks by capturing eye and head movements. A classification accuracy of 77% was obtained for multiclass classification and binomial classification showed an accuracy of 83%.

There are two modules in this chapter. Diagnosis is covered in the first module, and therapy and efficacy evaluation are covered in the second. Additionally, use federated learning (FL) to create a prediction model based on physiological [27] data and questionnaires. EEG and HRV data are collected using sensors and fed into a neural network along with the validation results of questionnaires. suitable machine learning algorithms are used to extract features and based on the patterns recognized prediction of schizophrenia is done. Virtual reality (VR)/Augmented reality (AR) is a therapeutic tool that is used to analyze cognitive and behavioral functions based on games designed. The activities performed by individuals are

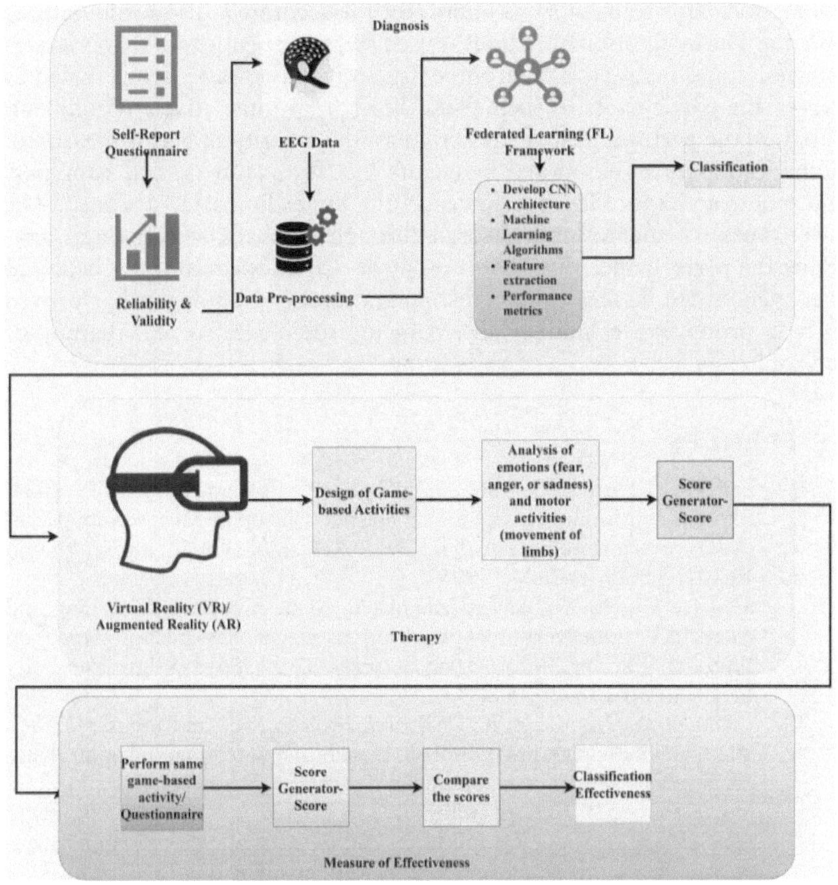

Figure 10.4 FL, VR/AR Integrated for Diagnosis and Therapy of Schizophrenia.

monitored and the effectiveness of therapy is analyzed. Figure 10.4 portrays the working of FL, VR and AR integrated for diagnosis and therapy of schizophrenia [28].

10.7 CONCLUSION

The integration of federated learning (FL) and AR/VR technology offers an innovative and immersive approach to the diagnosis and therapy of schizophrenia. Federated learning decentralizes data processing and preserves patient privacy by training ML models on EEG, clinical, and other physiological data. This method does not require large storage and training time and preserves data privacy thus improving model generalization across the population. This framework is important for accurately diagnosing schizophrenia. The integration of AR/VR is used as a therapeutic tool that provides immersive and interactive environments. Game-based tasks are designed to expose the participants to their fears through an interactive environment. Based on the performance of the activities, the severity of fear is measured. Activities based on emotional behaviors like fear, sadness, and happiness and motor activities like movements in the upper limbs are designed. The effectiveness of therapy is measured through feedback sessions and analyzing the performance. In the future, more activities can be designed, and effectiveness can be measured. This integration of technologies has proven to be a promising technology in enhancing the diagnosis and therapy of schizophrenia.

REFERENCES

[1] Earl, R.J., Ford, T.C., Lum, J.A., Enticott, P.G. and Hill, A.T., 2024. Exploring aperiodic activity in first episode schizophrenia spectrum psychosis: A resting-state EEG analysis. *Brain Research*, 149052, https://doi.org/10.1016/j.brainres.2024.149052..

[2] Sun, L., Wu, J., Xu, Y. and Zhang, Y. 2023. A federated learning and blockchain framework for physiological signal classification based on continual learning. *Information Sciences*, 630, 586–598 https://doi.org/10.1016/j.ins.2023.02.003.

[3] Ciampelli, S., Voppel, A. E., De Boer, J. N., Koops, S., and Sommer, I. E. C. 2023. Combining automatic speech recognition with semantic natural language processing in schizophrenia. *Psychiatry Research*, 325, 115252, https://doi.org/10.1016/j.psychres.2023.115252.

[4] Li, B., Wang, J., Guo, Z., and Li, Y. 2023. Automatic detection of schizophrenia based on spatial–temporal feature mapping and LeViT with EEG signals. *Expert Systems with Applications*, 224, 119969, https://doi.org/10.1016/j.eswa.2023.119969.

[5] Nwoye, E., Fidelis, O., Umeh, K., Fadipe, B., Umeh, C., Akano, T., Jesuoluwa, Z., and Woo, W. L. 2021. Detecting hidden patterns in EEG waveforms of schizophrenia patients using convolutional neural network. *International Journal of Automation, Artificial Intelligence and Machine Learning*, 2(2), 1–19, https://doi.org/10.61797/ijaaiml.v2i2.103.

[6] Mostafavi, M., Ko, S.B., Shokouhi, S.B., and Ayatollahi, A. 2024. Transfer learning and self-distillation for automated detection of schizophrenia using single-channel EEG and scalogram images. *Physical and Engineering Sciences in Medicine*, 1–16, https://doi.org/10.1007/s13246-024-01420-1.

[7] Almaghrabi, N., Hussain, M., and Alotaibi, A. 2024. CALSczNet: Convolution neural network with attention and LSTM for the detection of schizophrenia using EEG signals. *Mathematics*, 12(13), 1989, https://doi.org/10.3390/math12131989

[8] Misgar, M.M., and Bhatia, M.P.S. 2024. Utilizing deep convolutional neural architecture with attention mechanism for objective diagnosis of schizophrenia using wearable IoMT devices. *Multimedia Tools and Applications*, 83(13), 39601–39620, https://doi.org/10.1007/s11042-023-17119-6.
[9] Yu, R., Pan, C., Fei, X., Chen, M., and Shen, D. 2023. Multi-graph attention networks with bilinear convolution for diagnosis of schizophrenia. *IEEE Journal of Biomedical and Health Informatics*, 27(3), 1443–1454, https://doi.org/10.1109/JBHI.2022.3229465.
[10] Nguyen, D.K., Chan, C.L., Li, A.H.A., Phan, D.V., and Lan, C.H. 2022. Decision support system for the differentiation of schizophrenia and mood disorders using multiple deep learning models on wearable devices data. *Health Informatics Journal*, 28(4), 14604582221137537, https://doi.org/10.1177/14604582221137537.
[11] Sancho, M.L., Ellis, C.A., Miller, R.L., and Calhoun, V.D. 2024. Identifying reproducibly important EEG markers of schizophrenia with an explainable multi-model deep learning approach. *bioRxiv*, https://doi.org/10.1101/2024.02.09.579600.
[12] Hua, Y., Blackley, S.V., Shinn, A.K., Skinner, J.P., Moran, L.V., and Zhou, L. 2024. Identifying psychosis episodes in psychiatric admission notes via rule-based methods, machine learning, and pre-trained language models. *medRxiv*, https://doi.org/10.1101/2024.03.18.24304475.
[13] Jakobsen, P., Garcia-Ceja, E., Stabell, L.A., Oedegaard, K.J., Berle, J.O., Thambawita, V., Hicks, S.A., Halvorsen, P., Fasmer, O.B., and Riegler, M.A. 2020, July. Psykose: A motor activity database of patients with schizophrenia. In *2020 IEEE 33rd International Symposium on Computer-Based Medical Systems (CBMS)* (pp. 303–308). IEEE, https://doi.org/10.1109/CBMS49503.2020.00064.
[14] Yi, C., Li, F., Wang, J., Li, Y., Zhang, J., Chen, W., Jiang, L. et al. 2024. Abnormal trial-to-trial variability in P300 time-varying directed eeg network of schizophrenia. *Medical & Biological Engineering & Computing*, 1–15, https://doi.org/10.1007/s11517-024-03133-9.
[15] Mondal, H., Hassan, M.M., Nag, A., and Bairagi, A.K. 2024. The integration of federated deep learning with internet of things in healthcare. In Federated Deep Learning for Healthcare (pp. 143–159). CRC Press.
[16] Menon, N.G., Bhavana, N.D., and Deva Hema, D. 2022. Towards better intelligent implementation of Schizophrenia prediction using federated deep learning framework. *International Journal of Health Sciences* III, 5631–5645, https://doi.org/10.53730/ijhs.v6nS3.7207.
[17] Santoro, V., Hou, M. D., Premoli, I., Belardinelli, P., Biondi, A., Carobin, A., and Puledda, F. et al. 2024. Investigating cortical excitability and inhibition in patients with schizophrenia: A TMS-EEG study. *Brain Research Bulletin*, 212(4), 110972, https://doi.org/10.1016/j.brainresbull.2024.110972.
[18] Zhang, J., Wang, Q., Wang, X., Qiao, L. and Liu, M. 2024. Preserving specificity in federated graph learning for fMRI-based neurological disorder identification. *Neural Networks*, 169, 584–596, https://doi.org/10.1016/j.neunet.2023.11.004

[19] Kanyal, A., Mazumder, B., Calhoun, V.D., Preda, A., Turner, J., Ford, J., and Ye, D.H. 2024. Multi-modal deep learning from imaging genomic data for schizophrenia classification. *Frontiers in Psychiatry*, 15, 1384842, https://doi.org/10.3389/fpsyt.2024.1384842.

[20] Ranjan, R., and Sahana, B.C. 2024. Multiresolution feature fusion for smart diagnosis of schizophrenia in adolescents using EEG signals. *Cognitive Neurodynamics*, 1–29, https://doi.org/10.1007/s11571-024-10120-1.

[21] Desai, A.B., Gangodkar, D.R., Pant, K., and Pant, B. 2024, January. Harnessing the potential of light gradient boosting machine for accurate diagnosis of schizophrenia from EEG signals. In *2024 14th International Conference on Cloud Computing, Data Science & Engineering (Confluence)* (pp. 568–574). IEEE, 10.1109/Confluence60223.2024.10463450.

[22] Srinivasan, S., and Johnson, S.D. 2024. A novel approach to schizophrenia detection: Optimized preprocessing and deep learning analysis of multi-channel EEG data. *Expert Systems with Applications*, 246, 122937, https://doi.org/10.1016/j.eswa.2023.122937.

[23] Altukhaim, S., Sakabe, N., Nagaratnam, K., Mannava, N., Kondo, T., & Hayashi, Y. 2024. Immersive virtual reality enhanced reinforcement induced physical therapy (EVEREST). Available at SSRN: https://ssrn.com/abstract=4898128 or http://dx.doi.org/10.2139/ssrn.4898128.

[24] Gomaa, Y.S., Awad, M.I., Emara, T., Elbokl, A., Al-Yahya, E., and ElMeligie, M.M. 2024. Role of virtual reality in examining the effect of fear of falling (FOF) on postural stability in individuals without and with Parkinson's disease in Egypt: a mixed-methods feasibility study protocol. *BMJ Open*, *14*(5), e080592. https://doi.org/10.1136/bmjopen-2023-080592.

[25] Reddy, K.K., Anisha, P.R., Mohd Hanafiah, M., Pragathi, Y.V.S.S., Ramana Murthy, B.V., Madana Mohana, R. 2023. An intelligent optimized cyclone intensity prediction framework using satellite images. *Springer Earth Science Informatics*, https://doi.org/10.1007/s12145-023-00983-z

[26] Candela, F., Romeo, S., Faundez-Zanuy, M., and Ferrer-Ramos, P. 2024. Cognitive impairment detection based on frontal camera scene while performing handwriting tasks. *Cognitive Computation*, 1–18, https://doi.org/10.1007/s12559-024-10279-z.

[27] Reddy, C.K.K., Anisha, P.R., Reddy, T., Srinivasulu, B., and Rambabu, D. 2022. *Light-Weight Real Time Weather Forecasting Simulation over Bangladesh using Deep Learning*. INT-JECSE, 449–465.

[28] Reddy, C.K.K., Anisha, P.R., Reddy, T., and Rambabu, D. *Early Monitoring of Social Distancing using Opencv and Deep Learning*. INT-JECSE, 2022, 1275–1283.

Chapter 11

Harnessing deep learning for the early diagnosis of dementia

A transformative approach in neurological health

Avula Mahathi, Kishor Kumar Reddy C, Srinath Doss, and Shenson Joseph

11.1 INTRODUCTION

The word "dementia" is a catch-all for a group of neurodegenerative diseases marked by a loss of cognitive functions like language, memory, thinking, and problem-solving. When it comes to individuals sixty years of age and above, dementia most often results from Alzheimer's disease (AD) [9]. With Alzheimer's disease accounting for 60–70% of cases, it is the most prevalent type of dementia. Lewy body dementia, frontotemporal dementia, and vascular dementia are among more forms [13]. While it is not a typical aspect of aging, dementia primarily affects older persons. Over time, the disease progressively deteriorates, significantly affecting a person's capacity to carry out everyday tasks and preserve their independence. Early diagnosis is essential for treating symptoms, reducing the rate at which the disease progresses, and enhancing the quality of life for both patients and carers because the condition is progressive.

This work proposes a new deep learning paradigm for the initial screening of dementia patients in order to increase the accuracy of diagnoses and timeliness. As a result, we propose a clear and straightforward comparison between usual diagnostic methods and modern deep learning techniques and show the advantages of AI solutions. The paper describes comprehensive research arising from real data; the results highlight strategies that may be used by healthcare professionals to improve early identification of dementia. The proposed framework is fully scalable and can be used in any healthcare context, which makes it useful in clinical practice for early intervention. The results of our study provide a basis for subsequent studies on the application of AI in neurology, including dementia diagnosis and therapy.

This chapter is organized as follows. We include an extensive assessment of the literature on the influence of deep learning techniques in the field of dementia diagnosis early in Section 11.2. In Section 11.3, the technique is described with special attention to the deep learning models and datasets used in this investigation. The trials we conducted are presented in Section 11.4, which shows how effective the suggested strategy is. Section 11.5

DOI: 10.1201/9781003591085-11

delves into the ramifications of the results and draws comparisons with existing methodologies. The chapter's conclusion, included in Section 11.6, provides a summary of the main findings and research directions.

11.1.1 The global impact of dementia

Dementia has become a major public health issue that is defining the aging population in various groups of people and diverse cultural backgrounds. Currently, more than 55 million of the global population suffers from dementia and this figure has been predicted to rise to 152 million by mid-2050 due to increased life expectancy and increased proportion of the aging population. About 10 million people are newly diagnosed with cancer annually as evidenced by a new diagnosis every three seconds. Dementia is most common among the elderly, but the early forms of dementia are also possible, in people under the age of 65 years. Most patients with dementia are found in LMICs [1–3], and the dementia burden is also significantly higher among these nations. The study also estimated that by the year 2050, about 71% of the people living with dementia will be found in LGICs and these countries usually have underfunded healthcare that cannot support the needs of the patient. The following countries are experiencing a rise in dementia rates alongside numerous problems with a low level of awareness, late diagnosis, and a lack of adequate specialized healthcare. This rising NTD requires international action plans on dementia and other care disparities and to improve healthcare delivery systems. Alzheimer dementia is one of the most common causes of disability and dependence in the elderly, and it affects not only the patient [4]. Those who suffer from dementia are predominantly dependent on their families as more than 80% of people with the condition receive care from 'informal carers'; unpaid and mostly relatives. This particular type of caregiving can be stressful and tiring and many of the caregivers end up being burnt-out and develop depression and financial woes. Sadly, in most situations, caregivers are forced to scale down their working hours or even pull out of the market altogether which is an added cost to households and, in extension, the overall economy.

As shown, the economic burden of dementia is enormous. WHO noted that the global cost of dementia was $1.3 trillion in 2020, or 1% of the global GDP, including direct medical and nursing care costs and the cost of the care provided by informal caregivers. Such costs are expected to increase to over $2.8 trillion by 2030 depending on the prevalence of as much as the affected persons. These costs are funded through taxes in high-income nations through the facility of formal healthcare systems while in LMICs they are funded by families or communities [3] and are very limited in access to formal healthcare provisions. Dementia also has large social and psychological implications within the needy economic context besides the above-specified burdens within the nuclear family members. Individuals with dementia are discriminated against in society; they are isolated, and discriminated against, and this will escalate the dementia symptoms and lower the quality of life of the sufferers. This puts a lot of pressure, especially, on those with such a condition since society tends to look at dementia patients as of lower value, this makes such patients delay seeking a diagnosis and treatment, especially in regions with low levels of awareness and literacy. This underlines the importance of more effective dementia communication, in order to raise awareness about the condition and promote timely assessment.

However, as life expectancy increases, more people fall prey to dementia. Dementia is not a prerogative of aging; however, it is more frequent among the elderly. That is why early diagnostic and therapeutic management is important, as while it helps to prevent further disease evolution and allows early intervention, it also enables consultation with a patient on how best to prepare for the future. Unfortunately, the most common diagnostic procedures do not differentiate diseases in their initial stages; thus, prompt intervention is impossible, and additional requirements for care are required further down the line. It is for this reason that there is a need to move forward with the diagnostic technologies and therefore the consideration of enhanced technologies such as deep learning for early diagnosis.

11.1.2 Importance of early diagnosis

A good understanding of dementia at an early stage can be of great importance to both the patients and the caregivers plus the health sector. Dementia is a chronic disease that gets worse as time progresses and therefore identifying parameters early on is crucial to its management. As with most diseases, however, there is no cure for dementia so detection methods enable treatment that may slow the worsening of symptoms, improve the patient's overall quality of life, and buy precious time to help with further consultations. Pharmacological and non-pharmacological treatments can be managed early provided there is a correct diagnosis [5]. Some drugs, such as cholinesterase inhibitors and memantine, are not a cure but are most beneficial when given shortly after the disease begins. These medications actually alleviate symptoms like memory loss and regulate confusion and deteriorate the thinking process thereby enabling patients with dementia to lead a more productive functional life. Like with drug interventions, non-pharmacological measures such as cognitive stimulation therapy, physical exercises, and changes in diet also fared better when given early in dementia.

On this level, early onset also allows patients and their families to make better choices regarding treatment and support, legal issues, and finance. The planning includes drawing up the advance directives, establishing the financial Powers of Attorney and debating the long-term care, which in turn grants people more control over the future. These services involve counseling, dementia care programs and other specialty services enabling early access to more appropriate services, to help both patient and carer in terms of emotional and practical coping strategies. Receiving early intervention support helps to reduce the caregiving burden and enables families to manage the new challenges posed by dementia care better. A wider implementation of early diagnosis can lead to saving much of the healthcare cost in the long run. In this manner, the idea of controlling the disease before it advances too far can help healthcare systems reduce costly, lifetime stays in the hospital or nursing homes. On the other hand, early diagnosis encourages home care, but implies the absolutization of institutional care, and suggests independence for longer time intervals.

Also, the issue of timely diagnosis is important in the prevention of dementia's progression. Screening for new treatments frequently involves patients who have early-stage dementia and early incidence of the disease consequently leads to a large population of early-stage patients. They may point to progress in what could be referred to as a disease-modifying intervention, or be useful in helping gain insights into early biomarkers of dementia. Such insights are essential in the improvement of other diagnostic techniques and in future treatments. Lastly, from the social and psychological point of view, the early diagnosis means orientation for people who have some early signs of the severe form. It is helpful because it gives them the facts about the condition and makes it easier for them to know what to expect and receive therapy for the emotional side of the disease. This in turn means that employing early diagnosis also allows patients to perform mentally stimulating tasks, hence delaying their cognitive decline and living a better life for ever-increasing periods.

11.1.3 Limitations of traditional diagnostic methods

Clinical interviews and examinations, rating scales, cognitive and neuropsychological tests, magnetic resonance imaging (MRI) and positron emission tomography (PET) have been used in diagnosing dementia as well as characterizing the clinical and pathological features of the disease [6]. However, these techniques are frequently diagnostic after major neurodegeneration suggesting that these techniques are less useful for early diagnosis of dementia. Since these methods largely depend on symptoms to measure, they often identify the condition at the advanced stage when Alzheimer's has started interfering with the affected individual's ability to carry out activities. As a kind of dementia that affects cognition, memory, and behavior, Alzheimer's disease (AD) is not a natural part of aging [7]. This delay may cost exactly those priceless moments after which significant opportunities to intervene early are lost permanently. Neuropsychological tests are those that check memory recall, problem-solving authority, etc., which means that they can contain biased answers according to the patient's education standards, culture, or slight mood swings. Although these assessments provide positive measures of cognition, they are sometimes not sufficient to identify early signs of dementia. Likewise, neuroimaging is expensive and cannot be used for early detection of Alzheimer's disease-related brain atrophy and protein deposition in large populations living in developing countries. These scans usually come into more force once there are clinical signs and therefore are not very useful for early diagnosis.

Moreover, the utilization of clinical imaging techniques, such as PET scans, as useful in showing amyloid plaques, may have problems in differentiating between the dementias [8]. For example, amyloid plaques can show up in a person who has no dementia, thus, the use of these scans in the diagnosis of dementia is quite challenging. However, other types of dementia including frontotemporal dementia or Lewy body dementia that are shown in other types of dementia do not adhere to the patterns of changes observed in Alzheimer's disease where it is relatively easy to diagnose with the help of the mentioned activities. The other disadvantage that traditional methods possess is scalability of problems that organizations are facing. Cognitive assessments that are currently conducted include those of short interval, and these may be tiresome, and they need a specialist to conduct them, which renders them inadequate for mass screen tests. Furthermore, procedures like CTZ analysis which require lumbar puncture cannot be used on a large scale, especially finding CSF is very painful for the patients and the techniques used are also dangerous. This is an implication that most early-stage dementia patients and those who are within the high-risk category do not receive a diagnosis until symptoms worsen.

The disadvantages of conventional procedures explain why there is a strong call for new procedures to diagnose this disease in its preclinical stage. There is great promise in new technologies such as deep learning and artificial intelligence to solve these issues. Whereas humans are apt to notice only gross deviations, these technologies can find hidden patterns in the physiological brain scans or a patient's genome. This breakthrough could potentially help save early dementia cases, providing an active and timely approach to simply managing the illness.

Cerebrospinal fluid (CSF) analysis, MRIs, PET scans, cognitive testing, and clinical evaluations are among the most often utilized conventional diagnostic methods for dementia which are summarized in Table 11.1. Based on its goals, benefits, and drawbacks, each approach is assessed, especially in relation to dementia early detection. Nowadays neuropsychological tests are commonly used to diagnose cognitive impairment, yet such assessments allow detection of dementia solely in the late stage and can be influenced by various factors such as education and mood of the patient. CT scans and EEG provide good imaging, but MRI and PET are more specific but expensive and only show differences once a large amount of brain tissue has been lost. CSF analysis is accurate, but the procedure is invasive and cannot be

Table 11.1 Comparison of Traditional Diagnostic Techniques and Their Limitations

Diagnostic Technique	*Description*	*Advantages*	*Limitations*
Neuropsychological Testing	Cognitive assessments (e.g., memory recall, problem-solving) to evaluate decline	Useful for identifying cognitive deficits in later stages	Subjective, influenced by education, mood, and cultural background; detects dementia after symptoms appear
MRI (Magnetic Resonance Imaging)	Imaging technique that provides detailed brain structure images	Identifies brain atrophy linked to dementia	Expensive, not suitable for routine screening, detects structural changes only after significant neurodegeneration
PET (Positron Emission Tomography) Scans	Imaging technique to detect abnormal protein deposits (e.g., amyloid plaques)	Effective in identifying amyloid plaques and tau tangles associated with Alzheimer's	High cost, may detect plaques in individuals without cognitive symptoms, limited distinction between dementia types
Cerebrospinal Fluid (CSF) Analysis	Analysis of biomarkers (e.g., amyloid-beta, tau proteins) in CSF	High accuracy in detecting Alzheimer's-related biomarkers	Invasive, lumbar puncture required, not feasible for large-scale screening
Clinical Assessment	General observation of symptoms and patient history	Easy to administer, non-invasive	Highly subjective, dependent on visible symptoms; often late-stage diagnosis

used for screening purposes. Unlike clinical assessments, surveys are simple to conduct but are totally biased which only targets a practical approach distinguishing dementia among patients; they only work with Residual symptoms but rarely diagnose the early stages of the disease.

This comparison reveals the importance of diagnostics that can detect dementia before severe cognitive decline where new approaches like deep learning come in handy.

11.2 THE ROLE OF DEEP LEARNING IN MEDICAL DIAGNOSIS

The use of DL as a technique in diagnostic medicine is transforming medical diagnosis by offering solutions that go beyond conventional diagnostic methods, especially in complex and large-scale medical data. Thanks to deep learning's capacity for analyzing various datasets, diagnostic accuracy is increased, early-stage disease biomarkers are detected, and individualized treatment is developed. In dementia diagnosis, DL can be very useful as it provides an additional opportunity to find early changes in the structures that are often hard to notice in other ways. While in classical machine learning, one has to extract features using one's own expertise and knowledge, deep learning methods are capable of learning from raw data and detecting subtle patterns in neuroimaging and genetic data as well as patient records. This capability allows for dementia identification before substantial cognitive loss is perceptible. Also, as deep learning models learn from more data, they refine their performance; these approaches screen the population scale. Some of the benefits of deep learning in medical practice are as follows:

Scalability: Historically, diagnostics for dementia involve time-consuming examinations and expensive imaging procedures and equipment that call for professional medical personnel. However, the present paper illustrates that DL-based systems could be used more widely and effectively, enabling first-stage screening to be available to significantly more at-risk individuals. This tends to enable healthcare provision agencies to offer early enough interventions so as to help arrest the further deterioration of dementia and thus reduce the general social cost. Multimodal data fusion is also well-handled by deep learning which is crucial in comprehending severe diseases such as dementia. Being based on neuroimaging data and integrated with genetic and clinical information, deep learning models output an accurate comprehensive diagnosis. This will enhance the specificity of the differentiation of various types of dementia including Alzheimer's, frontotemporal dementia, and Lewy body dementia to adequately practice early treatment. Although deep learning has enormous potential, there are obstacles in the way of its widespread implementation, such as the requirement for sizable, high-quality datasets and making sure AI is used ethically in healthcare contexts. Deep learning is a crucial component of future medical diagnostic procedures, particularly for the early diagnosis of dementia, as a result of ongoing research and technology breakthroughs that are overcoming these obstacles.

11.2.1 Deep learning vs. traditional machine learning

The techniques of traditional machine learning (ML) and deep learning (DL) are of great beneficial use in the medical diagnosis field, but they work in different ways to learn from data. Conventional techniques like support vector machines (SVM), decision trees, etc., require prior selection of features; a process known as feature selection from the raw data. This process involves the use of considerable information on the particular field, and may take a lot of time. That is why these models are good for simple data and do not work well with large, high-dimensional data, which are distinctive for neuroimaging and genomics, and critical for the early diagnosis of dementia. However, deep learning models, particularly neural networks, are capable of learning features independently without any intervention from the programmer. Deep learning is particularly suitable for analyzing medical imaging data such as MRI [9] and PET scans, especially when changes are minimal; early-stage dementia, for instance, may be identified from a scan. Using deep learning models, patterns that could be obscure even to a machine learning algorithm might be discovered hence improving diagnostics. Although neuroimaging methods like positron emission tomography (PET) and magnetic resonance imaging (MRI) offer precise insights into the structure and function of the brain, they are hampered by their high cost, limited accessibility, and requirement for specialized equipment [10].

It is also important to shed light on the handling of multimodal data as one more distinction between the two. Conventional ML approaches in oncology are challenging for data amalgamation, i.e., imaging, genomic markers, or cognitive tests. Nevertheless, deep learning is well-equipped for multimodal data treatment because it integrates these dissimilar sources into one model [11]. That lets one get a broader view and increases the prognostic accuracy of the early dementia diagnosis, which is a crucial advantage for the concept understanding of the disease. Furthermore, deep learning models have remarkable scalability. Traditional machine learning techniques can be resource-intensive since they frequently need a large amount of manual labor to fine-tune and train the model for every new dataset. However, once trained, deep learning algorithms can be used on massive datasets, which makes them perfect for mass screening people at risk for dementia. The long-term strain on healthcare systems can be lessened by using this scalability to identify people who may benefit from preventative care early on. Deep learning has benefits, but it also has drawbacks. For example, large volumes of labeled data are required for models to be trained efficiently, and the interpretability of the outcomes is a source of concern. Deep learning is expected to outperform classical machine learning in the diagnosis of complicated medical disorders, such as dementia, with more efficiency and accuracy as research progresses and more extensive datasets become accessible. The main characteristics, advantages, and disadvantages of several deep learning architectures for dementia detection are contrasted in Table 11.2. This overview helps determine which models—such as CNNs, RNNs, and autoencoders—are most appropriate for a certain sort of dementia-related dataset and how they are used to detect anomalies in the brain.

Table 11.2 Comparison of Deep Learning Architectures in Dementia Detection

Deep Learning Architecture	*Key Features*	*Strengths*	*Limitations*	*Applications*
Convolutional Neural Networks (CNN)	Uses convolutional layers to detect patterns in images.	Excellent for processing image-based data (e.g., MRI scans).	May require large datasets to avoid overfitting.	Detecting brain abnormalities in MRI scans.
Recurrent Neural Networks (RNN)	Designed for sequential data and time series analysis.	Good for analyzing time-based data (e.g., EEG signals).	Can suffer from vanishing gradient problems.	Predicting disease progression over time.
Long Short-Term Memory (LSTM)	A type of RNN that addresses vanishing gradient issues.	Effective for long-range dependencies in data.	Computationally expensive.	Modeling disease trajectories in patients.
Autoencoders	Used for unsupervised learning.	Excellent for dimensionality reduction and anomaly detection.	Can be complex and hard to interpret.	Detecting subtle brain changes over time.

11.2.2 Advantages and ethical considerations of deep learning in dementia detection

Advantages: Three major advantages associated with deep learning include accuracy and efficiency in data analysis and the ability to handle large dataset characteristic of dementia patients. These models can recognize traits that can easily go unnoticed which is why they are best suited for preliminary detection [12]. They can analyze heterogeneous data, such as MRI, EEG, and genomics data which would help to get a better picture of the disease. These models help in quick diagnosis, thereby saving much time and cost since more of the activities run on autopilot. The idea that social engagement may influence overall health and well-being, as well as cognitive health and dementia risk, has generated interest. It has been shown to encourage healthy lifestyles, lower stress levels, and improve cognitive function [13].

Ethical Considerations: However, the advancement of AI and deep learning in dementia diagnosis has its own set of problems as discussed below. Another problem is related to data protectionism, which is crucial when dealing with dementia databases, as collections of data belonging to patients with dementia may contain rather personal information. Yet, it must be ensured that such data are personal and secure. The onset of dementia, depression, and higher death rates are among the health hazards linked to loneliness among older persons [14]. The ultimate concern is the capability of deep learning models, which are often categorized as black boxes. Thus, a lack of transparency may result in a conflict of trust between the patients and healthcare service providers. Finally, there are issues related to fairness and potential prejudice in AI models due to the fact that algorithms based on inadequate data give worse results to members of underrepresented groups. It is important for fairness, accountability, and transparency purposes, to practice some ethically reasonable approaches to AI diagnosis. The main ethical issues with AI-driven dementia diagnosis are listed in Table 11.3, along with data privacy, bias, interpretability, and regulatory compliance. It also draws attention to how these difficulties affect diagnosis and offers some possible fixes to guarantee the ethical application of AI in healthcare.

Table 11.3 Ethical Challenges in AI-Driven Dementia Diagnosis

Ethical Challenge	*Description*	*Impact on Diagnosis*	*Potential Solutions*
Data Privacy and Security	AI systems require access to sensitive patient data, including brain scans, genetic information, and clinical history.	Breaches of patient data privacy can lead to misuse of personal health information and loss of trust.	Implementing strict data anonymization, secure data storage, and compliance with privacy laws (e.g., GDPR, HIPAA).
Bias and Fairness	Deep learning models can inherit biases present in training data, leading to unfair treatment of certain groups.	Can result in discriminatory outcomes and unequal access to diagnosis, especially for minorities or underserved populations.	Using diverse datasets, employing bias detection methods, and ensuring equitable model development.
Lack of Interpretability	AI models, especially deep learning systems, are often criticized for being "black box" models.	Lack of understanding about how a model arrives at its conclusions can erode trust among healthcare providers and patients.	Development of explainable AI (XAI) to make models more transparent and understandable for medical professionals.
Regulatory Compliance	AI technologies in healthcare must adhere to medical device regulations, including safety and efficacy standards.	Failure to comply with regulations can delay the approval and adoption of AI tools in clinical settings.	Establishing clear regulatory frameworks for AI in healthcare, and regular monitoring for ongoing compliance.

Table 11.3 (Cont.)

Ethical Challenge	*Description*	*Impact on Diagnosis*	*Potential Solutions*
Informed Consent	Patients must understand how AI will be used in their diagnosis and provide consent for data usage.	Without clear consent, patients may feel their privacy is violated or they are being diagnosed without full understanding.	Ensuring transparent communication and clear consent processes regarding the use of AI in diagnosis.
Accountability	In the case of AI-driven errors, it is unclear who holds responsibility—the developer, the healthcare provider, or the AI system itself.	Ambiguity around accountability may complicate the resolution of medical errors and legal issues.	Establishing legal frameworks to define accountability between AI developers and healthcare providers.
Job Displacement	The increasing reliance on AI could reduce the demand for certain healthcare jobs, especially in diagnostic roles.	This can lead to job loss and disruption within healthcare professions, particularly in diagnostic imaging.	AI should be viewed as a support tool, with a focus on retraining healthcare professionals to work alongside AI systems.

11.3 KEY DEEP LEARNING ARCHITECTURES FOR DEMENTIA DIAGNOSIS

The most successful deep learning architectures for dementia diagnosis will be discussed in this section. In order to detect early indicators of dementia, these structures make use of cutting-edge methods for handling complicated medical data, including MRI scans, EEG signals, and genetic data. We'll talk about each architecture's advantages and particular uses. PET, MRI, and CT scans are three neuroimaging methods used to diagnose dementia [15].

Convolutional Neural Networks (CNNs)

Convolutional neural networks (CNNs) are commonly used in image diagnostics and therefore applicable in analyzing imaging derived from the brain such as MRI and PET. CNNs are particularly good at preserving the 2D spatial structure of images and detecting spatial hierarchies predicting areas of brain atrophy in dementia.

Applications: CNNs are applied to categorize the brain images, divide the brain into areas of the interested region of interest, and identify possible early signs of the disease associated with dementia.

Strengths: The high accuracy in image-based tasks, and the fact that features such as spatial relationships can be learned without the need for specifying them beforehand.

Recurrent Neural Networks (RNN)

Recurrent neural networks (RNNs) are named as such because they need to remember some previous information and they are very suitable for analyzing temporal data: for instance, EEG signals or repeated patient observations. Sequential data such as progression trends in dementia could be tracked effortlessly because RNNs, especially LSTM networks, can capture temporal dependencies in data.

Applications: The use of RNNs is in EEG data analysis; in early identification of decline in cognition; in disease progression.

Strengths: Houses excellent performance for sequential data, can recognize temporal effects, and is ideal for monitoring the evolution of a disease.

Autoencoders

An autoencoder is an unsupervised learning neural network that is used to model an input space of a dataset by encoding it and decoding it thus being useful in cases where the dimension of data desires to be reduced. In dementia diagnosis, autoencoders are applied to access features such as MRI or genetic data by decoding and filtering through noise from the data.

Applications: Segmentation of the MRI images of the brain and characterization of some distinct patterns and classification of neurodegenerative diseases.

Strengths: Traditional for unsupervised learning, scales down the number of features while maintaining them relevant, useful for outlier detection.

Hybrid Models

Most of the combined models involve the integration of ideas from various deep learning to make the best out of each kind of model. For instance, a model in an image with patient records could involve the use of CNNs to interpret images and the use of RNNs to interpret a patient's record over time. This enables the construction of a more complete picture of the patient's dementia since the various data types for diagnosing dementia include brain imaging and anamnesis.

Applications: Adding MRI scans with genetic or behavioral data to make the approach to diagnosing dementia elaborate.

Strengths: This is a collection of various models to enhance věku accuracy and modifications of handling multimodal data.

Generative Adversarial Networks (GANs)

Generative adversarial networks (GANs) are employed in the production of training datasets for deep learning as most of the time annotated datasets are limited. Activities of GANs are equally applicable in dementia to increase the dataset, developing synthetic images of brain scans for training models in order to enhance model performance.

Applications: Overcoming cases when real patient data is not sufficient; improvements to the training process through data augmentation.

Strengths: Adaptable to produce high-quality synthetic datasets which is helpful for the situation of data insufficiency.

Deep learning architectures play a crucial role in the improvement of timely diagnosis of dementia fully illustrated below. Due to the application of specific structures for various types of medical information, the models allow the creation of more precise, fast, and extensive diagnostics.

Figure 11.1 shows the different deep learning architectures for dementia diagnosis. It indicates the proportion of usage of each model in the field and reveals that CNNs are the most widely used out of all the models, mostly in interpreting brain imaging data, such as MRI scans. The following are recurrent neural networks (RNNs), which are useful in the case of the time-dependency nature of EEG signals and longitudinal patient records. Identified applications include dimensionality reduction / feature extraction using autoencoders, and hybrid models and GANs with less representation although promising as a way of leveraging different architectures to come up with a formidable one. This chart can show the recent concerns and topics related to the use of deep learning in the diagnosis of dementia.

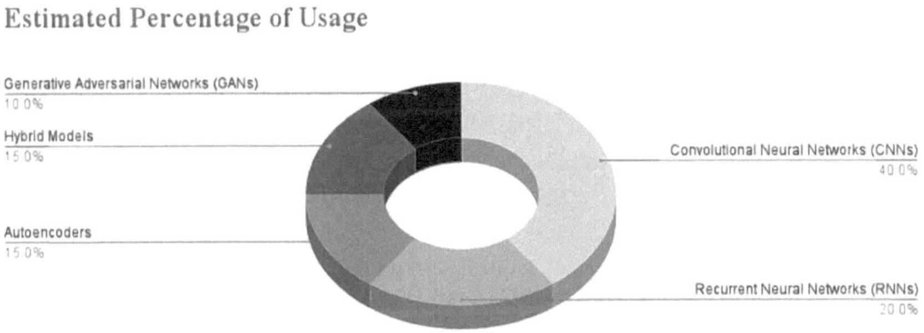

Figure 11.1 Distribution of Deep Learning Architectures in Dementia Diagnosis.

11.4 DATASETS AND TOOLS FOR TRAINING DEEP LEARNING MODELS

The datasets and resources necessary for deep learning model training for dementia diagnosis will be covered in detail in this section. Having access to high-quality data is essential to building and testing these models. Deep learning models can be effectively trained, validated, and benchmarked utilizing a number of publicly available datasets that have been generated especially for dementia research. The prediction power of these diagnostic tools has increased while analyzing complicated datasets thanks to the incorporation of artificial intelligence and machine learning algorithms [16].

11.4.1 Publicly available datasets

Making use of multimodal data collected from many cohorts [17], public dataset analysis helps researchers and practitioners to employ and experiment with deep learning models. Of all the databases for dementia diagnosis, both well-known datasets include ADNI (Alzheimer's Disease Neuroimaging Initiative) and OASIS (Open Access Series of Imaging Studies). These datasets consist of neuroimaging information, clinical parameters and genetic data, the collecting of which is crucial in the analysis of neurodegenerative diseases.

In Table 11.4 the researcher has described various datasets that are publicly available and widely incorporated in DL for diagnosing dementia. Both datasets are essential for designing and developing the models to detect AD, MCI, and further investigate other neurodegenerative diseases.

ADNI (Alzheimer's Disease Neuroimaging Initiative): ADNI dataset is one of the largest and most popular datasets for dementia study especially for Alzheimer's disease. It encompasses a vast amount of neuroimaging data (MRI, PET, etc.) together with clinical data (such as cognitive test results, age, gender, etc.). The dataset contains information from over 1,500 patients and contains both cross-sectional and follow-on data regarding the disease. figuration is vital in training deep learning models to identify potential symptoms of dementia and indeed, track the disease progression over time. The dataset for ADNI is deposited in publicly accessible repositories, but specific permission is needed to access the dataset.

OASIS (Open Access Series of Imaging Studies): Another well-known dataset in the diagnosis of dementia, especially Alzheimer's disease and MCI is the Open Access Series of Imaging Studies (OASIS). It comprises both imaging data mostly MRI and non-imaging data, and the former ranges across normal aging, MCI, and early Alzheimer's disease. It contains data from approximately 1,000

Table 11.4 Overview of Key Datasets for Dementia Diagnosis Using Deep Learning

Dataset Name	*Data Type*	*Size*	*Key Features*	*Availability*
ADNI	Neuroimaging (MRI, PET), Clinical Data	1,500+ Participants	Longitudinal data for Alzheimer's disease diagnosis	Publicly available upon request
OASIS	Neuroimaging (MRI), Clinical Data	1,000+ Participants	Data on Alzheimer's disease, mild cognitive impairment, and normal aging	Open access
UK Biobank	Neuroimaging (MRI, PET), Genomic Data, Clinical Data	500,000+ Participants	Large-scale dataset with comprehensive health data	Requires registration
MIRIAD	Neuroimaging (MRI), Clinical Data	200+ Participants	Focus on dementia subtypes (vascular dementia, Alzheimer's)	Publicly available
AIBL	Neuroimaging (MRI, PET), Clinical Data	1,000+ Participants	Longitudinal study focusing on Alzheimer's disease and mild cognitive impairment	Publicly available upon request

participants and has the advantage of being publicly available to anyone wishing to use it for non-commercial purposes. OASIS plays a great role in enabling researchers to construct models that can differentiate between healthy aging and early stages of neurodegenerative disease.

UK Biobank: The UK Biobank is very large-scale population-based and holds the data of more than 500,000 people. It contains not only neuroimaging data, such as MRI or PET or MEG or EEG, but also clinical data and even genomic data, so it is considered as a gold mine for developing models based on the deep learning approach. It is particularly helpful for researchers planning on including genetic data in the model for naming dementia. Nevertheless, the UK Biobank is not open to the public, anyone willing to get a hold of this resource must register and be approved as the use of this facility is reserved for researchers only.

MIRIAD (MRI in Alzheimer's Disease): The MIRIAD database is deliberately concerned with diagnosing Alzheimer's disease and vascular dementia from neuroimaging data, particularly MRI scans. It involves more than 200 people, and the data contain images of patients with various forms of dementia: early- and late-stage, as well as different subtypes that can be used for developing appropriate deep learning models. MIRIAD can be particularly helpful to investigators who are interested in comparing vascular dementia and Alzheimer's disease. A dataset with clinical annotations for the conditions is available. This dataset is available for use by the public.

AIBL (Australian Imaging, Biomarkers and Lifestyle Study of Aging): The AIBL dataset contains MRI/PET neuroimaging data and clinical covariate data (cognitive tests, lifestyle information, etc.) in well over 1,000 individuals. As people age, many experience memory loss, and some develop dementia [18]. It follows people for a long time allowing researchers to investigate the development of Alzheimer's disease and mild cognitive impairment. The dataset is of much use to deep learning in the diagnosis of dementia and can be provided with public access if desired. This makes the dataset important where the context of interest is age-related cognitive decline in people with dementia while controlling for healthy aging data.

11.4.2 Data preprocessing techniques and tools for deep learning models

The essential subjects of data preparation methods and resources for deep learning model training in dementia diagnosis will be covered in this section. Deep learning models cannot be successfully trained without proper data preparation since raw data frequently contains noise, missing values, and irrelevant information. Additionally, these models' performance and efficiency can be greatly increased by using the appropriate frameworks and tools.

11.4.2.1 Data preprocessing techniques for dementia diagnosis

Building precise machine learning and deep learning models for gait identification requires careful consideration of both feature selection and data preprocessing [19]. Data preprocessing is a crucial step inclusive of data cleaning, data transformation as well as data reduction before feeding into the ML models. For the case of diagnostic models for dementia, preprocessing is critical to enhance the proper identification of early AD, MCI, and other related diseases. Common techniques for preprocessing data in dementia research include:

11.4.2.2 Normalization and standardization

Normalization standardizes the data with a particular range stretching from 0 to 1 and guarantees that no feature prejudices the model just because it is larger in magnitude [20]. This is especially valuable for neuroimaging data sources such as MRI scans, as pixel intensities may differ a lot.

Z-score normalization is another technique in which values of a dataset are made to adjust the average to zero and a variable to one on the scale. This helps to avoid models that assign certain features a preferential status, for example, when working with clinical data (numerical, for example, results of cognitive tests).

11.4.2.3 Handling missing data

Empty entries within datasets especially in clinical data (age, test scores, medical history, etc.) can be managed by way of imputation (where missing values are substituted using the mean, median or mode) or by excluding such samples from the dataset.

There are also more sophisticated methods that are gradually being adopted for imputing missing neuroimaging data or longitudinal data, for example, generative models, or nearest-neighbor imputation.

11.4.2.4 Feature extraction and selection

Feature extraction is the process of deriving only important features from the data. When dealing with more complex neuroimaging data, such as MRI scans, useful features include Principal Component Analysis (PCA), wavelet or PCA transforms or texture features.

Feature selection covers the process of selecting the best features that will be used for the training of deep learning models. In dementia diagnosis, such information may be in the form of choosing either clinical variables associated with worse cognition or brain areas that show signs of degeneration.

11.4.2.5 Data augmentation

Neuroimaging data such as MRI and PET scans our data augmentation can be used to oversample the existing dataset. It can / This may involve simple transformations like rotation, scaling, cropping or even flipping of the images at random. This in turn avoids overfitting and strengthens the model.

11.4.2.6 Tools and frameworks for deep learning models

Accurate dementia diagnosis requires the use of proper tools for creating scalable deep learning models [21]. Several popular deep learning libraries and frameworks are widely adopted in the research community for medical image analysis and clinical prediction:

TensorFlow and Keras
TensorFlow is an open-source machine learning framework, created by Google, to provide both algorithms and components for deep learning. Keras is an application programming interface that is on top of TensorFlow. It is used for deep learning, especially for beginners. Both are best suited to medical AI applications due to their versatility, modularity, and good documentation.

PyTorch
PyTorch is another deep learning framework created by the Facebook company. It has become popular in research because of its ability to have a more flexible computation graph than TensorFlow. PyTorch is preferred specifically for experimentation-related work and is implemented in the diagnosis of dementia using medical images and time series.

Scikit-**learn**
Scikit-learn is not a deep learning library but rather a powerful high-level tool set for machine learning in Python used for data preprocessing, feature selection, model validation, etc. This is commonly used together with deep learning libraries, for instance, in operations such as Keras and TensorFlow for purposes of data partition and model testing.

SimpleITK
Originally, SimpleITK was developed for the purpose of medical image processing. As such it is particularly useful for image registration, image segmentation and image resampling, processes which are characteristic of neuroimaging data, for example MRI or PET scans used in dementia diagnosis.

MONAI (Medical Open Network for AI)
MONAI is a deep learning framework that was created to be used in medical imaging. It has image preprocessing, data augmentation, and evaluation tools for deeper medical applications such as neuroimaging applications. Specifically, MONAI is optimized for MRI CT and PET and thus is suitable to be used to train models for dementia diagnosis.

Fastai

If the reader has never heard of this before, Fastai is a deep learning library that is based on PyTorch and is designed to be simple. This entails that deep learning model development is abstracted at high levels and does not require much coding by the researcher in the medical domain to enhance the deep learning models for dementia detection.

Applying suitable tools and frameworks and data preprocessing strategies, deep learning models for dementia diagnosis can be made accurate and efficient by researchers and practitioners. Prior processes like normalization, feature extraction and data augmentation mentioned above are crucial to the quality of the data—the tools that are used in the building of advanced models include TensorFlow, PyTorch and MONAI. Together with the preprocessing, such tools significantly contribute to the improvement of the performance and robustness of deep learning models in dementia studies.

The following is a simple table that elaborately describes some of the dominating data preprocessing methods that are crucial in enhancing the efficiency of deep learning models while diagnosing dementia. Data preprocessing is the process of preparing raw data to feed into the model-making process and this is done in the right way due to its importance in improving model accuracy, minimizing overfitting and improving model generalization.

Table 11.5 shows the summary of data preprocessing steps used in deep learning models for dementia diagnosis. Normalization and standardization

Table 11.5 Common Data Preprocessing Techniques for Deep Learning in Dementia Diagnosis

Preprocessing Technique	*Description*	*Applications in Dementia Diagnosis*
Normalization	Adjusts the scale of data to a specific range, usually [0, 1], ensuring all features are treated equally during training.	Used in neuroimaging data (e.g., MRI and PET scans) to standardize pixel intensities, preventing certain features from dominating the model due to large differences in scale.
Standardization	Transforms data to have a mean of 0 and a standard deviation of 1.	Applied to clinical data such as cognitive scores and demographic features to ensure they are on a similar scale, aiding in model convergence.
Data Augmentation	Involves generating additional data points by applying transformations such as rotation, flipping, and cropping.	Frequently used in neuroimaging to artificially increase dataset size by applying random rotations, flips, and zooms on MRI/PET images to prevent overfitting and increase model robustness.
Denoising	Involves removing noise (irrelevant information) from the data. For images, techniques like Gaussian filtering or wavelet transforms are used.	Essential for MRI scans or EEG data, where noise can obscure important features. Denoising helps in better highlighting regions of the brain affected by dementia.

(continued)

Table 11.5 (Cont.)

Preprocessing Technique	*Description*	*Applications in Dementia Diagnosis*
Imputation of Missing Data	Replaces missing values in the dataset with statistical values (mean, median, mode) or uses advanced methods like k-nearest-neighbor imputation.	Applied to clinical and longitudinal data when certain records are missing, ensuring that incomplete patient profiles do not reduce the training dataset's size.
Feature Extraction	Involves transforming raw data into a set of relevant features that better represent underlying patterns. Techniques like PCA (Principal Component Analysis) and LDA (Linear Discriminant Analysis) are common.	Used to extract key features from neuroimaging data, such as brain regions or connectivity patterns that are indicative of Alzheimer's or other forms of dementia.

reduce the impact of different features thus helping in improving algorithms in the deep learning model. For instance, rotating or flipping MRI images constitutes data augmentation to simulate a large dataset especially when there is little data.

A denoising process is employed to eliminate redundant noise in the images or signals which plays a critical role in medical imaging like MRI scans for the initial stage of dementia. It was also important to note that using imputation for the missing data means that records where information may be missing from patient records cannot hinder the use of the remaining information for training the models which is often a challenge in large datasets. Last but not least, uniformly in all the articles, feature extraction methods such as PCA also play a crucial role when it comes to feature reduction in neuroimaging, thus making it easier to model these features without much loss of information.

Each of these preprocessing techniques is important in that it not only allows the deep learning models for dementia detection to be trained on the best dataset but also improves the performance of such models.

The usage percentages of several deep learning frameworks in dementia diagnosis are visually represented in Figure 11.2. While the x-axis will list the deep learning frameworks—TensorFlow, Keras, PyTorch, and Fastai—the y-axis will show the proportion of usage. This graph shows how popular TensorFlow and Keras are in the industry, with PyTorch gaining ground because of its adaptability and application in educational settings.

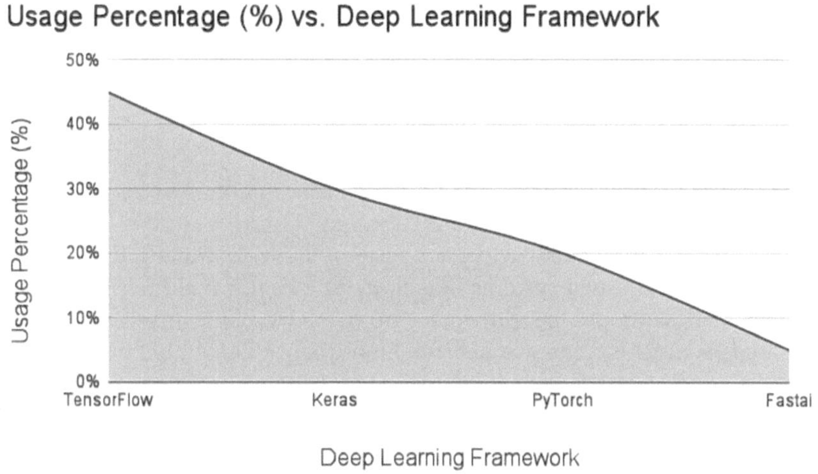

Figure 11.2 Popular Deep Learning Frameworks for Dementia Diagnosis.

11.5 CHALLENGES AND FUTURE DIRECTIONS IN DEMENTIA DIAGNOSIS USING DEEP LEARNING

Using deep learning for the early diagnosis of dementia has been promising; however, its implementation is faced with a number of challenges that need to be solved before deep learning is embraced in clinical practice. The issues can be seen to largely stem from factors within the four major subject areas of model interpretability, clinical implementation, future advancements, and directions in model development. These hurdles will have to be surmounted in order for artificial intelligence solutions in dementia diagnosis to be more efficient, open, and practical.

Model Interpretability and Transparency

A major problem of employing deep learning for identifying dementia is the black box nature of the network structures. Artificial neural networks used in applications like analysis of MRI images or pattern detection in neuroimaging are called deep neural networks and are often labeled as black box models. Although these models may give high accuracy their predictions are not very helpful as they do not explain how they reached the conclusion. For many applications in healthcare, especially diagnosing dementia, it is more important for models to be interpretable because clinicians have to understand the logic behind the artificial intelligence's decision before it can be applied in their practice.

This problem will therefore require future advancement in explainable AI (XAI) [22]. Scientists are working on making model interpretability by representing the activity of a neural network or creating saliency maps that point out the dominant image features to which an AI pays attention during classification. The aim is to generate value by delivering better, more actionable data to clinicians so that, in addition to being accurate, AI-based tools are accessible, consistent, and safe for use in medicine.

Integration into Clinical Practice

In contrast, the existing literature points to the potential of deep learning in dementia diagnosis, adoption of AI tools in clinical workflows continues to pose a major challenge. AI-based systems have to function in parallel with already established systems like electronic health records (EHRs) and be integrated with the instruments employed by clinicians [23]. As the presented sections indicate, to achieve high-quality hospitable models even the most sophisticated deep learning-based systems can turn useless and inconceivable in actual clinical settings if they are not part of an integrated system.

Furthermore, once implemented, the task of artificial intelligence entails shifts in the health profession training and clinical reasoning process. Clinicians need to not only know how to apply the AI tools but also know what the results mean in their clinical setting. There is also a need to engage AI manufacturers and healthcare consumers and systems so that deep learning paradigms meet clinical needs and suit current regulations. Large-scale patient trials are required to prove the diagnostic accuracy and safety of AI models in dementia diagnosis as well as to enhance popular trust in these models.

Future **Research** and Technological Trends

Many real-world issues have found automated solutions thanks to the combined efforts of artificial intelligence (AI) and machine learning (ML) [24]. In the future, a number of promising directions in deep learning research for dementia diagnosis and interesting technological trends can be predicted. One of the major research fields is the integration of the data coming from various modalities using deep learning models: neuroimaging, genomic, and clinical data about patients will provide a more comprehensive view of the disease. With this approach, there will be enhanced diagnosis accuracy, especially of the early stage dementia that is important in the early intercessions. Many different conditions fall under the category of neurological illnesses, including brain tumors, head injuries, epilepsy, and syndrome disorders [25].

Another exciting possibility is to provide individualization of the AI models. Most current deep learning models are trained on general data which excludes the variation in patients' disease progression. In the future, new models will probably use individual identification to create diagnostic tools that would describe how dementia would progress in a given subject. Individualized approaches could also improve the treatment procedures making the treatment plans much better. The role of edge computing in personal monitoring together with the development of wearable gadgets is also an interesting topic for further investigation. These devices may be capable of delivering constant reports on the patient's mental and physical well-being, which may be entered into deep learning algorithms to allow early assessment and action to be taken. Smart applications that track mental health status via mobile interfaces may benefit both patients and clinicians in the context of disease progression by pointing to new approaches to more tailored and anticipatory care. Through the provision of cutting-edge technologies for improving diagnostic precision, customizing treatment regimens, and forecasting patient outcomes, artificial intelligence (AI) is transforming modern healthcare [26].

Finally, the important cooperation among shareholders of practical knowledge including researchers, doctors, and designers of AI will be indispensably significant again. Also, we anticipate that large collaborative datasets across different demographic and geographical characteristics will be crucial to enhancing the generality of AI models. Collaboration between computer scientists and medical practitioners working collectively will promote the enhancement of new models that are not only precise, but also accountable for the outcomes they provide, and will seem legitimate and logical to the healthcare practitioners and patients.

Overall, the potential and future of advanced dementia diagnosis through deep learning techniques hold a lot of promise [27]; however, there lie many challenges as well. From this paper's findings, it will be imperative to provide solutions to constraints concerning model interpretability, model incorporation into practice, and future research direction. Indeed, it will help to improve the effectiveness of diagnosis and treatment of patients with dementia [28], as well as the overall acceptance of AI technologies in clinical practice when the aforementioned challenges cease to exist or become less significant as deep learning techniques improve.

The deep learning trends shown in Table 11.6 have the potential to completely transform the diagnosis of dementia. For the purpose of overcoming obstacles relating to restricted data availability and privacy issues, transfer learning and federated learning are particularly crucial [29]. Reinforcement learning and self-supervised learning offer innovative approaches to model development by reducing reliance on labeled data. Finally, the capacity of generative adversarial networks (GANs) [30] to produce synthetic data may contribute to enhancing the resilience of training datasets, especially when it comes to uncommon dementias. Regarding neurodegenerative disorders, each of these changes offers a different chance to improve AI systems' capacity for diagnosis [31].

Table 11.6 Emerging Trends in Deep Learning for Dementia Diagnosis

Emerging Trend	*Description*	*Potential Applications in Dementia Diagnosis*
Transfer Learning	Transfer learning involves taking a pre-trained model and fine-tuning it on a new dataset. This reduces the amount of data required for training and speeds up the model development process.	Transfer learning can be used to leverage pre-existing models trained on large datasets for neuroimaging, then fine-tuned with specific datasets of dementia patients to improve accuracy in early diagnosis.
Federated Learning	Federated learning allows multiple institutions to collaborate on model development without sharing sensitive patient data. Data remains decentralized, ensuring privacy.	In dementia diagnosis, federated learning can facilitate collaborative research while maintaining patient privacy, allowing models to be trained across various healthcare institutions and datasets.
Reinforcement Learning	Reinforcement learning is an area of machine learning where agents learn by interacting with an environment to achieve a goal. It's used for optimization tasks.	This approach could optimize AI diagnostic tools over time by improving their decision-making ability as they interact with patient data, refining the predictive accuracy of dementia diagnosis models.
Self-Supervised Learning	A type of learning where the model is trained on unlabeled data, with the system creating its own labels by finding structure in the data.	In dementia diagnosis, self-supervised learning could be applied to neuroimaging datasets, where the model learns useful features without relying on labor-intensive manual annotations.
Generative Adversarial Networks (GANs)	GANs are used for generating new data that is similar to real-world data by pitting two networks against each other in a "game" to improve accuracy.	GANs could be used to augment neuroimaging datasets, creating synthetic brain scans that simulate different stages of dementia, thus improving the training data for deep learning models.

11.6 CONCLUSION

This paper has benchmarked deep learning applications in diagnosing dementia at an early stage, its barriers, and trends in the future. For instance, it is worth mentioning the neuroimaging analysis with the aid of which deep learning models have shown high efficiency as well as increased diagnostic accuracy when using multimodal data analysis. Nonetheless, there are questions regarding model interpretation, data privacy, and clinical implementation. The way forward for dementia diagnosis is to overcome these hurdles where transfer learning and federated learning are among key promising solutions to steer up dementia diagnosis models while keeping the identities of the patients concealed. In a nutshell, AI within healthcare can enable early diagnosis as well as individual treatment but proper training for the clinicians and ethical issues should be addressed.

Thus, deep learning has the potential to change the current situation in dementia treatment and improve diagnostics. The next activities require enhancing AI explanatory models, increasing interdisciplinary research, and applying the presented technologies to optimize the treatment of dementia patients.

REFERENCES

[1] Mukherjee, M. B. (2024). The role of neuro-imaging biomarkers in the early detection of dementia and Alzheimer's disease. In: *Exploring Medical Biotechnology-In Vivo, In Vitro, In Silico* (pp. 112–118). Boca Raton: CRC Press. https://doi.org/10.1201/9781003423007-11

[2] Noroozi, M., Gholami, M., Sadeghsalehi, H., Behzadi, S., Habibzadeh, A., Erabi, G., ... & Deravi, N. (2024). Machine and deep learning algorithms for classifying different types of dementia: A literature review. *Applied Neuropsychology: Adult*, 1–15. https://doi.org/10.1080/23279095.2023.1307195

[3] Mondal, H., Hassan, M. M., Nag, A., & Bairagi, A. K. (2024). The Integration of Federated Deep Learning with Internet of Things in Healthcare. In Federated Deep Learning for Healthcare (pp. 143–159). CRC Press.

[4] Park, C. Y., Kim, M., Shim, Y., Ryoo, N., Choi, H., Jeong, H. T., ... & Youn, Y. C. (2024). Harnessing the power of voice: A deep neural network model for Alzheimer's disease detection. *Dementia and Neurocognitive Disorders*, 23(1), 1. https://doi.org/10.0000/dnd.2024.001

[5] Frederiksen, K. S., Arus, X. M., Zetterberg, H., Gauthier, S., Boada, M., Pytel, V., ... & Mattke, S. (2024). Focusing on earlier diagnosis of Alzheimer's disease. *Future Neurology*, 19(1), FNL77. https://doi.org/10.2217/fnl-2024-0005

[6] Chouliaras, L., & O'Brien, J. T. (2023). The use of neuroimaging techniques in the early and differential diagnosis of dementia. *Molecular Psychiatry*, 28(10), 4084–4097. https://doi.org/10.1038/s41380-023-02290-8

[7] Santhiya, M., Praveenraj, H., & Madhuvarshini, N. A. (2024, February). A study on multimodal approach for early detection of dementia using deep learning. In: *2024 IEEE International Conference for Women in Innovation, Technology & Entrepreneurship (ICWITE)*, Chennai, India, pp. 384–388. https://doi.org/10.1109/ICWITE.2024.0001

[8] Nwamekang Belinga, L., Espourteille, J., Wepnyu Njamnshi, Y., Zafack Zeukang, A., Rouaud, O., Kongnyu Njamnshi, A., ... & Richetin, K. (2024). Circulating biomarkers for Alzheimer's disease: Unlocking the

diagnostic potential in low-and middle-income countries, focusing on Africa. *Neurodegenerative Diseases*, 24(1), 26–40. https://doi.org/10.1159/000532345

[9] Knight, J. E., Yoneda, T., Lewis, N. A., Muniz-Terrera, G., Bennett, D. A., & Piccinin, A. M. (2023). Transitions between mild cognitive impairment, dementia, and mortality: the importance of olfaction. *The Journals of Gerontology: Series A*, 78(7), 1284–1291. https://doi.org/10.1093/gerona/glac179

[10] Moya, J. A. B. (2024). Addressing the gaps in early dementia detection: A path towards enhanced diagnostic models through machine learning. arXiv preprint arXiv:2409.03147.

[11] Lyall, D. M., Kormilitzin, A., Lancaster, C., Sousa, J., Petermann-Rocha, F., Buckley, C., ... & Ranson, J. M. (2023). Artificial intelligence for dementia—Applied models and digital health. *Alzheimer's & Dementia*, 19(12), 5872–5884. https://doi.org/10.1002/alz.12918

[12] Warren, A. (2023). An integrative approach to dementia care. *Frontiers in Aging*, 4, 1143408. https://doi.org/10.3389/fragi.2023.1143408

[13] Sommerlad, A., Kivimäki, M., Larson, E. B., Röhr, S., Shirai, K., Singh-Manoux, A., & Livingston, G. (2023). Social participation and risk of developing dementia. *Nature Aging*, 3(5), 532–545. https://doi.org/10.1038/s43587-023-00310-9

[14] Budak, K. B., Atefi, G., Hoel, V., Laporte Uribe, F., Meiland, F., Teupen, S., ... & Roes, M. (2023). Can technology impact loneliness in dementia? A scoping review on the role of assistive technologies in delivering psychosocial interventions in long-term care. *Disability and Rehabilitation: Assistive Technology*, 18(7), 1107–1119. https://doi.org/10.1080/17483107.2023.2236345

[15] Ozkan, D., Katar, O., Ak, M., Al-antari, M. A., Ak, N. Y., Yildirim, O., ... & Acharya, U. R. (2024). Deep learning techniques for automated dementia diagnosis using neuroimaging modalities: A systematic review (2012–2023). *IEEE Access*. https://doi.org/10.1109/ACCESS.2024.3065879

[16] Etekochay, M. O., Amaravadhi, A. R., González, G. V., Atanasov, A. G., Matin, M., Mofatteh, M., ... & Praticò, D. (2024). Unveiling new strategies facilitating the implementation of artificial intelligence in neuroimaging for the early detection of Alzheimer's disease. *Journal of Alzheimer's Disease* (Preprint), 1–20. https://doi.org/10.3233/JAD-240001

[17] Xue, C., Kowshik, S. S., Lteif, D., Puducheri, S., Jasodanand, V. H., Zhou, O. T., ... & Kolachalama, V. B. (2024). AI-based differential diagnosis of dementia etiologies on multimodal data. *Nature Medicine*, 1–13. https://doi.org/10.1038/s41591-024-00001

[18] Hashmi, A., & Barukab, O. (2023). Dementia classification using deep reinforcement learning for early diagnosis. *Applied Sciences*, 13(3), 1464. https://doi.org/10.3390/app13031464

[19] Parashar, A., Parashar, A., Ding, W., Shabaz, M., & Rida, I. (2023). Data preprocessing and feature selection techniques in gait recognition: A comparative study of machine learning and deep learning approaches. *Pattern Recognition Letters*, 172, 65–73. https://doi.org/10.1016/j.patrec.2023.07.015

[20] Nag, A., Das, A., Sil, R., Kar, A., Mandal, D., & Das, B. (2022, December). Application of artificial intelligence in mental health. In International Conference on Intelligent Systems Design and Applications (pp. 128–141). Cham: Springer Nature Switzerland.
[21] Rodriguez, R. V., Kannan, H., Shaikh, K., & Bekal, S. (Eds.). (2024). *Deep Learning Approaches for Early Diagnosis of Neurodegenerative Diseases*. New York: IGI Global. https://doi.org/10.4018/9781799897784
[22] Jinad, R., Islam, A. B. M., & Shashidhar, N. (2024). Interpretability and transparency of machine learning in file fragment analysis with explainable artificial intelligence. *Electronics*, 13(13), 2438. https://doi.org/10.3390/electronics13132438
[23] Prabhakar, T., Gómez-Flores, W., & Reddy, C. K. K. (2022). Deep learning-based automatic detection of breast lesions on ultrasound images. In *Intelligent Systems and Machine Learning for Industry* (pp. 65–92). Boca Raton: CRC Press.
[24] Javeed, A., Dallora, A. L., Berglund, J. S., Ali, A., Ali, L., & Anderberg, P. (2023). Machine learning for dementia prediction: a systematic review and future research directions. *Journal of Medical Systems*, 47(1), 17. https://doi.org/10.1007/s10916-023-01916-9
[25] Khalid, U. B., Naeem, M., Stasolla, F., Syed, M. H., Abbas, M., & Coronato, A. (2024). Impact of AI-powered solutions in rehabilitation process: Recent improvements and future trends. *International Journal of General Medicine*, 943–969. https://doi.org/10.2147/IJGM.S422347
[26] Kale, M. B., Wankhede, N. L., Pawar, R. S., Ballal, S., Kumawat, R., Goswami, M., ... & Koppula, S. (2024). AI-driven innovations in Alzheimer's disease: Integrating early diagnosis, personalized treatment, and prognostic modelling. *Ageing Research Reviews*, 102497. https://doi.org/10.1016/j.arr.2024.102497
[27] Sohn, M., Yang, J., Sohn, J., & Lee, J. H. (2023). Digital healthcare for dementia and cognitive impairment: A scoping review. *International Journal of Nursing Studies*, 140, 104413. https://doi.org/10.1016/j.ijnurstu.2023.104413
[28] Nag, A. et al. (2024). TumorGANet: A transfer learning and generative adversarial network-based data augmentation model for brain tumor classification. *IEEE Access*, 12, 103060–103081. doi: 10.1109/ACCESS.2024.3429633..
[29] Rahman, A., Nag, A., & Bairagi, A.K. (2023). A Hybrid Model for Recognizing Human Activity Using Extreme Learning. In 2023 26th International Conference on Computer and Information Technology (ICCIT), Cox's Bazar, Bangladesh, pp. 1–6, doi: 10.1109/ICCIT60459.2023.10441574
[30] Kabir, S.R.R., Mondal, H., Nag, A., Jamil, S.M.H., Das, P. (2025). Identification of Lung Cancer Using Particle Swarm Optimization and Machine Learning Technique. In: Mahmud, M., Kaiser, M.S., Bandyopadhyay, A., Ray, K., Al Mamun, S. (eds) Proceedings of Trends in Electronics and Health Informatics. TEHI 2023. Lecture Notes in

Networks and Systems, vol 1034. Singapore: Springer. https://doi.org/10.1007/978-981-97-3937-0_29

[31] Reddy, C. K. K., & Vijaya Babu, B. (2017). ISLIQ-OC: Improved supervised learning in quest using optimal k-means clustering mechanism to nowcast snow/no-snow. *International Journal of Control Theory and Applications*, 10, 14.

Chapter 12

Federated learning-based diagnosis of epilepsy disease in healthcare 6.0

Monalisha Pattnaik, Deepti Rani Pattanaik, Sudev Kumar Padhi, Ashirbad Mishra, Alipsa Pattnaik, and Sadhu Charan Panda

12.1 INTRODUCTION

Epilepsy, one of the oldest diseases, is the second most common neurological condition, having a significant impact on individuals, families and healthcare systems. It is characterized by periodic seizures (two or more) due to abnormal electrical activity of the brain. It affects all ages. Around 50 million people suffer from it globally and 80% of them are from developing countries. Three-fourths of people afflicted with this problem in poor countries are not treated properly. Each year, 5 million people are diagnosed across the Globe. There are more than 12 million persons with epilepsy (PWE) in India. Fear, misunderstanding, stigma and discrimination prevent many of them from seeking treatment and it affects quality of life. Risk among epileptic patients is three times higher compared to the general population. Further, they are more vulnerable to bruises, fractures, anxiety and depression. If diagnosed and treated properly, up to 70% of them can lead life free of episodes of seizures. That's the reason why detection and treatment of epilepsy are significant to prevent seizures and associated complications and increase quality of life. Hence, identifying epilepsy with precision is of utmost significance to ensure better compliance and outcome.

As far as diagnosing epilepsy is concerned besides history-taking a physician depends on tools like "electroencephalography" (EEG), "magnetoencephalography" (MEG) and imaging procedures like "magnetic resonance imaging" (MRI) or "computed tomography" (CT) scans [1]. An EEG which is conducted commonly helps a physician to diagnose and monitor a patient with epilepsy. It detects patterns of episodes of seizures and facilitates real-time tracking. The information gathered from this tool is useful for making decisions on modalities of treatment [2]. Computerized techniques for the detection of epilepsy have been created to aid in the analysis and interpretation of EEG signals. "Machine Learning" (ML) algorithms are useful to categorize them into seizure automatically, to analyze EEG signals and non-seizure categories [3]. However, some machine learning models may not decipher the long-term time frame which is

DOI: 10.1201/9781003591085-12

important for "Epileptic Seizures" (EL). Further, pre- and post-ictal phases may not be captured [4].

This chapter proposes a federated learning-based neural network model for diagnosing epileptic seizures given a patient's EEG recordings. The aim is to differentiate EEG signals of a patient having seizures from other standardized brain test functions. This can help design a small tracking device to automatically monitor a patient's condition. The dataset in this study is for 500 patients and their 1-second EEG recording each containing 11500 data points with 178 features. We perform a random split of 70/30 of the dataset for training/testing and evaluate the models with metrics such as RMSE, CEL, and accuracy. Furthermore, using the DT analysis, we found that X_{121}, X_{123}, X_{144}, X_{145}, X_{156}, X_{160}, X_{161}, X_{167}, and X_{168} are sufficient to diagnose ED without depending on the rest 169 attributes of patients with RMSE of 0.2282669. We also propose PCA-LDA, ANN, five different DT-ANNs with one hidden layer and two hidden layers respectively, five and six different DNN and DT-DNN respectively, DWT-ANN and federated deep learning models that also perform well on the dataset. The DWT-ANN transforms the 178-dimensional mother signal into daughter wavelets using a Daubechies (Db4) wavelet pattern. This gives us variably scaled windowed forms of the signal that can now be used to better differentiate each 178-dimensional signal from another. Instead of using the resultant wavelet's coefficients directly, we use the aggregate characteristics of each wavelet such as min, max, mean, skew, and kurtosis among many others as input into a shallow multi-layer perception. This achieves a CE loss of 0.036 obtaining overall accuracy of 98.8% with 96% accuracy in the seizure category. The federated deep learning model has shown the finest results for diagnosing epilepsy disease with an accuracy of 0.997 and 0.9925 with train and test datasets, respectively which outperforms other models.

The reviewed studies provide a foundation for developing techniques such as PCA-LDA, DT, ANNs, DT-ANNs, DNNs, DT-DNNs, DWT-ANN, and federated deep learning models, for early prediction of ED patients. The rest of the chapter is organized into six sections. Section 12.2 explains the literature survey of the related topics. The Section 12.3 datasets include pre-requisite data analysis and the performance assessment metrics. Section 12.4 discusses the detailed conceptualization of the PCA-LDA, DT analysis, ANNs, DT-ANNs, DNNs, DT-DNNs, DWT-ANNs, and federated deep learning models. The experimental evaluation and outcomes of all the above models shown in Section 12.5 and Section 12.6 thoroughly discuss the results and practical significance along with concluding remarks.

12.2 LITERATURE SURVEY

Researchers explored advancements in epilepsy, including automated seizure detection, imaging analysis, pre-surgical planning, medication response prediction, and medical outcomes prediction, highlighting the use of machine learning (ML) approaches [5]. Machine learning techniques applied to predict epilepsy surgery outcomes using supervised classification data mining generated models predicting patients' recovery from epilepsy, with an accuracy of almost 90% [6]. They proposed to include specific psychological tests and machine learning tools besides classical analysis while evaluating epilepsy surgery clinically. A novel EEG feature extraction method using the Correlation Dimension (CD) determination is explored [7]. Their method achieves 100% accuracy in classification problems, using few features and a fast-running model. A dataset of 179 electroencephalography recordings is used to classify and predict ES [8]. They used traditional, ensemble, and deep machine learning techniques, including one-dimensional convolution neural networks, ensemble methods, and deep machine learning. The data is preprocessed using the Karl Pearson coefficient of correlation and manipulated using k-fold cross-validation methods. The convolution neural network and extra tree bagging classifiers showed better performance than all other classifiers. A classification method is applied for the epileptic seizure dataset revealing that the Random Forest classifier outperformed other classifiers with 97.08% accuracy [9]. Sensitivity analysis was performed, and feature selection based on attribute variance was performed. The study found that good classification accuracy can be achieved using only 148 features. For epileptic seizure prediction, a three-tier architecture is introduced using a "Federated Learning" (FD) model [10]. The architecture uses the "Spiking Encoder" and "Graph Convolution Neural Network" for local models, and the "Adaptive Neuro Fuzzy Inference System" for fine-grained personalization. The approach achieved 96.14% specificity and 96.33% sensitivity on the CHB-MIT EEG dataset, with FL enhancing accuracy by 96.28%. A "Brain-region Attention Network" (BANet) is developed to identify regions of interest (ROIs) in pre-processed SMRI data [11]. The method uses a brain template and self-supervised loss to generate attention maps. The method outperforms the high-tech methods, achieving mean accuracy rates of 85.69%, 63.34%, and 69.89% for "Alzheimer's disease" (AD) detection. A diagnostic model is proposed for AD using FL and hardware acceleration [12]. They used blood biosample datasets extracted from the ADNI website and introduced a hardware acceleration approach to speed up the training and testing of the datasets. The model achieved 89% accuracy and 87% sensitivity for early detection of the disease, with less training time and power consumption. It also had lower inference latency. Again a classification model is explored by applying edge computing, cloud computing and adaptive ML to classify EEG signal data efficiently for prediction of epileptic seizures [13]. The model includes a global adaptive classifier and local light classifiers, handling missing values. Implemented on CHB-MIT, it achieved high accuracy rates. The integration of machine learning and neuroimaging in epilepsy prognosis and diagnosis is discussed

[14]. They explored two machine learning methods: conventional and deep learning. The study covered tasks related to epilepsy neuroimaging, segmentation, localization, and lateralization. The authors discussed current challenges, achievements and future directions in these fields. Supervised machine learning techniques are applied to detect epileptic seizures [15]. They used Naïve Bayes, Support Vector Machine, Logistic regression, kNN, Decision Tree, Linear Discriminent and ensemble learning methods, etc. The study achieved 100% performance, with SVM achieving 98.3% sensitivity, 97.7% specificity, and 98% accuracy. The ML method is used for detecting epileptic seizures in EEG signals [16]. They used a public dataset from the University of Bonn, extracted meaningful statistical features, and trained models using hyperparameter optimization. The method achieved 98.4% accuracy, proving effective and practical in detecting seizures. A natural language processing (NLP) application is validated for assigning epilepsy surgery candidacy scores [17]. The application was trained on notes from patients with epilepsy, history of surgery, and seizure-free patients. The performance metrics were compared with surgical candidacy status from an expert chart review. The model improved with new patients added to the training set. The prospective AUC was 0.79%. A model is developed for preprocessing and feature extraction of epileptic seizures, predicting seizure duration and achieving a higher true positive rate of 92.23% [18]. The model uses empirical mode decomposition for preprocessing and feature extraction. The Extreme Gradient Boosting (XG Boost) algorithm is explored to classify 55 participants as healthy or epilepsy patients [19]. The analysis used neurophysiological features in five language regions and fMRI for phonological and semantic tasks. The subset SEM_LH BA_47-21 provided the best discrimination, highlighting the debates surrounding language reorganization in focal epilepsy. ML algorithms are applied to diagnose epileptic seizures in EEG [20]. They extracted EEG frequency components using DWT and AR model, applying them to classification algorithms like ANN, Naive Bayesian, k-NN, SVM, and k-Means. Results showed k-NN, ANN, and SVM were the most efficient. ML algorithms are used to diagnose epileptic seizures in EEG, revealing k-NN, ANN, and SVM as the most efficient [21]. Unsupervised machine learning is analyzed to estimate latent relations from 3T multimodal MRI features in 82 TLE patients [22]. They identified four latent disease factors, characterized by ipsilateral hippocampal alterations, loss of myelin, bilateral paralimbic and hippocampal gliosis, bilateral neocortical atrophy, and bilateral white matter microstructural alterations, supporting their specificity. Unsupervised machine learning is introduced to identify clusters of epilepsy patients with unique psychosocial characteristics [23]. They segregated the population into three clusters using k-means++ and multinomial regression. Post-hoc analysis revealed three clusters: high, intermediate, and poor. Failing to achieve seizure freedom predicted placement in the intermediate cluster. A review provided an overview of

various seizure detection techniques, focusing on 'black box' and 'nonblack box' techniques [24]. It offers new perspectives for data scientists working on epileptic seizure detection using EEG signals. Machine learning algorithms are applied to EEG data to find the best ensemble model for better learning [25]. They used classical techniques like Logistic regression, Naive Bayes, and Random Forest, with Random Forest and Long Short-Term Memory performing best.

12.3 DATA AND PRELIMINARY ANALYSIS

To diagnose the epileptic seizures of an individual, the electroencephalogram (EEG) recordings of the individual are investigated. In this dataset, each EEG recording is at a different point in time. The recording data points are only useful if the seizures are occurring during the EEG recording. A futuristic device can be invented that directly generates EEG recordings and interprets the recordings to determine if the current state of the individual is a seizure or not. Once an EEG pattern can be determined, there is also a possibility of identifying certain pre-seizure conditions. There are several data points pertaining to an individual during the epileptic seizure and during standard testing where the seizure isn't happening. The goal of this study is to identify which EEG recording pertains to seizures and others that don't. The dataset under consideration is imbalanced with 20% of the instances annotated with the seizures. There are 178 predictors to diagnose ED of patients. Table 12.1 presents the descriptive statistics of different variables related to ED of patients.

12.3.1 Performance measurement metrics

The RMSE is applied for measuring performance for various models with the disease datasets. For the performance evaluation metrics, the formula is expressed as follows:

$$RMSE = \sqrt{\frac{1}{n}\sum_{i=1}^{n}\left(w_i - \hat{w}_i\right)^2} \qquad 12.1$$

Where n represents the number of data points in the time series, w_i is true value, while $\hat{w}_i$ is an estimated value. The performance metric's minimum value shows the better performance of the model.

12.4 METHODOLOGY

Federated learning is increasingly utilized to enhance machine learning models while preserving data privacy and security. In traditional approaches,

Table 12.1 Descriptive Statistics of the Variables of ED

Variable	*Minimum*	*Q1*	*Median*	*Mean*	*Q3*	*Standard Deviation*	*Skewness*	*Kurtosis*
X1	-1839.00	-54.00	-8.00	-11.58	34.00	165.627	-0.454	22.061
X2	-1838.00	-55.00	-8.00	-10.91	35.00	166.066	-0.432	21.293
X3	-1835.00	-54.00	-7.00	-10.19	36.00	163.524	-0.603	21.402
X4	-1845.000	-54.000	-8.000	-9.143	36.000	161.269	-0.549	21.376
X5	-1791.00	-54.00	-8.00	-8.01	35.00	160.998	-0.304	20.737
X6	-1757.000	-54.000	-8.000	-7.003	36.000	161.328	-0.016	21.376
X7	-1832.000	-54.000	-8.000	-6.502	35.000	161.467	0.121	22.146
X8	-1778.000	-55.000	-8.000	-6.687	36.000	162.119	-0.170	23.721
X9	-1840.000	-55.000	-7.000	-6.558	36.000	162.033	-0.455	25.800
X10	-1867.000	-54.000	-7.000	-6.168	35.250	160.436	-0.093	23.158
X11	-1765.000	-54.000	-8.000	-5.827	36.000	160.471	0.301	20.685
X12	-1803.000	-54.000	-8.000	-6.042	35.000	161.181	0.196	20.369
X13	-1833.000	-54.000	-8.000	-6.687	36.000	165.071	-0.314	22.413
X14	-1867.000	-54.000	-8.000	-7.089	37.000	169.198	-0.809	25.090
X15	-1870.000	-53.000	-7.000	-7.211	37.000	170.641	-1.039	25.927
X16	-1839.000	-53.000	-7.000	-7.088	38.000	168.930	-1.114	25.807
X17	-1867.000	-53.000	-6.000	-6.807	37.000	164.646	0.959	23.835
X18	-1856.000	-52.000	-7.000	-6.745	38.000	162.062	-0.897	23.871
X19	-1844.000	-53.000	-6.000	-6.485	38.000	162.571	-0.684	21.881
X20	-1717.000	-53.000	-6.000	-6.448	39.000	162.339	-0.433	20.375
X21	-1764.000	-53.000	-7.000	-6.355	39.000	162.823	-0.282	20.049
X22	-1856.000	-53.000	-6.000	-6.543	38.000	163.909	-0.361	22.215
X23	-1844.000	-53.000	-6.000	-6.884	37.000	165.844	-0.356	23.854
X24	-1866.000	-52.000	-7.000	-6.883	38.000	166.009	-0.365	23.166
X25	-1863.000	-52.000	-7.000	-6.119	37.000	164.715	-0.502	24.577
X26	-1866.000	-52.000	-6.000	-5.159	38.000	162.774	-0.303	22.296
X27	-1781.000	-51.000	-6.000	-4.786	37.000	162.902	-0.266	21.495

X28	-1860.000	-50.000	-6.000	-4.875	38.250	164.799	-0.532	22.520
X29	-1818.000	-50.000	-5.000	-5.394	38.000	165.391	-0.718	23.779
X30	-1867.000	-50.000	-5.000	-5.936	38.000	164.291	-0.823	25.327
X31	-1743.00	-51.00	-5.00	-6.35	38.00	163.165	-0.723	22.505
X32	-1517.000	-52.000	-6.000	-6.213	38.000	163.408	-0.447	19.527
X33	-1552.00	-52.00	-6.00	-5.86	38.00	163.561	-0.331	19.168
X34	-1720.0	-51.0	-6.0	-5.3	38.0	162.548	-0.436	20.168
X35	-1864.000	-51.000	-6.000	-4.956	39.000	160.813	-0.565	20.614
X36	-1814.000	-51.000	-6.000	-5.278	39.000	160.441	-0.691	20.567
X37	-1829.000	-51.000	-6.000	-6.162	39.000	162.881	-0.838	21.075
X38	-1851.000	-51.000	-6.000	-7.317	38.000	166.235	-1.032	22.052
X39	-1840.000	-52.000	-7.000	-7.998	38.000	166.314	-0.870	21.059
X40	-1673.000	-52.000	-7.000	-7.819	37.000	164.513	-0.664	19.339
X41	-1838.000	-52.000	-6.000	-6.964	37.000	161.197	-0.577	19.222
X42	-1865.000	-53.000	-7.000	-5.774	37.000	158.045	-0.280	19.645
X43	-1656.000	-52.000	-7.000	-4.701	38.000	157.490	-0.127	19.089
X44	-1825.000	-51.000	-7.000	-4.144	38.000	160.163	-0.366	21.318
X45	-1870.000	-51.000	-6.000	-4.546	38.000	163.996	-0.802	23.747
X46	-1868.000	-52.000	-6.000	-5.532	38.000	167.744	-0.985	24.738
X47	-1850.00	-52.00	-6.00	-6.67	37.00	171.232	-0.954	25.282
X48	-1869.000	-53.000	-6.000	-7.702	37.000	171.484	-0.754	26.613
X49	-1885.000	-53.000	-6.000	-7.895	38.000	169.299	-0.761	26.160
X50	-1871.000	-53.000	-6.000	-8.081	38.081	166.255	-0.846	27.888
X51	-1867.000	-53.000	-7.000	-7.818	37.000	163.005	-0.671	27.451
X52	-1848.000	-52.000	-7.000	-7.694	38.000	162.158	-0.522	25.638
X53	-1868.000	-52.000	-8.000	-7.211	36.000	163.590	-0.493	24.492
X54	-1788.000	-53.000	-7.000	-6.653	36.000	165.476	-0.485	23.856
X55	-1773.000	-53.000	-7.000	-6.183	35.000	166.026	-0.390	23.424
X56	-1862.000	-53.000	-7.000	-5.978	35.000	163.938	-0.584	25.122
X57	-1869.000	-52.000	-7.000	-6.607	35.000	161.045	-0.661	25.402

(continued)

Table 12.1 (Cont.)

Variable	*Minimum*	*Q1*	*Median*	*Mean*	*Q3*	*Standard Deviation*	*Skewness*	*Kurtosis*
X58	-1865.000	-53.000	-8.000	-7.999	36.000	160.418	-0.807	27.029
X59	-1863.000	-54.000	-8.000	-9.598	36.000	163.199	-1.021	26.511
X60	-1861.00	-54.00	-8.00	-11.03	36.00	167.047	-1.151	25.606
X61	-1868.00	-53.00	-8.00	-11.37	35.00	168.601	-1.068	24.065
X62	-1860.00	-53.00	-8.00	-10.92	35.00	166.266	-0.953	22.878
X63	-1627.000	-53.000	-8.000	-9.661	35.000	161.822	-0.731	21.029
X64	-1721.000	-53.000	-8.000	-8.283	35.000	160.504	-0.608	22.176
X65	-1866.000	-53.000	-7.000	-7.091	36.000	161.614	-0.332	21.662
X66	-1862.000	-53.000	-7.000	-6.071	37.000	162.712	-0.153	19.972
X67	-1844.000	-53.000	-7.000	-5.658	38.000	161.908	-0.256	20.895
X68	-1843.000	-53.000	-6.000	-5.487	38.000	160.499	-0.131	19.997
X69	-1559.000	-53.000	-7.000	-5.893	37.000	161.100	-0.124	20.018
X70	-1797.000	-53.000	-7.000	-5.862	37.000	163.143	-0.353	21.067
X71	-1844.000	-53.000	-7.000	-5.894	37.000	165.152	-0.518	22.378
X72	-1852.00	-53.00	-7.00	-5.66	37.00	165.974	-0.403	22.842
X73	-1849.000	-53.000	-7.000	-5.935	38.000	164.336	-0.327	22.089
X74	-1850.000	-53.000	-7.000	-6.492	37.000	161.642	-0.177	21.799
X75	-1852.000	-53.000	-7.000	-7.022	37.000	161.345	-0.227	22.402
X76	-1868.000	-53.000	-7.000	-7.328	37.000	163.910	-0.414	23.876
X77	-1799.000	-53.000	-7.000	-7.302	37.000	165.442	-0.235	22.707
X78	-1650.000	-54.000	-7.000	-7.186	36.000	165.302	0.052	23.153
X79	-1838.000	-54.000	-8.000	-7.415	36.000	164.559	-0.337	25.874
X80	-1872.000	-54.000	-8.000	-8.219	36.000	165.725	-0.955	25.770
X81	-1884.000	-55.000	-8.000	-9.351	37.000	168.732	-1.257	29.949
X82	-1884.00	-54.00	-8.00	-10.32	36.00	171.053	-1.408	30.013
X83	-1848.00	-55.00	-9.00	-10.86	36.00	167.843	-1.115	26.916
X84	-1866.00	-55.00	-8.00	-10.67	35.00	162.249	-0.619	23.002
X85	-1835.00	-55.00	-8.00	-10.56	35.00	159.117	-0.544	21.730

X86	-1678.00	-56.00	-8.00	-10.13	35.00	159.979	-0.507	20.921
X87	-1863.000	-55.000	-8.000	-9.482	36.000	163.027	-0.522	21.703
X88	-1858.000	-55.000	-8.000	-8.838	36.000	163.613	-0.544	22.391
X89	-1689.00	-53.25	-7.00	-8.34	36.00	162.712	-0.645	22.019
X90	-1849.000	-54.000	-7.000	-8.015	37.000	162.184	-0.673	21.711
X91	-1865.000	-53.000	-7.000	-7.645	38.000	163.136	-0.641	20.275
X92	-1838.000	-53.000	-7.000	-6.774	37.000	163.089	-0.641	21.243
X93	-1771.000	-53.000	-6.000	-6.113	37.000	160.536	-0.398	21.004
X94	-1849.000	-52.000	-7.000	-5.478	37.000	159.388	-0.239	21.141
X95	-1846.000	-53.000	-6.000	-5.321	37.000	161.800	-0.508	22.841
X96	-1815.000	-53.000	-6.000	-5.477	38.000	165.078	-0.455	23.548
X97	-1745.000	-54.000	-7.000	-5.803	37.000	168.474	-0.120	21.360
X98	-1837.000	-54.000	-8.000	-6.351	37.000	168.674	-0.041	21.841
X99	-1864.000	-54.000	-7.000	-6.875	38.000	168.423	-0.229	21.518
X100	-1747.000	-54.000	-6.000	-7.269	37.000	170.665	-0.708	23.338
X101	-1868.000	-54.000	-7.000	-7.087	37.000	172.439	-0.844	24.802
X102	-1869.000	-54.000	-6.000	-6.526	38.000	171.269	-0.609	24.400
X103	-1860.000	-54.000	-7.000	-6.482	38.000	169.317	-0.494	25.894
X104	-1744.000	-53.000	-7.000	-7.201	38.000	166.303	-0.319	22.608
X105	-1582.000	-54.000	-8.000	-8.295	38.000	166.433	-0.450	21.819
X106	-1784.000	-53.000	-7.000	-9.425	36.000	166.137	-0.775	21.872
X107	-1829.000	-54.000	-8.000	-9.956	36.000	163.949	-0.892	21.637
X108	-1768.00	-54.00	-8.00	-10.11	36.00	164.024	-1.005	22.930
X109	-1736.00	-54.00	-8.00	-10.28	36.00	165.777	-1.103	23.382
X110	-1789.00	-55.00	-7.00	-10.06	37.00	168.714	-0.978	22.710
X111	-1867.00	-55.00	-7.00	-9.57	38.00	168.569	-0.784	21.669
X112	-1841.000	-55.000	-8.000	-8.955	37.000	165.233	-0.527	21.724
X113	-1867.000	-54.000	-8.000	-8.705	36.000	161.406	-0.220	22.385
X114	-1858.000	-55.000	-7.000	-9.091	36.000	162.467	-0.211	22.750
X115	-1868.000	-55.000	-8.000	-9.476	36.000	165.307	-0.450	22.737

(continued)

Table 12.1 (Cont.)

Variable	*Minimum*	*Q1*	*Median*	*Mean*	*Q3*	*Standard Deviation*	*Skewness*	*Kurtosis*
X116	-1813.000	-54.000	-7.000	-9.636	36.000	164.527	-0.630	24.807
X117	-1829.000	-53.000	-7.000	-9.354	36.000	160.502	-0.559	24.507
X118	-1868.000	-53.000	-8.000	-8.893	36.000	158.666	-0.403	20.350
X119	-1793.000	-53.000	-8.000	-8.423	36.000	158.726	-0.235	25.053
X120	-1637.000	-54.000	-8.000	-7.759	37.000	156.523	0.035	22.668
X121	-1415.00	-54.00	-8.00	-7.65	37.00	153.881	0.175	20.140
X122	-1830.000	-54.000	-7.000	-8.141	37.000	156.329	-0.216	21.304
X123	-1877.000	-54.000	-8.000	-9.474	37.000	162.612	-0.888	24.016
X124	-1885.00	-55.00	-8.00	-10.51	36.00	167.159	-1.187	24.304
X125	-1839	-55	-8	-11	37	166.930	-1.014	22.101
X126	-1863.00	-55.00	-8.00	-10.68	37.00	164.017	-0.925	21.317
X127	-1863.00	-55.00	-8.00	-9.88	36.00	162.832	-0.897	20.104
X128	-1774.000	-55.000	-8.000	-9.234	-36.000	162.839	-0.812	21.150
X129	-1864.000	-55.000	-8.000	-8.237	36.250	160.990	-0.740	23.461
X130	-1847.000	-54.000	-7.000	-7.629	36.250	158.301	-0.424	21.054
X131	-1589.000	-53.000	-7.000	-7.374	36.000	157.214	-0.033	19.320
X132	-1719.00	-53.00	-7.00	-7.44	36.00	158.679	-0.148	23.070
X133	-1859.000	-53.000	-7.000	-7.592	37.000	160.183	-0.314	25.980
X134	-1824.000	-54.000	-7.000	-6.898	37.000	162.002	-0.045	24.848
X135	-1843	-53	-6	-6	37	164.260	-0.035	25.327
X136	-1784.000	-53.000	-7.000	-5.424	37.000	166.182	0.128	25.077
X137	-1585.000	-52.000	-7.000	-5.151	37.000	167.154	0.259	23.758
X138	-1765.000	-52.000	-6.000	-5.587	37.000	167.414	-0.091	24.730
X139	-1857.000	-53.000	-7.000	-6.282	37.000	168.020	-0.368	25.227
X140	-1867.000	-54.000	-7.000	-6.997	36.000	168.567	-0.265	24.203
X141	-1826.000	-55.000	-8.000	-7.339	35.000	168.662	-0.253	24.750
X142	-1866.000	-55.000	-8.000	-7.912	35.000	167.643	-0.136	25.741
X143	-1854.000	-56.000	-8.000	-8.177	35.000	167.414	0.056	24.412

X144	-1759.000	-56.000	-8.000	-8.609	35.000	167.922	-0.060	24.114
X145	-1872.000	-56.000	-8.000	-8.578	35.000	168.274	-0.100	24.920
X146	-1866.00	-55.00	-8.00	-8.24	35.00	167.808	0.044	24.106
X147	-1675.000	-57.000	-9.000	-7.691	35.000	166.739	0.106	23.024
X148	-1778.000	-55.000	-9.000	-7.356	34.000	165.678	0.062	23.110
X149	-1733.000	-55.000	-9.000	-7.229	35.000	167.130	-0.268	22.826
X150	-1862.000	-54.000	-8.000	-6.981	36.000	168.156	-0.509	23.130
X151	-1861.000	-54.000	-8.000	-6.757	36.000	167.459	-0.523	22.718
X152	-1857.000	-53.000	-7.000	-6.355	36.000	165.061	-0.298	22.269
X153	-1839.000	-53.000	-7.000	-6.424	37.000	164.248	-0.234	22.379
X154	-1860.000	-53.000	-7.000	-6.465	36.000	166.226	-0.592	25.936
X155	-1843.000	-52.000	-7.000	-6.316	36.000	168.143	-0.749	27.427
X156	-1863.000	-52.250	-7.000	-5.808	35.250	167.067	-0.517	23.988
X157	-1861.000	-52.000	-7.000	-5.256	36.000	166.446	-0.409	22.394
X158	-1845.000	-52.000	-7.000	-4.682	36.000	167.554	-0.367	22.037
X159	-1820.00	-53.000	-7.000	-4.639	37.000	169.418	-0.340	22.149
X160	-1864.00	-52.00	-6.00	-4.77	36.00	170.639	-0.418	22.860
X161	-1868.000	-52.000	-7.000	-5.651	36.000	170.817	-0.633	24.103
X162	-1855.00	-52.00	-7.00	-7.17	37.00	168.145	-0.607	24.078
X163	-1852.00	-53.00	-7.00	-8.76	35.00	166.817	-0.462	22.543
X164	-1870.000	-54.000	-8.000	-9.785	5.000	166.999	-0.692	24.328
X165	-1847.0	-54.0	-8.0	-10.1	34.0	167.756	-0.757	24.773
X166	-1578.000	-55.000	-9.000	-9.843	35.000	166.988	-0.482	22.816
X167	-1838.000	-55.000	-9.000	-91702	35.000	167.062	-0.470	23.683
X168	-1763.000	-55.000	-8.000	-9.351	34.000	166.606	-0.501	23.891
X169	-1860.000	-55.000	-8.000	-9.499	35.000	165.235	-0.390	23.877
X170	-1867.00	-55.00	-9.00	-10.15	34.00	164.652	-0.674	25.604
X171	-1865.00	-56.00	-10.00	-11.63	34.00	166.149	-1.026	25.547
X172	-1642.00	-56.00	-10.00	-12.94	33.00	168.554	-0.999	21.589
X173	-1723.00	-56.00	-10.00	-13.67	33.00	168.556	-0.863	20.586

(continued)

Table 12.1 (Cont.)

Variable	*Minimum*	*Q1*	*Median*	*Mean*	*Q3*	*Standard Deviation*	*Skewness*	*Kurtosis*
X174	-1866.00	-55.00	-10.00	-13.36	34.00	167.257	-0.769	21.412
X175	-1863.00	-56.00	-9.00	-13.04	34.00	164.241	-0.703	22.632
X176	-1781.00	-55.00	-9.00	-12.71	34.00	162.895	-0.699	24.638
X177	-1727.00	-55.00	-9.00	-12.43	34.00	162.886	-0.523	23.191
X178	-1829.0	-55.0	-9.0	-12.2	34.0	164.852	-0.483	22.014

data is centralized for training, which can pose significant risks related to sensitive information exposure [26] [27].

It can efficiently manage complex datasets. Its capability to offer insights into feature importance further enhances the interpretability of classification results, making it an important tool for medical data analysis and decision-making. We have employed various machine learning models like PCA-LDA, DT, ANN, DT-ANN, DNN, DT-DNN, DWT-ANN and federated deep learning. The suggested federated deep learning model outperforms all the studied models.

12.4.1 Principal component analysis and linear discriminant analysis

The "Principal Component Analysis" (PCA) is a potent dimensionality reduction method usually applied to streamline large datasets. Its primary objective is to transform an extensive array of variables into a more compact set while retaining a significant portion of the information embedded in the original dataset. Reducing the number of variables in a dataset inevitably involves a trade-off between simplicity and accuracy. While dimensionality reduction sacrifices some precision, it offers enhanced accessibility and visualization of smaller datasets. This streamlined approach smooths quicker analysis for machine learning algorithms, eliminating unnecessary variables and expediting data processing. In essence, PCA aims to simplify datasets by reducing the number of variables while preserving as much information as possible.

"Discriminant Analysis" (DA) involves classifying data by utilizing responses to questions represented as variables and predictors. Its objective is to identify the linear combinations of the selected variables which effectively contribute to the classification of the groups. This technique is vital for constructing models that determine group membership, consisting of discriminant functions based on linear relationships among predictor variables. DA relies on numerous assumptions, including sample independence, equivalent variance-covariance matrices and a multivariate normal distribution of predictor variables for each group. Also, it assumes that cases exclusively belong to a single group. "Linear Discriminant Analysis" (LDA) is a supervised approach and it predicts the class of the dependent variable. It assumes a normal distribution of independent variables with equal variance and covariance, and it supports classification as well as dimensionality reduction.

12.4.2 Decision tree analysis

For classification and prediction tasks, "Decision Tree" (DT) is a widely used tool. They function by recursively dividing the variable set or the instance space. A DT is developed as a tree structure, consisting of some nodes categorized as either leaf nodes or decision nodes. The leaf nodes indicate the value of the target attributes, while decision nodes specify rules based on attribute values. Based on a discrete function of the input attributes' values, each decision node divides the instance space into multiple sub-spaces. For numeric attributes, this condition often involves a range. After applying the rule at a decision node, the resulting sub-tree represents one possible outcome. Leaf nodes then generate a probability vector that indicates the likelihood of the target attribute taking on various values. To classify instances, one navigates from the tree's root to a leaf, following the decisions made at each node along the path. A major advantage of decision tree algorithms is that their flowchart-like structure is often presented in a human-readable format after the model is built. This transparency offers valuable insights into the model's functioning and helps explain why it performs well or poorly for a given task.

12.4.3 Artificial neural network

One of the well-known supervised ML approaches for complex nonlinear time series forecasting is the "artificial neural network" (ANN). Neural nets, based on straightforward mathematical models of the brain, are utilized for complex nonlinear predictions. The architecture of any neural network may be envisioned as a network of "neurons" organized into different layers, including input, hidden, and output layers, the weights that are chosen with the "learning algorithm" related to risk minimization, where information is passed from one layer to another layer are used [28].

12.4.4 Deep neural network

The "Deep Neural Network" (DNN) is a special type of ANN characterized by a multiple number of hidden layers located between the input layer and output layer, allowing them to model complex patterns in datasets. They excel at handling large volumes of data. By leveraging multiple hidden layers, DNNs can master data that is represented hierarchically, from low-level features to higher-level abstractions. This deep architecture allows them to capture complex relationships and subtleties within the data.

12.4.5 Discrete wavelet transformation-based ANN

Each data point in the dataset is a 1-second recording of EEG for an individual. EEG signals exhibit non-stationary and transient characteristics, making time-domain features insufficient for classification [29]. To address this, the "Discrete Wavelet Transformation-based ANN" (DWT-ANN) method is applied to EEG signals, as it is well-suited for analysing non-stationary signals. The wavelet transformation method processes the signal through low and high-pass filters to generate approximate and detail coefficients. The approximate coefficients are helpful to examine the signal at different scales. The "Discrete Wavelet Transform" (DWT) is a technique that discretizes the mother signal into a hierarchy of daughter signals. It requires a representative wavelet pattern to perform the filtering process. We use Daubechies (db4) which is widely used in biomedical signal processing. Db4 uses a filter length of 10 that are orthogonal and asymmetric. We use a deconstruction level of 4 that outputs daughter signals until 4 levels.

12.4.6 Federated deep learning

Federated learning is increasingly utilized to enhance machine learning models while preserving data privacy and security. In traditional approaches, data were centralized for training, which can pose significant risks related to sensitive information exposure. Federated learning addresses this by introducing models to be trained across multiple decentralized servers or devices, where only model updates, rather than raw data are shared. This decentralized approach not only enhances privacy but also enables collaboration across institutions without compromising individual data, making it especially appealing in fields such as healthcare where data sensitivity is paramount [30].

In the field of neurodegenerative disorders identification, federated learning offers a promising approach to improve diagnostic accuracy while maintaining patient confidentiality. By leveraging data from diverse sources—such as hospitals and research institutions—models can be developed from a rich variety of patient information, including neuroimaging and genetic data, without ever accessing the actual data itself. This collaborative model enables researchers to develop more robust algorithms for early detection and monitoring of disorders like Alzheimer's, epilepsy and Parkinson's, potentially leading to improved patient outcomes through personalized treatment strategies while ensuring compliance with data protection regulations.

In the context of epilepsy, federated learning has the potential to significantly enhance the identification and prediction of seizure patterns while safeguarding patient data privacy. By aggregating insights from diverse medical datasets across hospitals and clinics, researchers can develop more accurate machine learning models to analyze electroencephalogram (EEG) readings and other patient-specific factors. This collaborative approach allows for the integration of a wide variety of patient experiences and responses to treatment, ultimately improving the understanding of seizure triggers and individualizing management plans. Furthermore, as data remains decentralized, patients' sensitive health information is protected, addressing one of the primary concerns in medical data sharing while fostering innovation in epilepsy research.

12.5 EXPERIMENTAL EVALUATION AND RESULTS OF EPILEPSY DISEASE

Identifying the characteristics and features of the healthcare datasets is a challenging task. The current study concentrates on diagnosing ED using PCA-LDA, DT, ANNs, DT-ANNs, DNNs, DT-DNNs, DWT-ANN and federated deep learning models. The models of federated deep learning model outperformed in comparison to other related models for prediction and classification of this disease. It is the best to notify the scientific experts and government or public-policy makers, and for managing and controlling the ED. Table 12.2 shows the accuracy result to diagnose ED of the patients applying all the above mentioned models.

12.5.1 Model for diagnosing ED using principal component analysis and linear discriminant analysis

By applying "Principal Component Analysis" (PCA) with all 178 predictors of ED, the variances with respect to the Principal Components (PCs) are evaluated. Applying PCA, it is observed that only the top 39 PCs with eigen values of more than one are selected, which is giving nearly 95.326% of variance, explained. For obtaining the influence of the studied variables their loadings are taken into consideration. It investigates that 39 PCs are derived from 178 studied variables for which the eigen values are greater than one. A biplot simultaneously plots the variables in a multidimensional dataset and information on the observations. Figure 12.1 shows a biplot which can optimally represent any two of the following characteristics: distances between observations and the variables. Figure 12.2 shows a scatter plot of PC1 and PC2 in percentage which indicates the relationship between the two PC. Figure 12.3 shows the explained variance ratio, a measure of the proportion of the total variance in the original dataset explained by each principal component. The explained variance ratio of a principal component is the ratio of its eigen value to the sum of the eigen values of all the principal components. Figure 12.4 shows the cumulative explained variance plot that shows the proportion of the dataset's variance, cumulatively explained by each component. When we execute PCA, a new coordinate system with axes ranked after transforming the data by how well they capture the variance in the data. Considering the risk factor of ED, the influential variables are chosen from the selected 39 PCs. With these 39 PCs and the target variable linear discriminant analysis is conducted to diagnose the ED of the patients. The entire dataset is split into 70% and 30% to train and test the models respectively. Through the analysis of 39 PCs associated with ED, we aim to develop a predictive model for enhanced diagnosis. The scores can be plotted to show graphically in Figure 12.5. It indicates the distribution of the two groups using the discriminant function. These two

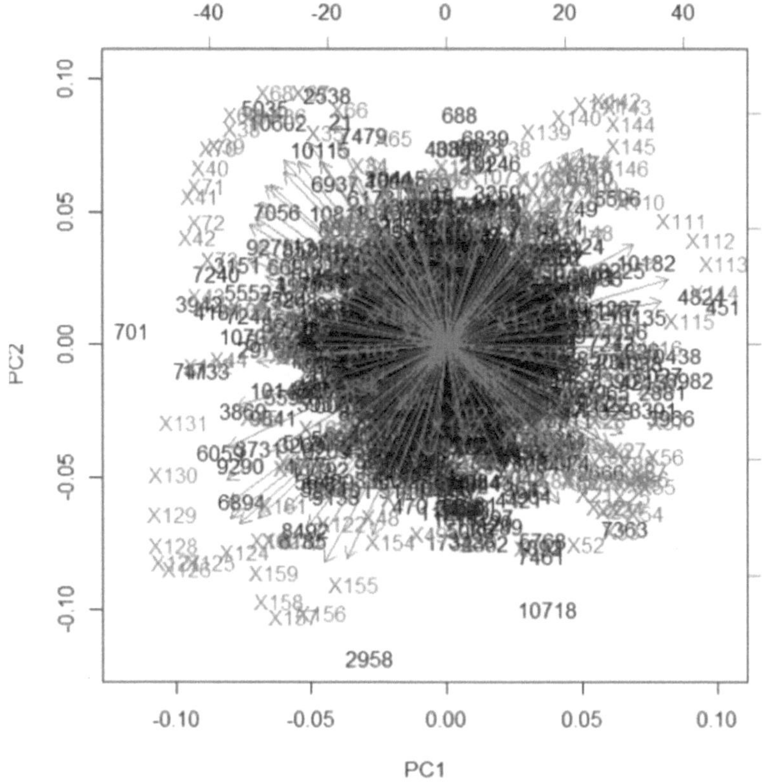

Figure 12.1 Biplot of distances between observations and the variables.

groups dwell in specifically different and disjoint regions. There is just one case of group 0 being close to 0 and group 1 being expanded from -5 to 5, so one can evidently state that this discrimination analysis has been successful. The effectiveness of the discriminant function in classifying the groups must be evaluated, and this is done by comparing the assignments calculated by using predict() function to the actual group assignments. Then the overall predictive accuracy of the test dataset, i.e. the proportion of cases that lie along the diagonal is calculated. Table 12.2 shows the accuracy result to diagnose ED of the patients applying PCA-LDA model is 0.8020319. Here the predictive accuracy of the test dataset is approximately 81%, quite a success. This approach measures the re-substitution error, it studies when all the samples are used to extend the discriminant function, how well the samples are classified. The classification of ED by the LDA classifier was moderately successful, with an "Area Under the Curve" (AUC) score of 0.54, see Figure 12.6.

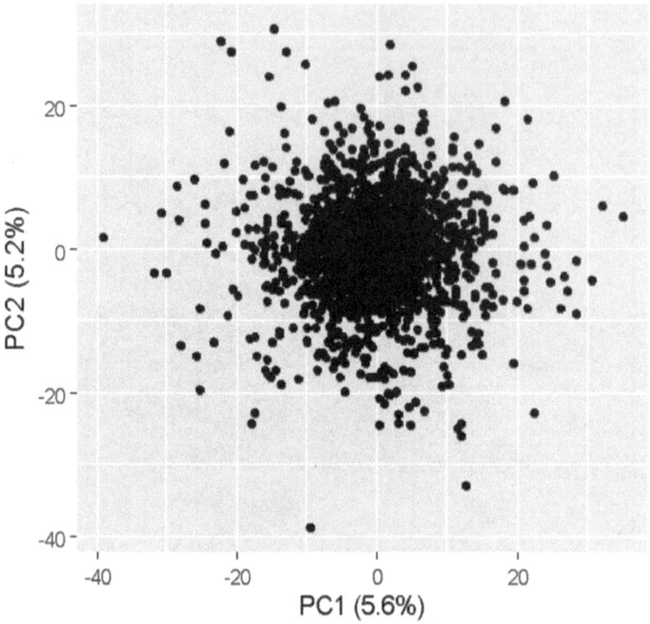

Figure 12.2 Scatter plot of PC1 and PC2 in percentage.

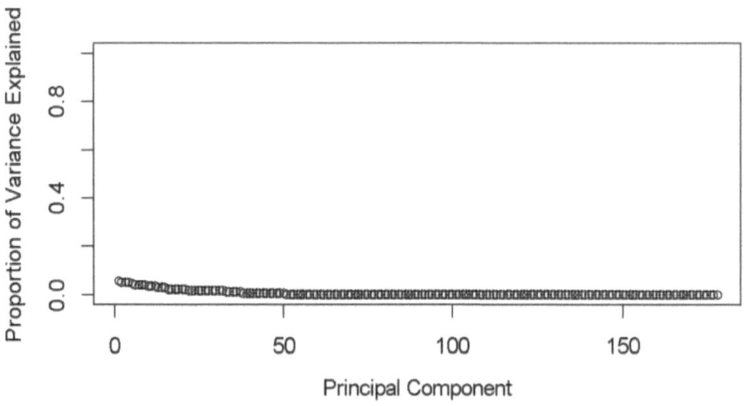

Figure 12.3 Proportion of the total variance explained by each principal component.

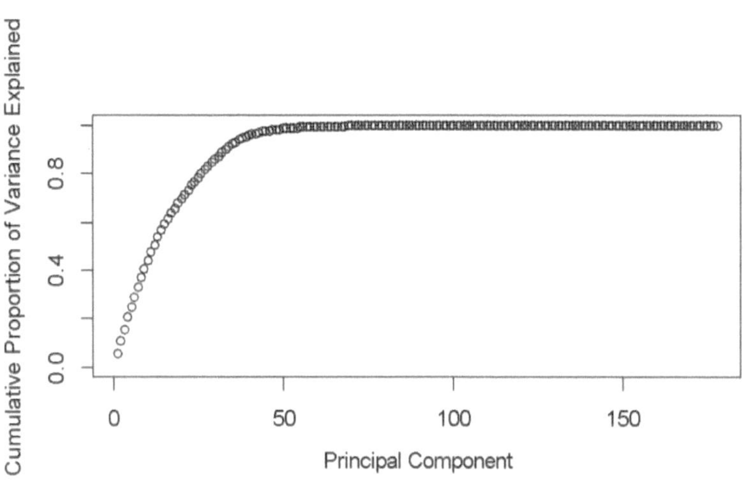

Figure 12.4 Cumulative proportion of variance explained by each principal component.

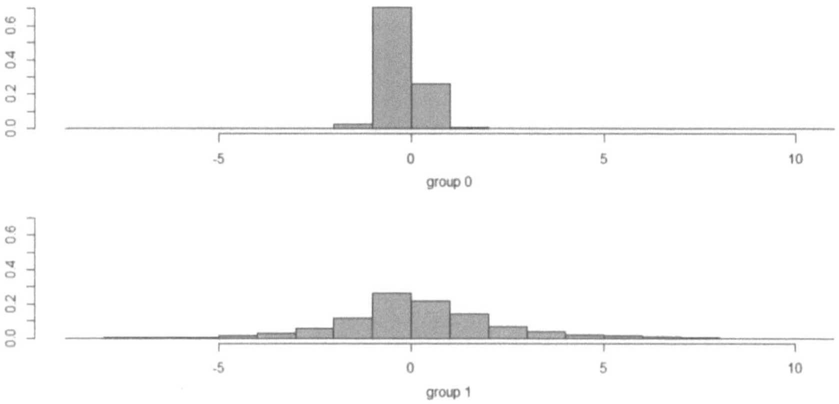

Figure 12.5 Plotting of linear discriminant model with binary classification of ED.

12.5.2 Decision tree analysis for diagnosing ED

The "Decision Tree" (DT) model is an influential classifier that uses a tree data structure to represent the relationships among potential outcomes and key features. When the final choice can be reached, the tree is concluded with leaf nodes (or terminal nodes) that indicate the action to be taken based on the sequence of decisions. For predictive models, these leaf nodes offer the anticipated outcome given the series of events processed through the tree. In

Table 12.2 Performance Measure of Different Models for Diagnosing Epilepsy Disease of the Patients

			Accuracy (%)	
Model	*Neurons in Hidden Layers*	*Predictors*	*Training*	*Testing*
PCA-LDA		39	--	0.8086854
ANN	64	178	0.8017124	0.7959895
ANN	64,32	178	0.994168	0.969195
DT-ANN	8,2	10	0.9630827	0.939508
DT-ANN	16,2	10	0.9708375	0.9387227
DT-ANN	8,4,2	10	0.9395563	0.9329689
DT-ANN	16,8,2	10	0.9399302	0.9332566
DT-ANN	32,16,2	10	0.9451645	0.9321059
DNN	64,2/200-32-0.2	178	0.9911188	0.9655172
DNN	128,2/200-32-0.2	178	0.99213088	0.9682000
DNN	128,64-2/200-32-0.2	178	0.99403358	0.9701881
DNN	128-0.4,64-0.3,32-0.1-2/200-32-0.2	178	0.99502796	0.9736614
DNN	128-0.4,64-0.3,32-0.2,16-0.1,2// 200-32-0.2	178	0.99403358	0.9727930
DT-DNN	128,2/200-32-0.28	10	0.9633210	0.9565598
DT-DNN	64,2/200-32-0.2	10	0.9618340	0.9553936
DT-DNN	32,16,2/200-32-0.2	10	0.9645601	0.9518951
DT-DNN	128,64,2/200-32-0.2	10	0.9806691	0.9448979
DT-DNN	128-0.4,64-0.3,32-0.1,2/200-32-0.2	10	0.97348201	0.9521866
DT-DNN	32-0.4,16-0.3,8-0.1,2/200-32-0.2	10	0.9542751	0.9460641
DWT-ANN	40,20	178	1.000	0.988
Federated Deep Learning	128, 64, 32, 64, 128	178	0.9967	0.9925

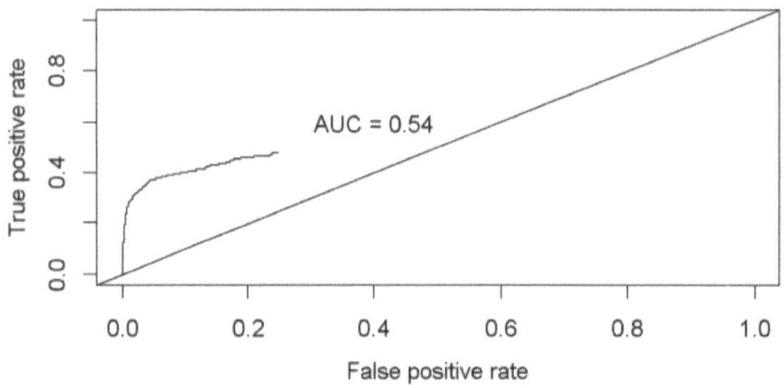

Figure 12.6 AUC of the true positive rate with respect to the false positive rate.

fact, decision trees are perhaps the single most widely used machine learning technique and can be applied to model almost any type of data—often with excellent out-of-the-box applications.

The decision to use a decision tree model for identifying significant input variables from 178 variables with the EEG recordings of the individual tested for diagnosing epilepsy stems from the model's simplicity, ease of interpretability, and high accuracy. At a different point in time each EEG recording is taken using this dataset. The recording data points are only useful if the seizures are occurring during the EEG recording. A futuristic device can be invented that directly generates EEG recordings and interpret the recordings to determine if the current state of the individual is a seizure or not. Once an EEG pattern can be determined, there is also a possibility of identifying certain pre-seizure conditions. There are several data points pertaining to an individual during the epileptic seizure and during standard testing where the seizure isn't happening. The objective of this study is to identify the significant EEG recording that pertains to seizures and others that don't. The dataset under consideration is imbalanced with 20% of the instance annotated with the seizures.

We applied an optimal decision tree model to a dataset comprising 11500 patients' data points to identify potential causal variables associated with epilepsy disease prediction. The DT was applied using the "rpart" package in R software, with a control parameter "minsplit" set to 10% of the total data. We evaluated the model's predictive performance evaluation using RMSE. The optimal DT, built with 9 input variables and a "minsplit" of 5, was created with the same costs for each variable. Figure 12.7 presents

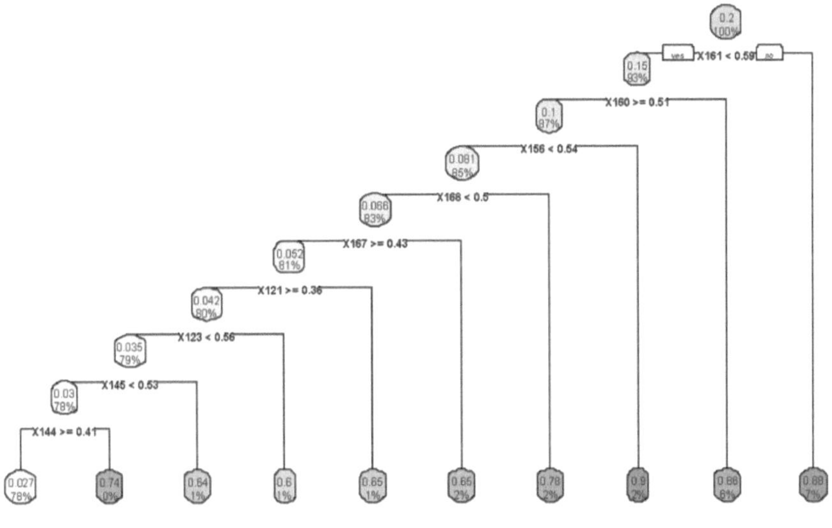

Figure 12.7 Decision tree for classification of ED.

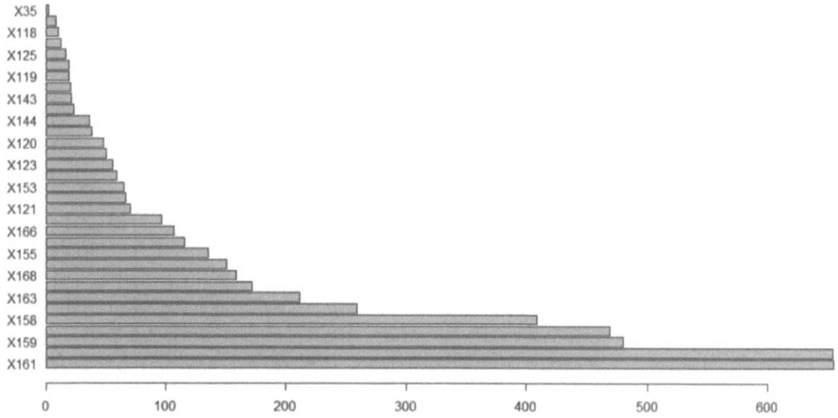

Figure 12.8 Variable importance for classification of ED.

the fitted tree and Figure 12.8 shows the variable importance list. From the decision tree analysis, it is concluded that nine out of the 178 potential input variables were found to be highly significant. But captivatingly, we captured nine essential causal variables like X121, X123, X144, X145, X156, X160, X161, X167, X168 can be managed to diagnose patients with epilepsy. By using the "rpart" package, we can evaluate the range of cost complexities. For comparing the errors for each of the cost complexity value, rpart performs cross-validation with 10-fold by computing the errors on the validation data. Figure 12.7 displays the optimal decision tree, which has 9 internal and 10 terminal nodes respectively, and partitions the data based on nine variables to develop its model. This tree can be expanded to a full tree with 10 terminal nodes by setting CP=0 shown in Figure 12.7. In Figure 12.9, the Y-axis represents cross-validation error, the upper X-axis indicates the number of terminal nodes and the lower X-axis displays cost complexity values. Beyond 10 terminal nodes, the reduction in error becomes less significant as the tree grows deeper. For predicting epilepsy disease, the decision tree identified nine key variables out of the 178 variables: X121, X123, X144, X145, X156, X160, X161, X167, X168. All 11500 patients' data points across 178 variables are processed through the decision tree illustrated in Figure 12.7, where each data point is evaluated at a node, proceeding left for a "Yes" answer and right for a "No" answer.

Firstly, 11500 data points of diagnosis of the ED in comparison to all data points of 178 variables where X161 is less than 0.59 go to the left branch, all other data points of diagnosing ED proceed to the right branch. All the patients with X161 less than 0.59 have X160 greater than or equal to 0.51, X156 less than 0.54, X168 less than 0.5, X167 greater than or equal to

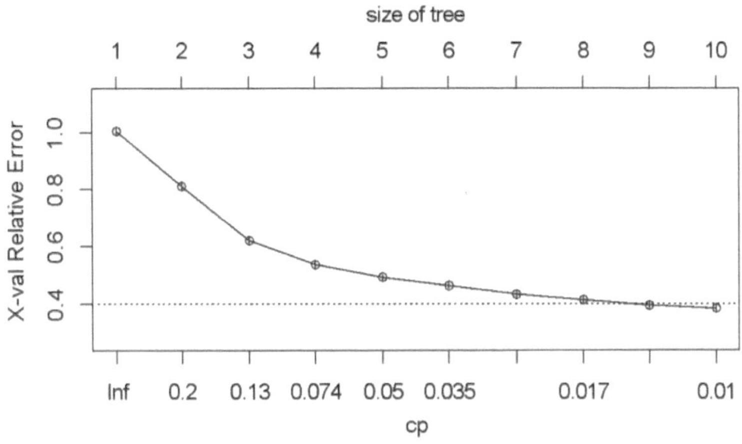

Figure 12.9 Complex parameter for classification of ED.

0.43, X121 greater than or equal to 0.36, X123 less than 0.56, X145 less than 0.53, and X144 greater than or equal to 0.41 have a 78% chance of not being diagnosed with ED. All the patients with X161 less than 0.59 have X160 greater than or equal to 0.51, X156 less than 0.54, X168 less than 0.5, X167 greater than or equal to 0.43, X121greater than or equal to 0.36, X123 less than 0.56, X145 less than 0.53, and X144 less than to 0.41 have a 0% chance if being diagnosed with ED. All the patients with X161 less than 0.59 have X160 greater than or equal to 0.51, X156 less than 0.54, X168 less than 0.5, X167 greater than or equal to 0.43, X121 greater than or equal to 0.36, X123 less than 0.56, X145 greater than or equal to 0.53 have a 1% chance of being diagnosed with ED. All the patients with X161 less than 0.59 have X160 greater than or equal to 0.51, X156 less than 0.54, X168 less than 0.5, X167 greater than or equal to 0.43, X121 greater than or equal to 0.36, X123 greater than or equal to 0.56 have a 1% chance of being diagnosed with ED. All the patients with X161 less than 0.59 have X160 greater than or equal to 0.51, X156 less than 0.54, X168 less than 0.5, X167 greater than or equal to 0.43, X121 less than 0.36 have a 1% chance of being diagnosed with ED. All the patients with X161 less than 0.59 have X160 greater than or equal to 0.51, X156 less than 0.54, X168 less than 0.5, X167 less than 0.43 have a 2% chance of being diagnosed with ED. All the patients with X161 less than 0.59 have X160 greater than or equal to 0.51, X156 greater than or equal to 0.54 have a 2% chance of being diagnosed with ED. All the patients with X161 less than 0.59 have X160 less than 0.51 have a 6% chance of being diagnosed with ED. All the patients with X161 greater than or equal to 0.59 have a 7% chance of being diagnosed with ED.

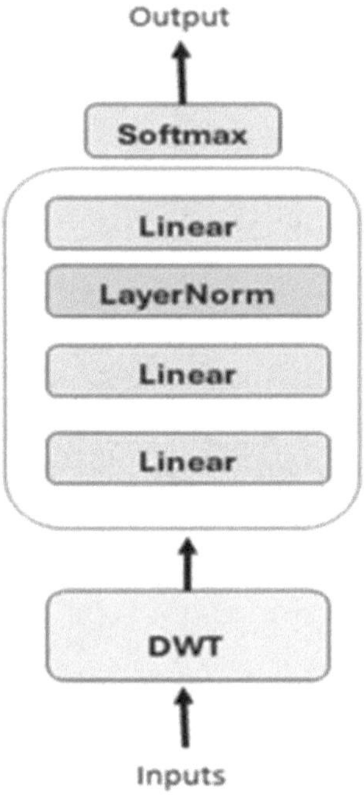

Figure 12.10 Neural architecture and the flow of the inputs including the discrete wavelet transformation.

The splitting process is continued, evaluating all the variables with each split, until the data points of ED are divided into 10 partitions. The predicted diagnosis of ED of the patients is (0, 1, 1, 1, 1, 1, 1, 1, 1, 1), based solely on nine variables. The RMSE result of this tree model for evaluating predictive performance is 0.2282669.

12.5.3 ANN and DT-ANN models for diagnosing ED

Analysis is conducted to diagnose ED of the patients. In the first ANN model, 178 input variables are fed into a three-layered feed-forward neural network having 64 hidden neurons and with one output neuron. Similarly, the second ANN model uses 178 input variables in a four-layered feed-forward neural network; it includes two hidden layers with 64 and 32 hidden neurons respectively, and with one output neuron. The third hybrid decision tree and ANN (DT-ANN) of five different models uses DT and 9 input variables in a three-layer feed-forward neural network, for diagnosing ED.

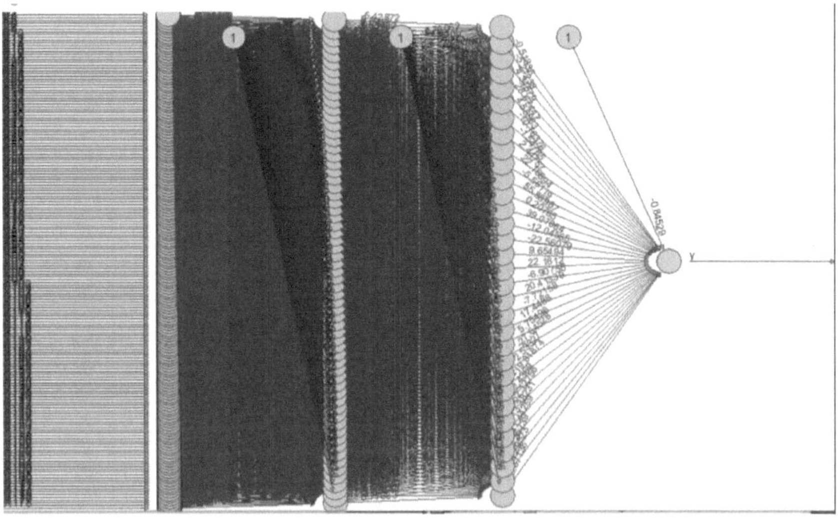

Figure 12.11 ANN model with two hidden layers to diagnose ED of the patients.

Artificial neural network disease prediction models can diagnose the ED of the patients. The entire dataset is split into 70% and 30% to train and test the models respectively. Two ANN models are developed: one with a single layer of 64 hidden neurons and another with two layers of 64 and 32 hidden neurons respectively. Figure 12.11 and Figure 12.12 show the best ANN with two hidden layers and DT-ANN models with one hidden layer for diagnosing ED of the patients with respect to the 178 inputs respectively. Table 12.2 shows the accuracy level for both train and test data to diagnose ED of the patients. It is investigated that the second ANN model shows better accuracy results with [0.994168 and 0.969195] for train and test data respectively to diagnose the ED of the patients. Similarly, a hybrid model with a single layer of 8 layers and of 16 layers of the predicted value of the decision tree model and nine identified risk factors namely X121, X123, X144, X145, X156, X160, X161, X167, X168 constituted DT-ANN prediction models can diagnose the ED. Two hybrid models with single layers of 8 and 16 hidden neurons and three hybrid models with two layers of 8 and 4 hidden neurons, 16 and 8 hidden neurons, and 32 and 16 hidden neurons respectively of the predicted value of the decision tree model and nine identified risk factors namely X121, X123, X144, X145, X156, X160, X161, X167, X168 constituted DT-ANN prediction models can diagnose the ED disease of the patients respectively. Table 12.2 shows the accuracy level for both train and test data to diagnose ED of the patients. It is investigated that the second DT-ANN model shows better accuracy results with [0.9708375

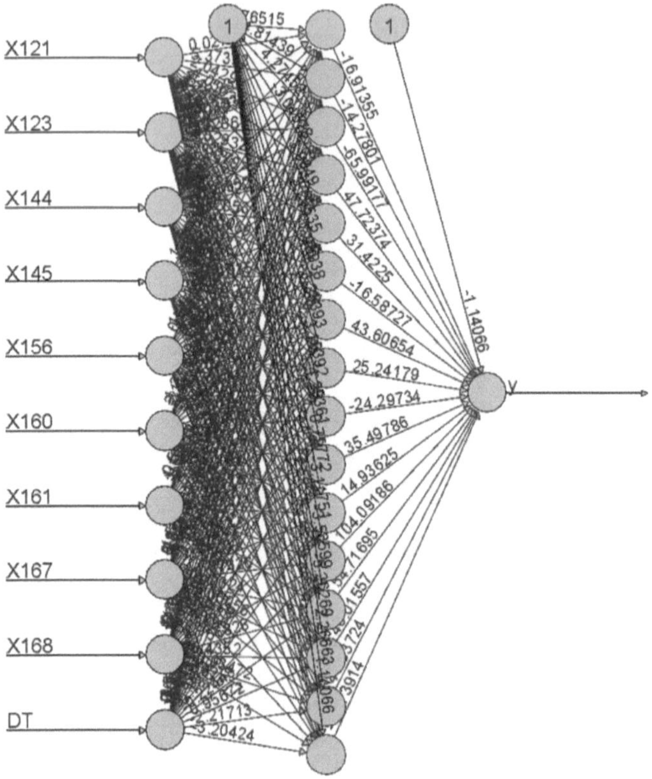

Figure 12.12 DT-ANN model with one hidden layer to diagnose ED of the patients.

and 0.9387227] for train and test data respectively to diagnose the ED of the patients.

10.5.3 DNN and DT-DNN models for diagnosing ED

Five different DNNs, and six different hybrid DT and DNN (DT-DNN) models, are developed to diagnose ED of the patients. We create 5 instances of the model; one can diagnose ED disease accurately. 70% of the total dataset is used for training these models, while the rest 30% is used for testing. Activation functions namely ReLU and Sigmoid are used for hidden layer and output respectively. Adam optimizer and binary cross entropy loss are applied as the matrix to train this hybrid model. The architecture of the five different DNN models are with [64, 2], [128, 2], [128, 64, 2], [128-0.4, 64-0.3, 32-0.1, 2] and [128-0.4, 64-0.3, 32-0.2, 16-0.1, 2] hidden layers and output respectively with respect to 178 inputs. Figure 12.13 and Figure 12.14

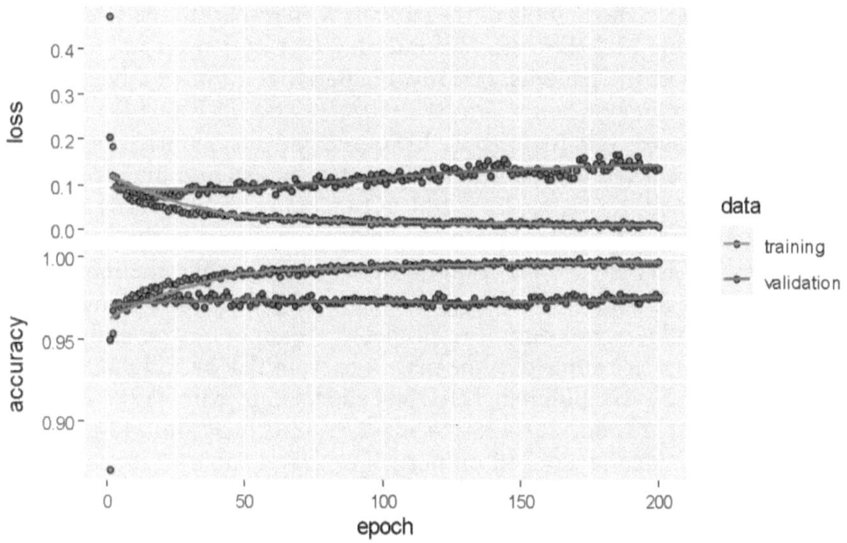

Figure 12.13 DNN with three-hidden layer model to diagnose ED of the patients.

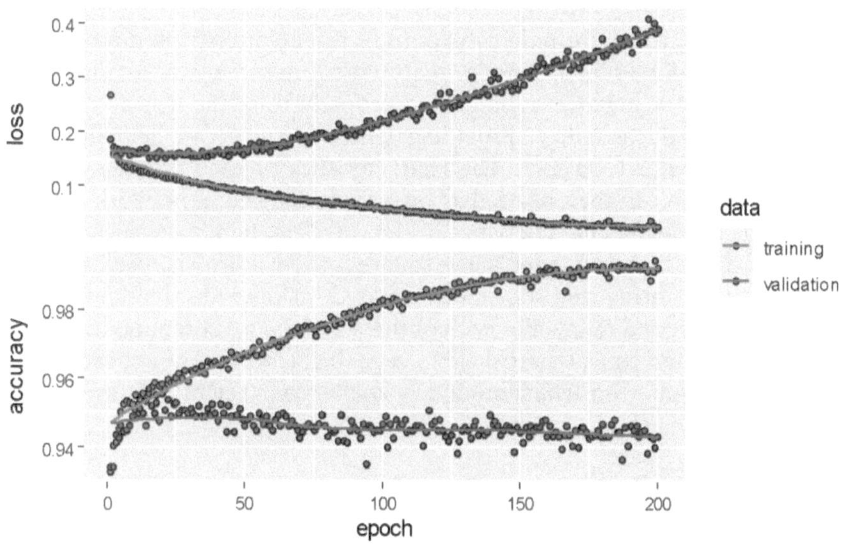

Figure 12.14 DT-DNN with three-hidden layers model to diagnose ED of the patients.

show the best DNN with two hidden layers and DT-DNN models with one hidden layer for diagnosing ED of the patients with respect to the 178 inputs respectively. Table 12.2 shows the accuracy level for both train and test data to diagnose ED of the patients. It is investigated that a fourth DNN model shows better accuracy results with [0.99502796 and 0.9736614] for train and test data respectively to diagnose ED of the patients. Similarly, a hybrid model of the predicted value of the decision tree model and nine identified risk factors namely X121, X123, X144, X145, X156, X160, X161, X167, X168 constituted DT-DNN prediction models can diagnose the ED. 70% of the total dataset is used for training these models, while the remaining 30% is used for testing. Activation functions namely ReLU and Sigmoid are used for hidden layer and output respectively. Adam optimizer and binary cross entropy loss are applied as the matrix to train this hybrid model. The architecture of the six different DT-DNN models are with [128, 2], [64, 2], [32, 16, 2], [128, 64, 2], [128-0.4, 64-0.3, 32-0.1, 2] and [32-0.4, 16-0.3, 8-0.1, 2] hidden layers and output respectively. Table 12.2 shows the accuracy level for both train and test data to diagnose ED of the patients. It is investigated that fourth DT-DNN model shows better accuracy results with [0.98104089 and 0.9510204] for train and test data respectively to diagnose ED of the patients.

12.5.4 DWT-ANN model for diagnosing ED

The feature extraction from the Db4 outputs can be directly used for binary classification. However, the model required to map the raw features can get quite complex making it difficult to properly train the neural network and achieve good accuracy. Providing better features can help differentiate each individual wavelet. The characteristics of each wavelet can be computed which can then be used as features to the neural network model. We use the following characteristics of the wavelets; min, max, mean, variance, standard deviation, root mean squared, skew, kurtosis, peak to root mean squared, normalized root mean squared, median absolute deviation, second moment, and range. For each of the wavelets, we compute the above characteristics and concatenate them to get a final feature. The concatenated feature dimension is 65 which are much smaller than the raw dataset's feature dimension (178).

Model Architecture

We use a shallow ANN architecture with one hidden layer with input and output dimensions of 40 and 20 respectively. The model is implemented using PyTorch and trained with a RTX GPU. We normalize the hidden layer's output by using the "*LayerNorm*" and the activation used by each neuron is ReLU. We run the training for 60 epochs along with the learning rate of 0.001 for the "Adam" optimizer. We use the "Cross Entropy Loss" (CEL) as it works well for imbalanced dataset. The CEL [31] requires a weighting of the classes such that it can weigh higher the class with lower number of instances. We provide a weight of 1 for class 0 and 10 for class 1. This helps us improve accuracy on class 1 i.e. seizure instances. Figure 12.10 shows the neural architecture and the flow [32] of the inputs including the discrete wavelet transformation.

We perform evaluation with a 70/30 split of the entire dataset. We achieved accuracy of 100% on the training dataset and an accuracy of 98.8% on the test dataset [33]. The accuracy for class 1 (seizure class) was 96% while the accuracy for class 0 was 99%. The minimum cross entropy loss was 0.036. The "Area Under the Curve" (AUC) for "Receiver Operating Characteristics" (ROC) was 0.9734.

12.5.5 Federated deep learning model for diagnosing ED

In the identification of epilepsy using federated learning, the approach can effectively leverage the epilepsy dataset comprising 11,500 data points categorized into five distinct clusters where each point has 178 features. By employing federated learning [34], we can train models on this diverse dataset without centralizing sensitive patient data. Each cluster may represent different patient demographics, seizure types, or responses to treatment, allowing the model to learn nuanced patterns in seizure identification and prediction. For instance, local models trained on data from each cluster can capture unique features that characterize specific groups, such as age-related differences or variations in EEG patterns. These local insights can then be aggregated to create a robust global model that enhances diagnostic accuracy while preserving patient privacy. This method not only improves the understanding of epilepsy's complexities but also promotes collaboration among healthcare institutions, leading to more comprehensive and personalized approaches to managing the condition.

- Data Preparation and Clustering
    - Feature Engineering: Before clustering, the 11,500 data points, each with 178 features, undergo preprocessing, which includes normalization, handling missing values, and possibly feature selection based on their relevance to seizure prediction.
    - Clustering: Using techniques of hierarchical clustering, the data points are partitioned into five clusters based on similarity metrics (e.g., Euclidean distance). Each cluster may represent specific patient characteristics, seizure types, or EEG patterns.
- Model Initialization
    - ANN Design: A deep ANN is structured with:
    - Input Layer: 178 neurons corresponding to input features.

- Hidden Layers: 5 hidden layers, each with varying numbers of neurons (i.e., 128, 64, 32, 64, 128) to capture complex patterns in the data.
- Output Layer: 2 neurons for the task of binary classification for seizure detection.
- Activation Functions: Common activation functions namely "Rectified Linear Unit" (ReLU) for hidden layers and softmax or sigmoid for the output layer are employed to introduce non-linearity and facilitate effective learning.

- Local Training
  - Model Initialization: Each local model is initialized with random weights, using techniques of Xavier initialization to promote effective convergence.
  - Forward Pass: Input data is fed through the network, generating outputs through each layer.
  - Loss Calculation: The loss is computed using a loss function appropriate for the task, which is binary cross entropy for binary classification.
  - Backward Pass: Back propagation is employed to calculate gradients for each weight based on the loss, adjusting weights using an optimization algorithm like Adam or SGD.
  - Batch Processing: Mini-batch gradient descent is typically used, with a chosen batch size (here 32) to enhance training stability and efficiency.
- Model Updates
  - Gradient Extraction: After local training, each local model computes the gradients and updated weights based on the back propagation results.
  - Model Compression: Updates may be compressed using techniques of weight quantization and sparsification to minimize bandwidth usage during transmission.
- Aggregation
  - Secure Transmission: Local updates are transmitted to a central server using secure communication protocols, ensuring that sensitive patient data remains confidential.
  - Weight Averaging: The central server aggregates the local model updates by computing a weighted average of the weights, each local model was trained on with weights proportional to the number of data points.
- Global Model Update
  - Model Synchronization: The global ANN model's weights are updated using the aggregated weights, which incorporate insights from all clusters into a single robust model.

  - Regularization: Regularization techniques (here L2 regularization) are employed to mitigate overfitting, particularly when exposed to diverse data distributions.
- Iteration
  - Communication Rounds: Steps 3 to 6 are repeated over multiple communication rounds (for 100 epoch), allowing the global model to iteratively improve as it learns from additional local updates.
- Evaluation and Fine-tuning
  - Model Evaluation: After training, the global model is evaluated using a held-out validation set.
  - Hyperparameter Tuning: Hyperparameters (such as number of hidden neurons, learning rate, and batch size) are fine-tuned based on validation results using different techniques of random search and grid search.

Using a 7-layer deep ANN within a federated learning framework enables effective seizure identification while prioritizing patient privacy. This architecture allows for capturing complex data patterns across diverse clusters, facilitating enhanced collaboration among healthcare institutions and ultimately leading to better management of epilepsy.

The outcomes of all models are exhibited in Table 12.2. A federated deep learning model for this disease shows higher values of accuracy both for training and testing than other models like ANNs, DNNs, DT-ANNs, DT-DNNs, and DWT-ANN models.

12.6 CONCLUSIONS

This study presents our experimentation with PCA and LDA models that we use to classify ED. From PCA 39 principal components are identified out of 178 predictors, and then using LDA, model binary classification of ED is conducted. It achieved 80.20% accuracy on the test dataset on ED. Multi-layer perceptrons were the best-performing models. We use 11500 patients' worth of data using a random split of 70/30 for train/test using RMSE for performance in the DT model. From the decision tree analysis, it is concluded that nine out of the 178 potential input variables were found to be highly significant with RMSE of 0.2282669. But captivatingly, we captured nine essential causal variables like X121, X123, X144, X145, X156, X160, X161, X167, X168 which may be applied to diagnose the patients with ED. Efficiency of diagnosis of this disease is tested by DT, ANN having hidden layer of one, ANN with two layers hidden, five different DT-ANN, five different DNN, six different DT-DNN, DWT-ANN and federated deep learning models. It is investigated that the second ANN model shows better accuracy results with [0.994168 and 0.969195] for train and test data respectively to diagnose the ED of the patients. Similarly, the second hybrid DT-ANN model shows better accuracy results with [0.9708375 and 0.9387227] for train and test data respectively to diagnose the ED of the patients. It is investigated that the fourth DNN model shows better accuracy results with [0.99502796 and 0.9736614] for train and test data respectively to diagnose ED of the patients. It is investigated that the fourth DT-DNN model shows better accuracy results with [0.98104089 and 0.9510204] for train and test data respectively to diagnose ED of the patients. We achieved an accuracy of 100% on the training dataset and an accuracy of 98.8% on the test dataset. The accuracy for class 1 (seizure class) was 96% while the accuracy for class 0 was 99%. The minimum cross entropy loss was 0.036. The AUC for ROC was 0.9734. The federated deep learning model has shown the finest results for this disease diagnosis with an accuracy of 99.67% and 99.25% with train and test datasets respectively which outperforms other models. Results showed improved accuracy in prediction and classification of the diagnosis of ED compared to all other models. The strategic diagnosis of ED ensured that the model received comprehensive data, enhancing its predictive capabilities. Challenges included managing communication overhead and ensuring consistent model updates. Adaptive algorithms and regular system checks addressed limitations such as data variability for feature identification and these are the scopes for future research ahead.

REFERENCES

1. Adams, C., Hwang, P. A., Gilday, D. L., Armstrong, D. C., Becker, L. E., & Hoffman, H. J. (1992). Comparison of SPECT, EEG, CT, MRI, and pathology in partial epilepsy. *Pediatric Neurology*, 8(2), 97–103. https://doi.org/10.1016/0887-8994(92)90028-w
2. Suryakala, V., Sree Vidya, T. R., & Ramakrishnans, S. H. (2024). Federated machine learning for epileptic seizure detection using EEG. *International Journal of Advanced Computer Science and Applications*, 15(4), 1048–1053.
3. Acharya, U. R., Vinitha Sree, S., Swapna, G., Martis, R. J., & Suri, J. S. (2013). Automated EEG analysis of epilepsy: A review. *Knowledge-Based Systems*, 45(0950–7051), 147–165. https://doi.org/10.1016/j.knosys.2013.02.014
4. Faust, O., Acharya, U. R., Adeli, H., & Adeli, A. (2015). Wavelet-based EEG processing for computer-aided seizure detection and epilepsy diagnosis. *Seizure*, 26(56–64), 56–64. https://doi.org/10.1016/j.seizure.2015.01.012
5. Abbasi, B., & Goldenholz, D. M. (2019). Machine learning applications in epilepsy. *Epilepsia*, 60(10), 2037–2047. https://doi.org/10.1111/epi.16333
6. Armananzas, R., Alonso-Nanclares, L., DeFelipe-Oroquieta, J., Kasta nauskaite, A., G.de Sola, R., De Felipe, J., Bielza, C., & Larranaga, P. (2013). Machine learning approach for the outcome prediction of temporal

lobe epilepsy surgery. *PLoS ONE*, 8(4), e62819. https://doi.org/10.1371/journal.pone.0062819

7. Brari, Z., & Belghith, S. (2021). A novel machine learning approach for epilepsy diagnosis using EEG signals based on correlation dimension. *IFAC-PapersOnLine*, 54(17), 7–11. https://doi.org/10.1016/j.ifacol.2021.11.018
8. Sahu, M., Verma, S., Nagwani, N. K., & Shukla, S. (2020). EEG signal analysis and classification on P300 speller-based BCI performance in ALS patients. *International Journal of Medical Engineering and Informatics*, 12(4), 375–400.
9. Almustafa, K. M. (2020). Classification of epileptic seizure dataset using different machine learning algorithms. *Informatics in Medicine Unlocked*, 21(100444), 100444. https://doi.org/10.1016/j.imu.2020.100444
10. Saemaldahr, R., & Ilyas, M. (2023). Patient-specific preictal pattern-aware epileptic seizure prediction with federated learning. *Sensors*, 23(14), 6578–6578. https://doi.org/10.3390/s23146578
11. Lei, B., Liang, Y., Xie, J., Wu, Y., Liang, E., Liu, Y., Yang, P., Wang, T., Liu, C., Du, J., Xiao, X., & Wang, S. (2024). Hybrid federated learning with brain-region attention network for multi-center Alzheimer's disease detection. *Pattern Recognition*, 153, 110423. https://doi.org/10.1016/j.patcog.2024.110423
12. Khalil, K., Khan Mamun, M. M. R., Sherif, A., Elsersy, M. S., Imam, A. A.-A., Mahmoud, M., & Alsabaan, M. (2023). A federated learning model based on hardware acceleration for the early detection of Alzheimer's disease. *Sensors*, 23(19), 8272. https://doi.org/10.3390/s23198272
13. Fatlawi, H. K., & Kiss, A. (2022). An adaptive classification model for predicting epileptic seizures using cloud computing service architecture. *Applied Sciences*, 12(7), 3408. https://doi.org/10.3390/app12073408
14. Yuan, J., Ran, X., Liu, K., Yao, C., Yao, Y., Wu, H., & Liu, Q. (2022). Machine learning applications on neuroimaging for diagnosis and prognosis of epilepsy: A review. *Journal of Neuroscience Methods*, 368(109441). https://doi.org/10.1016/j.jneumeth.2021.109441
15. Majed Alotaibi, S., Atta-ur-Rahman, Imran Basheer, M., & Adnan Khan, M. (2021). Ensemble machine learning based identification of pediatric epilepsy. *Computers, Materials & Continua*, 68(1), 149–165. https://doi.org/10.32604/cmc.2021.015976
16. Tran, L. V., Tran, H. M., Le, T. M., Huynh, T. T. M., Tran, H. T., & Dao, S. V. T. (2022). Application of machine learning in epileptic seizure detection. *Diagnostics*, 12(11), 2879. https://doi.org/10.3390/diagnostics12112879
17. Wissel, B. D., Greiner, H. M., Glauser, T. A., Holland-Bouley, K. D., Mangano, F. T., Santel, D. & Dexheimer, J. W. (2019). Prospective validation of a machine learning model that uses provider notes to identify candidates for resective epilepsy surgery. *Epilepsia*, 61(1), 39–48. https://doi.org/10.1111/epi.16398
18. Usman, S. M., Usman, M., & Fong, S. (2017). Epileptic seizures prediction using machine learning methods. *Computational and Mathematical Methods in Medicine,* 2017(9074759), 1–10. https://doi.org/10.1155/2017/9074759

19. Torlay, L., Perrone-Bertolotti, M., Thomas, E., & Baciu, M. (2017). Machine learning–XGBoost analysis of language networks to classify patients with epilepsy. *Brain Informatics*, 4(3), 159–169. https://doi.org/10.1007/s40708-017-0065-7
20. Karlik, B., & Bayrak, S. (2014). Comparison machine learning algorithms for recognition of epileptic seizures in EEG. In: International Work-Conference on Bioinformatics and Biomedical Engineering (IWBBIO 2014), Granada, Spain, 1–12.
21. Kadu, A., Singh, M., & Ogudo, K. (2022). A novel scheme for classification of epilepsy using machine learning and a fuzzy inference system based on wearable-sensor health parameters. *Sustainability*, 14(22), 15079. https://doi.org/10.3390/su142215079
22. Steriade, C. (2022). Entering the era of personalized medicine in epilepsy through neuroimaging machine learning. *Epilepsy Currents*, 22(3), 168–169. https://doi.org/10.1177/15357597221081627
23. Josephson, C. B., Jordan, Wang, M., Perera, K., Roach, P., Sajobi, T. T., & Wiebe, S. (2020). Psychosocial profiles and their predictors in epilepsy using patient-reported outcomes and machine learning. *Epilepsia*, 61(6), 1201–1210. https://doi.org/10.1111/epi.16526
24. Siddiqui, M. K., Morales-Menendez, R., Huang, X., & Hussain, N. (2020). A review of epileptic seizure detection using machine learning classifiers. *Brain Informatics*, 7(1). https://doi.org/10.1186/s40708-020-00105-1
25. Lekshmy, H. O., Panickar, D., & Harikumar, S. (2022). Comparative analysis of multiple machine learning algorithms for epileptic seizure prediction. *Journal of Physics: Conference Series*, 2161(1), 012055. https://doi.org/10.1088/1742-6596/2161/1/012055
26. Mammen, P. M. (2021). Federated learning: Opportunities and challenges. arXivpreprint arXiv:2101,05428. https://doi.org/10.48550/arXiv.2101.05428
27. McMahan, B., Moore, E., Ramage, D., Hampson, S., & Arcas, B. A. (2017). Communication-efficient learning of deep networks from decentralized data. In: *Proceedings of the 20 th International Conference on Artificial Intelligence and Statistics*, *JMLR* (pp. 1273–1282). https://doi.org/10.48550/arXiv.1602.05629
28. Chakraborty, T., & Ghosh, I. (2020). Real-time forecasts and risk assessment of novel coronavirus (COVID-19) cases: A data-driven analysis. *Chaos, Solitons & Fractals*, 135, 109850.
29. Postalcioglu, S. (2021). Wavelet transform based feature extraction for EEG signal classification. *WSEAS Transactions on Computers*, 199–206. https://doi.org/10.37394/23205.2021.20.21
30. Antunes, R. S., André da Costa, C., Küderle, A., Yari, I. A., & Eskofier, B. (2022). Federated learning for healthcare: Systematic review and architecture proposal. *ACM Transactions on Intelligent Systems and Technology*, 13(4), 1–23. https://doi.org/10.1145/3501813
31. Gangadhar Reddy, R., Srinivasa Reddy, M., Anisha, P. R., & Reddy, C. K. K. (2017). Identification of earthquakes using wavelet transform and clustering methodologies. *International Journal of Civil Engineering and Technology*, 8(8), 666–676.

32. Subbarayudu, B., Srija Harshika, D., Amareswar, E., Gangadhar Reddy, R., & Reddy, C. K. K. (2017). Review and comparison on software process models. *International Journal of Mechanical Engineering and Technology*, 8(8), 967–980.
33. Fatima, S., Kishor Kumar Reddy, C., Nag, A., Pullannagari, S.R. (2024). Leveraging Quantum Computing for Enhanced Decision Support in Disaster Management. In: Reddy, C.K.K., Nag, A., Ouaissa, M., Bhushan, B., Hanafiah, M.M. (eds) The Rise of Quantum Computing in Industry 6.0 Towards Sustainability. Advances in Science, Technology & Innovation. Springer, Cham. https://doi.org/10.1007/978-3-031-73350-5_6.
34. Rahman, A., Nag, A., Bairagi, A.K. (2023). A Hybrid Model for Recognizing Human Activity Using Extreme Learning. 2023 26th International Conference on Computer and Information Technology (ICCIT), Cox's Bazar, Bangladesh, pp. 1–6, doi: 10.1109/ICCIT60459.2023.10441574.

Chapter 13

Early detection of Alzheimer's

The evolving role of MRI in neuroimaging

Sumayya Afreen, Ayesha Nuzha, Noora Fatima Abdul Haleem, and Syeda Sadia Ahmed

13.1 INTRODUCTION

13.1.1 An Overview of Alzheimer's Disease

Alzheimer's disease is a degenerative neurological disorder that initially causes mild memory impairment and gradually leads to a complete decline in cognitive and physical functions. It is the leading type of adult-onset dementia, impacting millions of individuals globally. Early detection of AD is essential for prompt care, which can halt the disease's progression and enhance the affected person's general quality of life. While cognitive assessments such as the Mini-Mental Status Examination (MMSE) are frequently utilized for preliminary screening, a precise diagnosis typically depends on advanced imaging techniques like magnetic resonance imaging (MRI). Alzheimer's disease poses a significant challenge for the medical community considering the latter's complicated pathology and the impossibility of disease detection before formidable cognitive decline. Until recently, diagnosis relied primarily on medical assessment and elimination criteria, achieving an accuracy of approximately 85%. The diagnosis was confirmed after the post-mortem identification of the characteristic pathological signs of neurofibrillary tangles and amyloid deposits. The advancement in medical imaging and machine learning has recently started to transform the diagnostic process, thereby creating an earlier identification of AD by clinicians. Machine learning algorithms applied to MRI scans help identify subtle effects of changes in brain structure and predict the likelihood of disease progression by incorporating demographic and clinical data with imaging information [1].

First described by Dr. Alois Alzheimer in 1907, AD was first reported in a 51-year-old woman who was diagnosed with rapid loss of memory as well as severe dementia. With time, it was observed that the disease led to the degeneration of brain areas responsible for memory and judgment, including the hippocampus and entorhinal cortex [1]. Over time, there was marked atrophy of these areas due to this disease process, leading to clinical

 DOI: 10.1201/9781003591085-13

signs of loss of memory, poor judgment, and final dependency on caregivers. Though current treatments can only temporarily relieve symptoms, they are crucial in slowing disease progression, thereby delaying the onset of complete dependency. Several cognitive tests, among which was the 1975 MMSE, were developed to facilitate the diagnosis and tracking of Alzheimer's disease. The MMSE assesses multiple cognitions without special equipment or training, thus making it very common as a screening tool. The MMSE has limitations in monitoring disorder progression during advanced stages. Alternative cognitive assessments developed include the Clock Drawing Test (CDT) and the Clinical Dementia Rating (CDR); MRI still plays a crucial role as the actual changes in the structures in the brain are indicative of the progression of Alzheimer's. With MRI scans, doctors can see the brain and, more importantly, where there has been most loss from atrophy—the hippocampus and frontal cortex [1]. Besides MRI, other imaging techniques, such as PET, are utilized for assessing brain function and activity of some central proteins involved in AD pathology. Further development into amyloid-beta and tau protein indicators is expected to increase the diagnosis precision further. As knowledge about AD continues to grow, the development of new techniques and imaging approaches is helping and improving early detection, monitoring disorder progression, and refining treatment strategies, providing hope for more precise and effective management of the disease.

13.1.1 Overview of MRI in Neurodegenerative Diseases

A sophisticated non-invasive method for monitoring and diagnosing a wide range of illnesses, MRI is especially useful for neurodegenerative disorders. In contrast to X-rays or CT scans, MRI does not involve ionizing radiation, which makes it a safer choice for repeated assessments. Instead of ionizing radiation, MRI utilizes a strong magnetic field and radio waves to generate detailed, three-dimensional images of internal structures. It offers superior contrast, particularly for soft tissues like the brain, muscles, and organs [2].

The use of MRI is essential in the identification of physical alterations of the brain due to Alzheimer's and other neurodegenerative ailments such as atrophy in the hippocampus and other important regions including memory and cognitive activities. In its basic form, these volumetric changes can be followed up over time, making MRI so invaluable for purposes of early diagnosis but also as a marker for disease progression. With its high resolution and non-invasive nature, MRI represents one of the most excellent techniques to be used in studying neurodegenerative diseases, which usually present themselves early with subtle morphological changes. The association of MRI data with machine learning algorithms enhances diagnostic capabilities, allowing for the automated detection of subtle brain transformations and for more accurate, timely diagnosis. As technology becomes even more advanced, the potential use of MRI in combination with AI continues to widen its capabilities toward improved diagnostic accuracy and efficiency for clinical and research applications.

13.2.2 Statistical Analysis of Alzheimer's Disease

As of 2024, an estimated 6.9 million Americans aged 65 and older are living with Alzheimer's disease, with 74% of these individuals being 75 or older, as illustrated in Figure 13.1. With the advancement of AD, patients develop a dependency on caregivers because of deteriorating brain functions eventually leading to a loss of their intellectual and physical capabilities. According to the study, women had roughly 20% (1 in 5) lifespan chance of acquiring Alzheimer's dementia by the age of 45, while men had 10% (1 in 10) chance. This is shown in Figure 13.2.

This paper explores the evolving role of MRI in detecting and diagnosing Alzheimer's disease, highlighting techniques such as structural MRI (sMRI), diffusion tensor imaging (DTI), and functional MRI (fMRI). It covers their applications in early detection, particularly in patients with Mild Cognitive

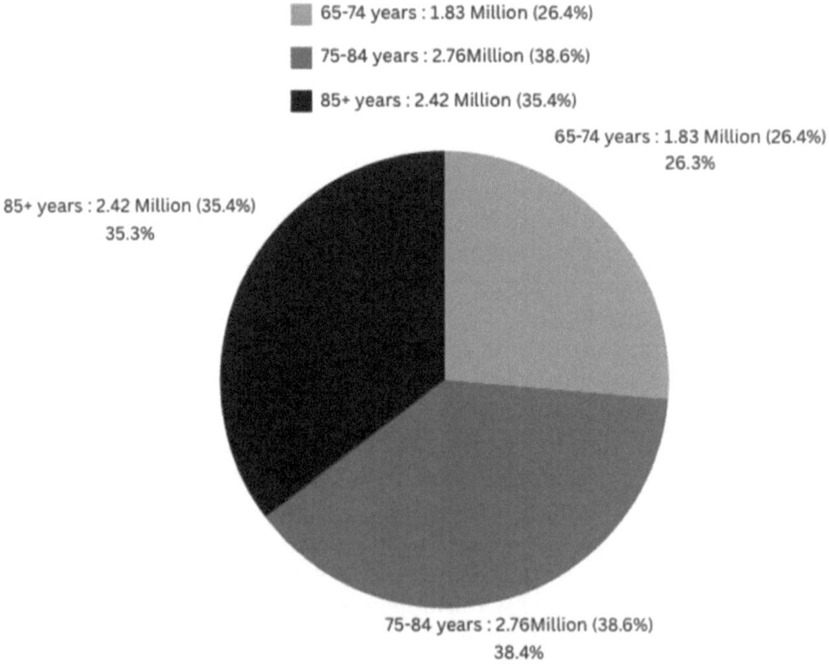

Figure 13.1 Data on the count and ages of individuals aged 65 and above with Alzheimer's disease in 2024.

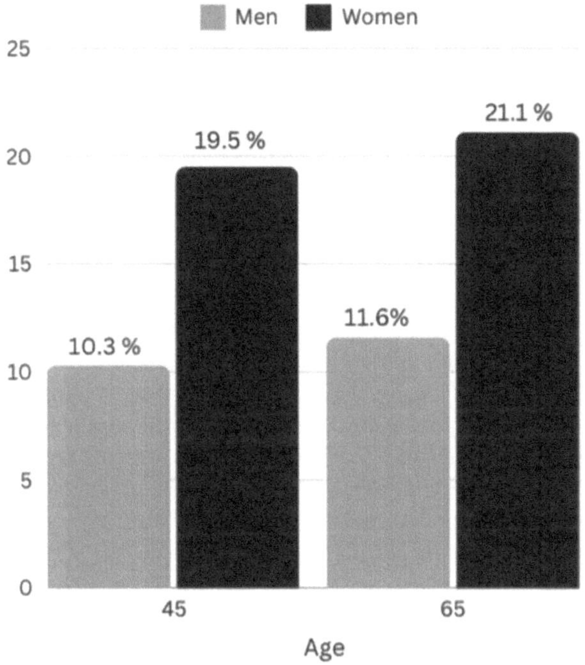

Figure 13.2 Gender-specific long-term risk estimates for Alzheimer's dementia in people aged from 45 to 65 years old.

Impairment (MCI), and discusses the integration of machine learning for enhanced assessment. Advanced MRI methods like Magnetization Transfer Imaging (MTI), Arterial Spin Labeling (ASL), and Magnetic Resonance Spectroscopy (MRS) are also reviewed, along with a comparison of MRI to other imaging modalities.

The paper is organized as follows: Section 13.2 gives a critical review of the use of sMRI for the diagnosis of AD, using the critical biomarkers of hippocampal atrophy, cortical thinning, and white matter degeneration. Section 13.3 discusses DTI and its ability to test the integrity of white matter, providing a pathway for measuring the early neurodegenerative changes in AD. Section 13.4 relates the functional MRI to studying aspects of functional connectivity including network functionality that may be compromised in AD, such as those that exist within the default mode networks. Section 13.5 focuses on the application of machine learning methods to MRI data so as to facilitate early diagnoses and classifications of AD. Section 13.6 discusses advanced techniques of MRI, including MTI, ASL, and MRS, which are then presented as state-of-the-art for the detection of early alterations in the course of AD. Section 13.7 Comparison with other neuroimaging techniques like PET and CT is also made; it has cleared out their complementary roles in the diagnosis of AD. Section 13.8 discusses future directions in MRI-based Alzheimer's research, including automated disease detection, multi-class classification, and how MRI can be combined with other biomarkers to achieve a more holistic approach to diagnosis.

13.2 STRUCTURAL MRI (SMRI) FOR DETECTING ALZHEIMER'S DISEASE

Structural MRI (sMRI) forms the backbone of neurodegenerative research and is a central aspect of clinical work, notably in the analysis and continued observation of Alzheimer's dementia. It offers high-resolution, non-invasive images of the brain, thus letting clinicians see structural changes that are the hallmarks of neural deterioration. When compared to alternative imaging techniques, like CT, structural MRI (sMRI) provides multiple advantages, including the identification of brain lesions, assessment of atrophy patterns, and evaluation involving vascular burden [3]. Such characteristics have made it an important tool in studying diseases like AD where prior identification of brain changes is sought for interventions. Detection of hippocampal atrophy is the first practical use of sMRI in patients with AD, and it is among the first indicators of the ailment. Subtle changes in the brain permitted to be delineated by sMRI scans help in substantiating the concept of decline in cognition, a biomarker that seems indispensable for early diagnosis of AD. Cortical thinning and white matter atrophy are crucial information provided by the methodological capabilities of sMRI once the disease advances. The study would also correlate with other tools used in cognitive assessment, like the clinical dementia rating, by relating structural brain changes to clinical symptoms, for a general understanding of the disease.

The past two years of development in machine learning have included providing a way to improve upon the diagnostic potential of sMRI. Models of device learning facilitate earlier and more accurate diagnoses of AD with enhanced speed at which clinicians can obtain an improved estimate of the progression of the disease. Therefore, sMRI is still a well-established instrument for preliminary diagnosis and extended monitoring of AD.

Hippocampal Atrophy: One of the primary uses of structural MRI in diagnosing Alzheimer's disease (AD) is assessing the reduction in hippocampal volume. The hippocampus, which plays a vital role in memory formation, undergoes shrinkage that stands as one of the earliest and most important signs of AD. Research has confirmed that hippocampal atrophy is closely linked to cognitive decline and the advancement of Alzheimer's. Therefore, hippocampal atrophy is regarded as one of the key biomarkers for diagnosis and monitoring of the disease [4].

Cortical Thickness: Additionally, sMRI is increasingly being utilized to assess cortical thickness, particularly in areas where AD-caused degeneration is most prominent, such as the cortical area and parietal lobes. Depletion of cortical thickness in these regions represents neuronal loss and is indicative of disease progression. The monitoring of cortical thinning with sMRI indicates how neurodegeneration follows in the brain, thus helping clinicians detect AD even in its early stages [5]. These structural changes in the cortex often precede noticeable cognitive impairment, making cortical thickness measurement a valuable tool for early detection.

White Matter Atrophy: Besides the deterioration of gray matter, sMRI is used to mark changes in white matter integrity, another feature of Alzheimer's progression. White matter atrophy, particularly within the temporal and parietal regions, has been associated with the progression of the disease. MRI can capture those changes in the white matter tracts, which connect different parts of the brain, and these connections, when AD progresses, degrade and further impair cognitive function [6]. This ability to continuously monitor white matter degeneration adds to the measurement of gray matter atrophy, providing a holistic perspective of how the disease impacts brain structure.

Applications in Mild Cognitive Impairment (MCI)

Structural MRI has significant applications in forecasting the likely progression from MCI to AD. Though MCI is essentially a transitional period from natural aging to Alzheimer's dementia, not everyone diagnosed with MCI will ultimately develop Alzheimer's dementia. However, sMRI can identify individuals who are at greater risk because the early stages of hippocampal atrophy and cortical thinning can predict progression to AD [7]. Prognostic longitudinal studies with MRI have shown that patients with considerable brain atrophy have an increased likelihood of progressing from MCI to AD; hence, sMRI can provide an early opportunity for intervention.

13.3 DIFFUSION TENSOR IMAGING (DTI)

Diffusion Tensor Imaging (DTI) is a sophisticated MRI method that is sensitive to microstructural changes within white matter, which consists of the axonal pathways connecting different regions in the brain. It assesses the circulation of water molecules within biological tissues, with a focus on anisotropic diffusion, where water predominantly moves in a single direction, such as along the white matter pathways. However, in cerebrospinal fluid or gray matter, the movement of water is uniform in all directions, resulting in isotropic diffusion. By interpreting diffusion, DTI enables a detailed quantification of white matter integrity that traditional MRI scans may not detect. White matter degeneration often occurs before gray matter loss, making DTI particularly valuable for identifying early neurodegenerative changes in diseases such as Alzheimer's.

DTI in Alzheimer's Diagnosis
In Alzheimer's, DTI is highly sensitive to disruptions in the microstructure of white matter, particularly pertaining to the medial temporal lobe, where essential memory mechanisms and cognition are found. Structural disruptions can manifest as early as the preclinical phase of AD, initially impacting the medial temporal limbic association tracts. With the progression of the disease, white matter degeneration further involves the temporal and parietal areas. Studies have demonstrated that white matter tracts such as hippocampal cingulum and fornix are degraded in AD, which DTI can detect even before any signs become clinically apparent [8] [9]. To assess the integrity of white matter loss, DTI measurements including mean diffusivity and fractional anisotropy are employed: typically, FA decreases while MD increases in AD patients, reflecting the breakdown of white matter integrity [10]. These metrics make DTI a valuable tool for detecting early pathological changes and tracking the disease's progress in AD.

Gray Matter Correlation with Pathology
DTI-detected white matter changes have a close correlation with gray matter atrophy in Alzheimer's. With the progression of AD, degeneration in white matter tracts eliminates connectivity between regions in the brain, contributing to further functionality loss in areas affected by gray matter atrophy. For example, white matter tracts from the hippocampus to other regions involved in memory degradation and breakage occur in accordance with the typical hippocampal atrophy seen in AD [11]. This close relationship between white matter disruption and gray matter atrophy is believed to reflect the involvement of neurofibrillary tangle (NFT) tau pathology, a hallmark of AD [8]. The interplay between white and gray matter degeneration emphasizes the role of DTI in providing a comprehensive view of brain deterioration in AD.

Limitations of DTI
Despite its advantages, DTI has limitations. One of the key challenges is the assumption that each voxel (3D pixel) contains a single tissue type, which can lead to inaccuracies when voxels contain multiple tissue types, such as a mix of CSF and brain matter. Moreover, DTI fails to incorporate the non-Gaussian diffusion properties of complex biological structures including cell membranes and myelin sheaths, and therefore reduces its ability to detect detailed microstructural changes, particularly in gray matter. Finally, the oversimplified DTI model of brain anatomy fails to capture crossing white matter fibers, ubiquitous in the voxels composing most adult brains [11].

This has the potential to limit the validity of DTI in regions of complex architecture.

13.4 FUNCTIONAL MRI (FMRI)

Introduction to fMRI

Functional MRI (fMRI) detects activity in the brain by means of blood flow changes and depends on the BOLD (blood-oxygen-level-dependent) indication in it. In living subjects, the more neurons fired, the more blood rich in oxygen is sent to the active areas of the brain in real time. This contrasts with structural MRI, which uses the static anatomical features of the brain for imaging. The atrophy or lesions can be detected in the case of structural MRI, but when it comes to observing patterns of brain function and connectivity during rest or cognitive tasks, fMRI is better suited for this purpose [12].

Functional Connectivity in AD

Functional changes in connectivity are crucial in the progression of Alzheimer's. DMNs are the networks the most affected by AD. The posterior cingulate cortex, medial prefrontal cortex, and hippocampal regions are among those included in these networks, posterior cingulate cortex. Research on resting-state connectivity in Alzheimer's patients showed down-regulation in the Default Mode Network's areas, which is linked to memory impairment and cognitive decline. Functional degradation typically associated with AD can be assessed by identifying early disturbances in this network using fMRI [13].

Resting-State fMRI

Resting-state fMRI (rs-fMRI) pertains to the examination of brain activity in which the subject does not perform any specific task. This allows rs-fMRI to detect significant network disruptions, particularly in a network such as the Default Mode Network. These disturbances can be present at the early stages of the ailment, including mild cognitive decline. Being non-invasive and detecting functional changes that have not yet progressed to the structural level, rs-fMRI could become an important tool in making early diagnoses and monitoring the development of AD [14] [15].

13.5 MACHINE LEARNING AND MRI IN ASSESSMENT OF ALZHEIMER'S

Application of Machine Learning on Structural MRI

Structural MRI would be one of the modalities used via machine learning algorithms in the assessment of Alzheimer's. Several researchers have utilized k-nearest Neighbors, Support Vector Machines, and Backpropagation Neural Networks for the categorization task to identify structural brain abnormalities from the scans. These ML approaches have been proven to be able to distinguish between AD, MCI, and healthy individuals based on identifying certain types of anatomical changes in areas such as the hippocampus. For instance, SVM trained for classification tasks on sMRI data has been shown to attain outstanding classification accuracy regarding identifying early structural alterations in AD patients. Table 13.1 provides a few examples of ML and Deep learning approaches used in studies for detecting and categorizing Alzheimer's using MRI images.

Table 13.1 Deep Learning Approaches in Alzheimer's Detection Using MRI

Approach	*Insights*	*Results*
CNN Utilization	A 6-layer CNN model is proposed for the classification of Alzheimer's based on MRI scans. The model improves diagnostic accuracy by automatically extracting key MRI features.	Achieved 98.83% accuracy, outperforming traditional CNN models on the ADNI dataset [16].
Alzheimer's MRI Recognition via CNN	This CNN-based approach effectively categorizes MRI images into different stages of Alzheimer's disease, offering enhanced clinical decision support for disease progression.	The model successfully classifies brain MRI images into four Alzheimer's stages [17].
VGG16 Architecture	This approach combines Machine Learning and Deep Learning techniques, utilizing VGG16 for predicting Alzheimer's, providing significant accuracy in identifying dementia stages.	Achieved 80.8% accuracy, outperforming other ML and DL models [18].
Automated Diagnosis via VGG16	Utilizes VGG16 for automated feature extraction and preprocessing, enhancing diagnostic accuracy and efficiency. This approach integrates clinical recommendations.	The automated system achieves high accuracy in Alzheimer's prediction and suggests treatments [19].
CNN with Explainable AI for Enhanced Classification	A CNN model is integrated with explainable AI to improve transparency and interpretability in Alzheimer's detection, using both real and synthetic MRI data to enhance classification accuracy.	Achieved 97.50% accuracy with real and synthetic datasets; 88.98% accuracy with real data alone [20].

Feature Extraction and Classification
Extracting features is a crucial step in training machine learning algorithms for detecting AD. From MRI scans, measures of hippocampal volume, cortical thickness, or white matter integrity may be extracted that are typically involved in the illness to differentiate between patients. Hippocampal atrophy is among the first observable characteristics and thus represents a major indicator for early diagnosis of AD. These features are further reduced in dimensionality using advanced methods such as PCA and ICA, which preserve essential diagnostic information, thereby allowing classifiers to more effectively differentiate between AD and non-AD individuals.

Accuracy and Predictive Value
Some research reports that the discrimination between AD patients and healthy individuals can reach up to 90% accuracy. Integrating sMRI data with other biomarkers, including CSF markers and adding genetic factors, such as the APOE genotype, considerably improves the accuracy. Moreover, the inclusion of neuropsychological tests, like the MMSE in combination with features of MRI enhance the predictability of the model to MCI progresses to AD.

13.6 ADVANCED MRI TECHNIQUES FOR DETECTION OF ALZHEIMER'S

13.6.1 Magnetization Transfer Imaging (MTI)

Advanced MRI techniques have shown promise in the early identification of Alzheimer's. MTI has a higher sensitivity for myelin-related changes that are critical in AD. This technique can determine subtle early changes in myelin during the early phase of the disease when compared to typical MRI methods [21] [22]. By highlighting aspects of the magnetization transfer ratio, MTI identifies specific changes associated with the extent of disease progression in the brain and aids in evaluating pathology linked to myelination.

13.6.2 Arterial Spin Labeling (ASL)

Using magnetically labeled blood plasma as a marker, ASL is an endogenous, non-invasive MRI method that quantifies cerebral blood flow (CBF). Modifications in CBF detect vascular changes caused by the neurodegenerative process of AD [23] [24]. The capability of early detection through ASL of such vascular changes has enormous potential for connecting to clinical symptoms of cognitive decline. Regional deficits of perfusion mapped with ASL are significantly useful additional information besides traditional structural MRI.

13.6.3 Magnetic Resonance Spectroscopy (MRS)

Magnetic Resonance Spectroscopy (MRS) allows the assessment of metabolic changes in the brain by measuring the concentration of certain metabolites, and in AD it can identify alterations in certain important metabolites, like N-acetyl aspartate (NAA), choline, and myoinositol which indicate some aspects of changing neuronal health and glial activity [25] [26]. Increased choline may indicate increased synthesis or degradation of membrane-related neurodegenerative changes, providing a view unique from classical neurochemistry approaches into the biochemical processes underlying AD. The new techniques developed with MRI are landmark progresses in an early Alzheimer's diagnosis, in the detection and monitoring of the ailment, providing information beyond what conventional imaging modalities may permit.

13.7 COMPARING MRI WITH OTHER IMAGING MODALITIES

13.7.1 A Comparison Between Positron Emission Tomography (PET) and Magnetic Resonance Imaging (MRI)

Positron Emission Tomography (PET) and Magnetic Resonance Imaging (MRI) share one purpose with high value toward the assessment and study of Alzheimer's, yet differ in their functions and complementary points of view. Their main job is to detect the pathogenic characteristics that form the foundation of AD, such as tau tangles and amyloid plaques. These protein aggregates are visualized by radioactive tracers in PET imaging and can be detected at very early stages of the disease when its clinical symptoms are still not apparent [27]. Amyloid PET scans can show deposition of amyloid-beta peptides in the brain, whereas tau PET imaging focuses on abnormalities of the tau protein. PET constitutes a central component for identifying molecular alterations in AD, and therefore, it is a potent tool in making early assessments and in studying disease progression. While MRI is sensitive to the anatomical detail of changes, including hippocampal atrophy, cortical thinning, and white matter degeneration, PET scans are more sensitive to detecting molecular pathology. While PET excels at detailing molecular changes, MRI has a superior spatial resolution for putting in context structural damage to the brain. The two are complementary: PET identifies the protein abnormalities that are the leading causes of AD, while MRI shows the structural and volumetric consequences of those changes. It integrates the scanning of PET and MRI, offering a more comprehensive approach toward AD, its early detection, and the tracking of both molecular and structural changes of the brain.

13.7.2 A Comparison of Computed Tomography (CT) and Magnetic Resonance Imaging (MRI)

The visualization of brain structures is a dramatically different outcome between CT and MRI scans, especially regarding their capacity to detect subtle changes that would account for neurodegenerative diseases like Alzheimer's. Computed Tomography scans create cross-sectional images of the brain using X-rays, making them particularly beneficial in emergency situations due to their speed and ease of use compared to MRI. On the other hand, CT cannot capture detail or soft tissue in the brain because it lacks the spatial resolution to distinguish between smaller types of tissue such as gray and white matter for subtle changes.

In contrast, MRI offers excellent soft tissue visualization and high-resolution images that would allow detection of early AD signs, which include shrinkage of the hippocampus, cortical atrophy, and white matter changes. Such fine structural changes are often critical to the identification of Alzheimer's at its onset, and CT does not scan. Furthermore, MRI does not employ ionizing radiation; thus, repeated applications in long-term follow-up of a disease process are safer. Under most circumstances, therefore, such fine-grained analysis is impossible with CT scans for neurodegenerative diseases, with MRI proving far more effective [28].

13.8 FUTURE DEVELOPMENTS IN MRI FOR ALZHEIMER'S DISEASE IDENTIFICATION

Advancements in MRI technology open wide avenues for improving the detection and diagnosis of AD. To fully exploit these gains, some critical areas remain to be further explored.

13.8.1 Automated Extraction of Disease-Specific Information

Future studies should concentrate on establishing reliable, validated, and automated methods of disease-specific information extraction from both cross-sectional and longitudinal sMRI data. This may lead to considerable accuracy and efficiency in the diagnosis of AD during early stages by enabling objective analysis of MRI scans.

13.8.2 Validation Across Various Clinical Populations

Validating the generalizability of sMRI as a biomarker requires cohort populations whose diagnosis and treatment are clinically based and represent common pathologies and disorders. Most current studies rely on highly screened populations that would not accurately reflect the broader demographics of individuals with Alzheimer's and related conditions. An extension of these research studies, including those populations, will increase the applicability of findings.

13.8.3 Expanding to Multi-Class Classification

Research should explore multi-class classification problems to accurately predict the different stages of Alzheimer's disease. Creating larger, combined datasets from various sources can increase variability and improve model generalization. Focusing on studies with patients exhibiting high clinical dementia rating (CDR) scores is essential for understanding disease trajectories more comprehensively [29].

13.8.4 Exploration of Advanced Imaging Techniques:

Advanced MRI techniques, including 7T MRI, enable detailed volumetric analysis of hippocampal subfields, but high-resolution volumetry is limited due to the small size of the medial temporal lobe. Further research studies should be dedicated to early changes in specific regions, like CA1 and the subiculum, as possible markers for early diagnosis and differentiation between different stages of AD [30].

13.8.5 Integration with Other Biomarkers

Integrating sMRI measurements with other clinical assessments, including cerebrospinal fluid (CSF) and PET biomarkers, is also crucial to explore. This integration is expected to offer a deeper understanding of disease progression and treatment options, thereby improving the clinical applicability of MRI-based markers for Alzheimer's [30].

13.8.6 Adoption of Surface-Based Imaging Techniques

Upcoming research should incorporate surface-based imaging as input for deep learning frameworks, which could enhance detection capabilities. Additionally, utilizing posthumous neuropathological data, regarded as the definitive standard for diagnosing Alzheimer's disease, could help validate MRI findings and improve their clinical significance [30].

13.8.7 Assessment of Iron Deposition

Future studies should integrate cutting-edge MRI techniques, such as QSM, to quantify iron deposition in the brain. Studies have indicated that elevated or deficient levels of iron are associated with dementia progression and could serve as a supplementary indicator for diagnosing and tracking the progression of Alzheimer's dementia [31].

13.8.8 Data-Centric Approaches

Utilizing data-centric machine learning models along with demographic MRI features can further improve the classification accuracy of AD patients. It would be essential to provide a comprehensive performance analysis incorporating longitudinal MRI features with advanced preprocessing techniques to handle missing data and develop a more robust model.

13.9 CONCLUSION

MRI plays a crucial role in diagnosing and monitoring AD. Its non-invasive, high-resolution imaging allows for the evaluation of alterations in brain anatomy and function associated with AD. Techniques like DTI, fMRI, and sMRI provide valuable information on brain connectivity changes, hippocampal atrophy, and the condition of white matter. These methods are instrumental in early detection and disease progression tracking, enhancing the management and treatment of AD. As the understanding of Alzheimer's evolves, there is a pressing requirement for further advancements in MRI techniques. Integrating emerging technologies such as machine learning and artificial intelligence possesses the capability to boost the accuracy and predictive value of MRI in detecting early signs of AD. Additionally, combining MRI with biomarkers from genetic and cerebrospinal fluid analyses may provide a more comprehensive approach to diagnosis. Continued research in this area is essential to refine these techniques and improve patient outcomes, ultimately contributing to more effective interventions and therapies for those affected by Alzheimer's disease.

REFERENCES

1. Saratxaga, C. L., Moya, I., Picón, A., Acosta, M., Moreno-Fernandez-de-Leceta, A., Garrote, E., & Bereciartua-Perez, A. "MRI deep learning-based solution for Alzheimer's disease prediction," *Journal of Personalized Medicine*, 11, 2021, https://doi.org/10.3390/jpm11090902.
2. Brown, R. W., Cheng, Y. C. N., Haacke, E. M., Thompson, M. R., & Venkatesan, R. *Magnetic Resonance Imaging: Physical Principles and Sequence Design*. New Jersey, USA: John Wiley & Sons, 2014, https://doi.org/10.1002/9781118633953.
3. Young, P. N., Estarellas, M., Coomans, E., Srikrishna, M., Beaumont, H., Maass, A., & Schöll, M. "Imaging biomarkers in neurodegeneration: current and future practices," *Alzheimer's Research & Therapy*, 12, 2020, https://doi.org/10.1186/s13195-020-00612-7.

4. Frisoni, G. B., Fox, N. C., Jack, C. R., Scheltens, P., & Thompson, P. M. "The clinical use of structural MRI in Alzheimer disease," *Nature Reviews Neurology*, 6(2), 67–77, 2010, https://doi.org/10.1038%2Fnrneurol.2009.215.
5. Thompson, P. M., Hayashi, K. M., De Zubicaray, G., Janke, A. L., Rose, S. E., Semple, J., & Toga, A. W. "Dynamics of gray matter loss in Alzheimer's disease," *Journal of Neuroscience*, 23(3), 994–1005, 2003, https://doi.org/10.1523/JNEUROSCI.23-03-00994.2003.
6. Kantarci, K., Weigand, S. D., Petersen, R. C., Boeve, B. F., Knopman, D. S., Gunter, J., ... & Jack, C. R. "Longitudinal 1H MRS changes in mild cognitive impairment and Alzheimer's disease," *Neurobiology of Aging*, 32(12), 2103–2115, 2011, https://doi.org/10.1016%2Fj.neurobiolaging.2006.06.018.
7. Jack, C. R., Knopman, D. S., Jagust, W. J., Shaw, L. M., Aisen, P. S., Weiner, M. W., ... & Trojanowski, J. Q. "Hypothetical model of dynamic biomarkers of the Alzheimer's pathological cascade," *The Lancet Neurology*, 9(1), 119–128, 2010, https://doi.org/10.1016%2FS1474-4422(09)70299-6.
8. Kantarci, K., Murray, M. E., Schwarz, C. G., Reid, R. I., Przybelski, S. A., Lesnick, T., & Dickson, D. W. "White-matter integrity on DTI and the pathologic staging of Alzheimer's disease," *Neurobiology of Aging*, 56, 172–179, 2017, https://doi.org/10.1016/j.neurobiolaging.2017.04.024.
9. Magalhães, T. N. C. Biomarcadores moleculares e de neuroimagem em pacientes com comprometimento cognitivo leve: estudo transversal e longitudinal. Doctoral Dissertation, Universidade Estadual de Campinas (UNICAMP), Faculdade de Ciências Médicas, 2021, https://hdl.handle.net/20.500.12733/1641683.
10. Agosta, F., Pievani, M., Geroldi, C., Copetti, M., Frisoni, G. B., & Filippi, M. "Resting state fMRI in Alzheimer's disease: Beyond the default mode network," *Neurobiology of Aging*, 33(8), 2012, 1564–1578, 2012, https://doi.org/10.1016/j.neurobiolaging.2011.06.007
11. Kamagata, K., Andica, C., Kato, A., Saito, Y., Uchida, W., Hatano, T., Lukies, M., Ogawa, T., Takeshige-Amano, H., Akashi, T., et al. "Diffusion magnetic resonance imaging-based biomarkers for neurodegenerative diseases," *International Journal of Molecular Sciences*, 22, 5216, 2021, https://doi.org/10.3390/ijms22105216.
12. Wang, K., Liang, M., & Wang, L. "Altered functional connectivity in early Alzheimer's disease: A resting-state fMRI study," *Human Brain Mapping*, 28(10), 967–978, 2007, https://doi.org/10.1002%2Fhbm.20324.
13. Greicius, M. D., Srivastava, G., Reiss, A. L., & Menon, V. "Default-mode network activity distinguishes Alzheimer's disease from healthy aging: evidence from functional MRI," *Proceedings of the National Academy of Sciences*, 101(13), 4637–4642, 2004, https://doi.org/10.1073/pnas.0308627101.
14. Biswal, B. B., Mennes, M., Zuo, X. N., et al. "Toward discovery science of human brain function: The human connectome project and beyond," *Nature Reviews Neuroscience*, 12(12), 732–742, 2010. https://doi.org/10.1073/pnas.0911855107

15. Zhang, H. Y., Wang, S. J., Liu, B., et al. "Resting brain connectivity: Changes during the progression of Alzheimer's disease," *Radiology*, 256(2), 598–606, 2010, https://doi.org/10.1148/radiol.10091701
16. Nag, A., Hassan, M.M., Rony, M.A.T., Das, B., Sil, R., Saha, P., Sarker, P. and Bairagi, A.K. (2025). Fusing Sentiment Analysis with Hybrid Collaborative Algorithms for Enhanced Recommender Systems. In B. Bhushan, A. Khanday, K. Aurangzeb, S.K. Sharma and P. Nand (eds) Wellness Management Powered by AI Technologies. https://doi.org/10.1002/9781394287024.ch13
17. Mingjun, W. Alzheimer's MRI Recognition Based on Convolutional Neural Networks. Transactions on Materials, Biotechnology and Life Sciences, 3rd International Conference on Biotechnology, Life Science and Medical Engineering (BLSME 2024), vol. 3. DOI: https://doi.org/10.62051/0xherm33
18. Manimuthu, A., Peter Jose, P., Gangadevi, E., Udhaya Kumar, U., & Anandaraj, M. D. Prediction of Alzheimer's disease from Magnetic Resonance Images (MRI). In: 2024 IEEE International Conference on Computing, Power and Communication Technologies (IC2PCT), IEEE, Greater Noida, India, 2024. https://doi.org/10.1109/ic2pct60090.2024.10486545
19. Nag, A. et al., TumorGANet: A Transfer Learning and Generative Adversarial Network- Based Data Augmentation Model for Brain Tumor Classification. In: IEEE Access, vol. 12, 103060–103081, 2024, doi: 10.1109/ACCESS.2024.3429633
20. Mansouri, D., Echtioui, A., Khemakhem, R., & Hamida, A. B. „Explainable AI framework for Alzheimer's diagnosis using convolutional neural networks." Proceedings of the 2024 IEEE 7th International Conference on Advanced Technologies, Signal and Image Processing (ATSIP), Sousse, Tunisia, 2024, https://doi.org/10.1109/atsip62566.2024.10639037
21. Kavroulakis, E., Simos, P. G., Kalaitzakis, G., Maris, T. G., Karageorgou, D., Zaganas, I., Panagiotakis, S., Basta, M., Vgontzas, A., & Papadaki, E. Myelin content changes in probable Alzheimer's disease and mild cognitive impairment: Associations with age and severity of neuropsychiatric impairment. *Journal of Magnetic Resonance Imaging*, 47, 1359–1372, 2018, https://doi.org/10.1002/jmri.25849
22. Makovac, E., Serra, L., Di Domenico, C., Marra, C., Caltagirone, C., Cercignani, M., & Bozzali, M. Quantitative magnetization transfer of white matter tracts correlates with diffusion tensor imaging indices in predicting the conversion from mild cognitive impairment to Alzheimer's disease. *Journal of Alzheimer's Disease*, 63(2), 561–575, 2018, https://doi.org/10.3233/JAD-170995
23. Wierenga, C. E., Hays, C. C., & Zlatar, Z. Z. Cerebral blood flow measured by arterial spin labeling MRI as a preclinical marker of Alzheimer's disease'. *Journal of Alzheimer's Disease*, 2014, S411–S419, 2014, https://doi.org/10.3233/JAD-141467
24. Bangen, K. J., Restom, K., Liu, T. T., Wierenga, C. E., Jak, A. J., Salmon, D. P., & Bondi, M. W. Assessment of Alzheimer's disease risk with functional

magnetic resonance imaging: an arterial spin labeling study. *Journal of Alzheimer's Disease*, 31(s3), S59–S74, 2012, https://doi.org/10.3233/JAD-2012-120292

25. Swathi Sree, M., Reddy, C. K. K., Mohd Hanafiah, M., & Lippert, K. "Smart education systems using the Internet of behavior-based computational intelligence," IGI Global Internet of Behavior-Based Computational Intelligence for Smart Education Systems, October 2024, https://doi.org/10.4018/979-8-3693-8151-9.ch008
26. Swathi Sree, M., Reddy, C . K. K., Mahathi, A., & Doss, S. "Behavior-based computational intelligence on the web for integrated educational systems." IGI Global Internet of Behavior-Based Computational Intelligence for Smart Education Systems, October 2024, https://doi.org/10.4018/979-8-3693-8151-9.ch010
27. Ganga, P. R., Reddy, C. K. K., Lippert, K. J., & Ranjan, A. "Aero metamorphosis in Industry 6.0 Pioneering structural adaptability in contemporary aviation using deep learning." Industry 6.0 Technology, Practices, Challenges, and Applications, CRC Press, October 2024, https://doi.org/10.1201/9781003517993
28. Ashritha, P., Reddy, C. K. K., Ozer, O., & Doss, S. "Identification of earthquake patterns for predictive modeling using decision tree classifiers to maintain sustainability." Industry 6.0 Technology, Practices, Challenges, and Applications, CRC Press, October 2024, https://doi.org/10.1201/9781003517993
29. Scheltens, P., Leys, D., Barkhof, F., Huglo, D., Weinstein, H. C., Vermersch, P., ... & Valk, J. (1992). Atrophy of medial temporal lobes on MRI in "probable" Alzheimer's disease and normal aging: Diagnostic value and neuropsychological correlates. *Journal of Neurology, Neurosurgery & Psychiatry*, 55(10), 967–972, 1992, https://doi.org/10.1136/jnnp.55.10.967.
30. Battineni, G., Hossain, M. A., Chintalapudi, N., Traini, E., Dhulipalla, V. R., Ramasamy, M., & Amenta, F. Improved Alzheimer's disease detection by MRI using multimodal machine learning algorithms. *Diagnostics*, 11(11), 2103, 2021, https://doi.org/10.3390/diagnostics11112103.
31. Lu, B., Li, H. X., Chang, Z. K., Li, L., Chen, N. X., Zhu, Z. C., ... & Yan, C. G. A practical Alzheimer's disease classifier via brain imaging-based deep learning on 85,721 samples. *Journal of Big Data*, 9(1), 101, 2022, https://doi.org/10.1186/s40537-022-00650-y.

Chapter 14

Federated learning-enabled CNN for predicting and detecting brain tumors in healthcare 6.0

Boggarapu Srinivasulu, Srinivasa Rao Dhanikonda, Dammu Venkata Ravi Kumar, Ravega Venkata Gandhi, and Bonthala Prabhanjan Yadav

14.1 INTRODUCTION

The ability to think, move voluntarily, speak, judge, and perceive is all controlled by the brain, which is one of the body's most vital organs [1]. Movement, balance, and posture functions are under its control. We would behave like "walking puppets" without it [2]. The Latin term for "little brain" is where the word cerebellum originates. A brain tumor is defined as the development of a tumor in the brain which could either be benign (non-cancerous) or malignant (cancerous). It can metastasize from any other part of the frame or start inside the brain itself [3]. Primary brain cancers are less frequent than metastases in the brain. About 2,500,000 people worldwide are impacted by about 50% of breast or lung cancer metastases each year, which equals 2% or less than all cancer cases. The second most common kind of cancer in children and young adults below the age of 15 is a brain tumor. To investigate brain tumors, radiologists typically use magnetic resonance imaging (MRI) [4]. Deep learning algorithms are used to determine whether the brain is healthy or broken. Brain tumors and everyday brains prominently use neural networks [5]. A complicated synthetic neural network is made of several processing units with truthful controls. Typically, conversation hyperlinks related to a specific weight connect these components. The closest records, which are inputs obtained through connections, are concerned with manipulations by way of units. The interactions among the network's processing gadgets are what give synthetic neural networks their intelligent behaviors [6]. There might be one or more hidden layers further to both layers like an input and output layer. Throughout the mastering procedure (for output layers and hidden layers), weight and bias are given to every layer's neurons relying on the input features and previous layers. The muse for schooling a version is the activation functions applied to the input capabilities and the hidden layers [7], wherein extra mastering takes place to create the preferred output.

DOI: 10.1201/9781003591085-14

14.2 LITERATURE SURVEY

This section includes a literature survey of existing systems and problem formulation for detecting brain tumor detection. Research papers, journals, and publications have also been referred to in the preparation of this survey. Raymond v. Damadian invented the primary magnetic photograph in 1969. The primary MRI of the human body, the most current generation, turned advanced in 1977 [8]. Using MRI, we can study the interior structures of the brain in addition to the various kinds of tissues inside the human frame. The images produced by MRI are of superior quality compared to different types of medical imaging strategies like computer tomography (CT test) and X-ray[9]. The MRI technique is a useful approach for detecting human brain tumors. One-of-a-kind MRI, inclusive of "T1 weighted, T2 weighted, and flair (Fluid attenuated inversion recovery) weighted images", are used for mapping tumor-precipitated alteration. T1, T2.

Artificial neural network methods are employed primarily to identify tumor blocks within the MRI scans of different patients and class the form of tumor. The second stage uses numerous image-processing techniques to identify brain tumors in cancer patients' MRI images [10]. These techniques encompass characteristic extraction, morphological operations, picture segmentation, and histogram equalization. This look cautioned an automated brain tumor detection approach to boost precision and accelerate analysis instances [Figure 14.1].

14.2.1 Image Pre-processing

The system uses MRI as a noise input. Therefore, the first thing you want to do is to clean the noise of the input image. We use a higher pass filter for the noise removal and pre-processing, as represented in the system flow [11].

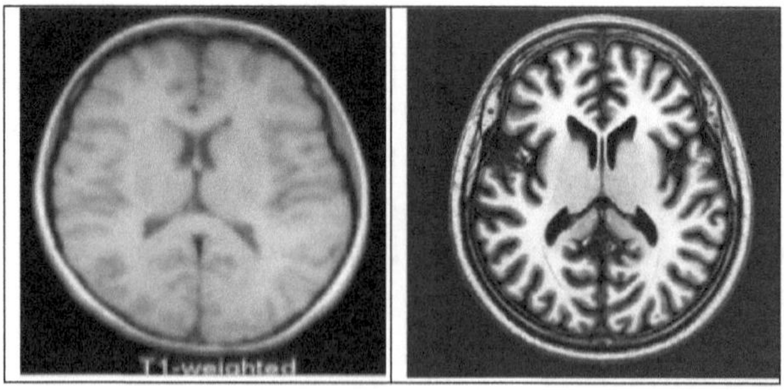

Figure 14.1 FLAIR, T1 and T2 weighted images.

14.2.2 Segmentation

Location expansion is an easy technique for region-based complete photograph segmentation. It is often called a pixel-based photograph segmentation approach since it consists of choosing initial seed points for photo segmentation [12].

14.2.3 Morphological Operation

The morphological operation is used to extract the boundary regions of brain photographs [27]. This procedure best affects the relative order of pixel values, no longer their real numerical values; consequently, it could only be useful for binary photographs. Erosion and dilation are morphology's primary tactics. Dilation involves adding pixels to an object's border whereas erosion involves removing pixels [13].

14.2.4 Feature Extraction

Feature extraction is used to find the snapshot edge detection. It involves collecting greater-intensity information about an image, shape, texture, color, and assessment.

14.2.5 Connected Component Labeling

Each group of connected pixels with identical gray-stage values is given an identical specific region name after the connected factors of an image have been diagnosed [14].

14.2.6 Tumor Recognition

In this stage, we are taking out characteristics from gathered brain MRIs. For comparison, a knowledge base is developed [15].

14.3 SOLUTION

The main 5 modules of the proposed tool are pre-processing, an information set to categorize and divide the information, constructing a CNN model, and training a deep neural network. We will use one MRI image as our input photograph out of many that we will use in the dataset. The labels become encoded and the image is resized through pre-processing. We divided the information into education and check agencies using a manner of setting the picture to 80 percent training and 20 percent testing. Constructing a CNN version and training a deep neural network for epochs follows. Following that, the facts are categorized, and a degree of accuracy is provided [16].

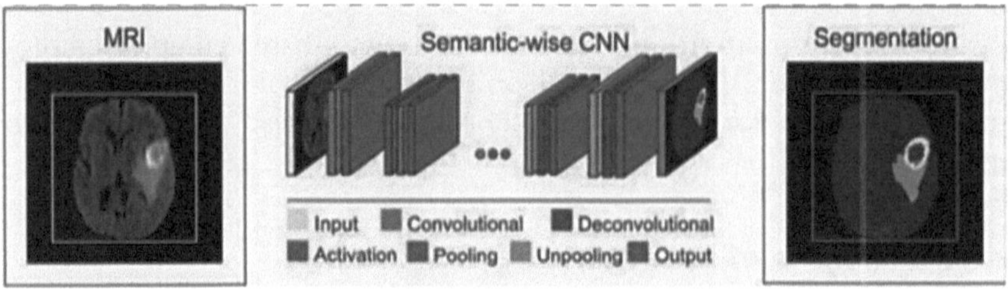

Figure 14.2 Working of CNN model for brain tumor detection.

14.3.1 Goals of the Proposed System

The objectives of the proposed architecture include the following:

- To detect brain tumors.
- To provide integrity and accuracy.
- To collect a dataset containing various brain images and do preprocessing on the dataset in order to train the model.

Convolution 2D: Figure 14.2 tells the extract of the featured part of the enter photo using convolution second. It offered the outcomes in matrix format [17].

MAX Poolig2D: MAX polling 2D uses the maximum element from the corrected feature map.

Flatten: Feed output values into a fully connected layer. Data lists are offered.

Dense: To merge the inputs and outputs coupled by weight using a linear procedure. The non-linear activation function came next. It employed the sigmoid function to activate and estimate the probabilities of 0 and 1. Because the compilation model has two levels, 0 and 1, we employed binary cross entropy. We employed the Adam optimizer when building the model [18]. Adaptive moment estimation, Adam, is easy to implement and useful for non-convex optimization problems. Low memory requirements are computationally efficient.

14.3.2 Working of VGG16 Model:

Constructing deep learning models requires less time, cash, and PC resources [19] and is an information-sharing approach for gaining and transferring knowledge of a pre-educated version's learning by transferring to a newborn model with the usage of switch learning. Switch-gaining knowledge

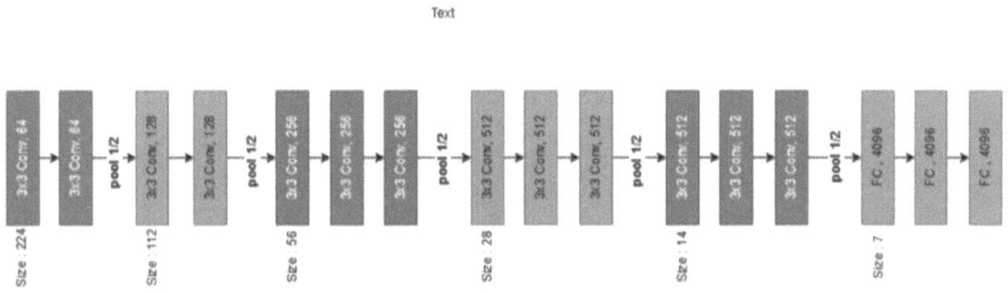

Figure 14.3 VGG16 layered architecture.

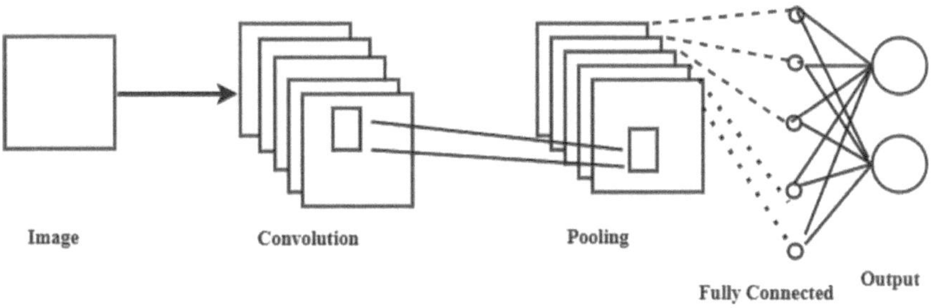

Figure 14.4 Working ofVGG16 version for brain tumor detection.

has been implemented to a variety of responsibilities, together with hobby recognition, sentiment evaluation, tumor categorization, and software fault prediction. Figures 14.3 and 14.4 compare the effectiveness of the proposed deep CNN model to the well-liked switch mastering technique VGG16. Figures 14.3 and 14.4 indicate VGG16 architecture and explain switch learning effectiveness clearly [20].

14.4 METHODOLOGY

Records Pre-processing: Pre-processing is an information-mining technique used to show the raw statistics in a layout that is both realistic and effective [21].

Deep Learning: Deep learning is a method of training processing machines to do what comes clearly to humans by way of example. Deep learning is a key technology behind driverless vehicles, making them able to, for example, react to a stop signal or distinguish a pedestrian from a lamppost. It is by far the key to voice management in person apparatuses like phones, tablets, TVs, and hands-free persons talking. Deep learning is receiving large amounts of interest these days and for good reason. It is enabling activities that were not possible before. In deep learning, a knowledge processing device is designed to learn to act at once from snapshots, textual content, or sound. Deep learning techniques can help accomplish new levels of accuracy, on occasion going over the limits of human capability.

Neural Network: A neural network is the order, organization, and lines of algorithms that try to take in relations in a collection of facts through a procedure that models how the human brain operates. In this sense, neural networks have a relation to structures of neurons, either an important part of a device or a synthetic nature [22]. Neural networks can adjust to converting input; so the network produces a great feasible outcome without needing to repeat the original examples and rules. The idea of neural networks, which has its roots in artificial information, is quickly and smoothly getting extra circumstance of having general approval within the development of trading structures.

Classification: Class is a supervised learning method utilized in machine learning and information wherein the PC application creates new observations or classes depending on the statistics that are given to it [23]. It is a method for grouping together a set of facts. Both dependent and unstructured statistics can be used with it.

Creating Model: The use of imaging to predict the future with move takes in the seeing who a person diseased growth (in body) biological qualities that make ready news given on the likely get help from process. The above complex parts around clear outlines of move are therefore equally related to the use of imaging to say what will take place in the future with move.

Python: Python was selected as the project's language of desire. For lots of reasons, this was an easy decision.

- There may be a sizeable network that supports the Python language. An easy visit to Stack Over float can restore any issues that could arise. Python is one of the most widely used computer languages, increasing the probability that any inquiry may have a clear answer.
- Python affords several sturdy pieces of equipment that are geared up for clinical computing.
- Python applications like NumPy, Pandas, and SciPy are completely documented and unfastened to use. Those kinds of applications will notably lessen and adjust the amount of code needed to create certain software program. This quickens generation.
- Python is a forgiving language that permits programs that look to be pseudo-code. While the tutorial papers' provided pseudo

code desires to be checked and implemented, this may be useful. This step can sometimes be finished quickly using Python. Python, even though, isn't without flaws. Packages are notorious for their Duck writing and the language is dynamically written. This will be traumatic if a bundling technique returns something that, as an example, resembles an array but isn't always one. Moreover, because the go-back form of a technique isn't constantly laid out in trendy Python documentation, this might result in a number of trials and errors that would no longer usually arise in a powerfully designed language. This can be traumatic whilst a package deal method returns some information that, as an example, re-assembles an array but it is not always an array. Additionally, because the method is not always specified in general Python software, this might bring about a number of trial-and-mistakes that could not generally occur in a powerfully designed language. This issue makes it more difficult than normal to learn how to make use of an alternative Python package.

Dataset Used in the Proposed System: Images of diverse data units are accrued from the source. Datasets are collections of more than a thousand images of the human brain. The dataset is subjected to statistics pre-processing techniques which are a good way to extract the important functions from the datasets which can be utilized to classify the tumor. Datasets contain photographs of brain scans. With this dataset, there can be a type to outline accuracy.

14.5 PROPOSED SYSTEM ARCHITECTURE

An architectural diagram shows (Figure 14.5) the parts of the system, their connections, and how the system works. A sizable dataset where the data has been pre-processed, CNN-classified [24] [25], and then the model has been trained. The information is submitted by programmers into the program, which concept according to the various types of detection and generates the various types of brain tumors. The final output is then sent to the user [26].

14.6 IMPLEMENTATION AND RESULTS

Step 1: Importing package
Step 2: Loading the dataset
Step 3: Loading classified datasets yes and no (Figure 14.6)
Step 4: Description
Step 5: Analyzing data
Step 6: Working of training model
Step 7: Test accuracy 0.71

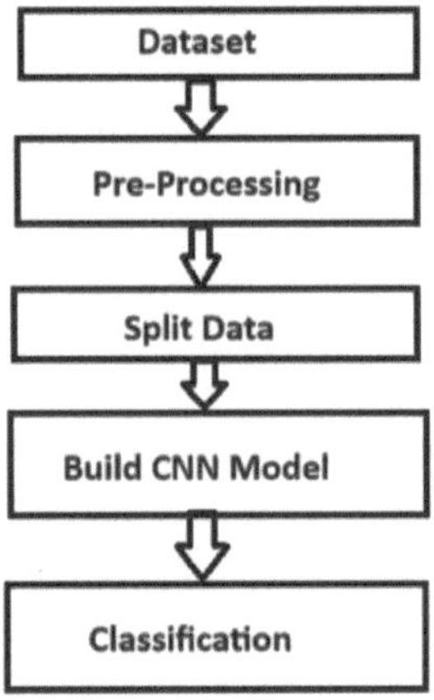

Figure 14.5 An architecture diagram.

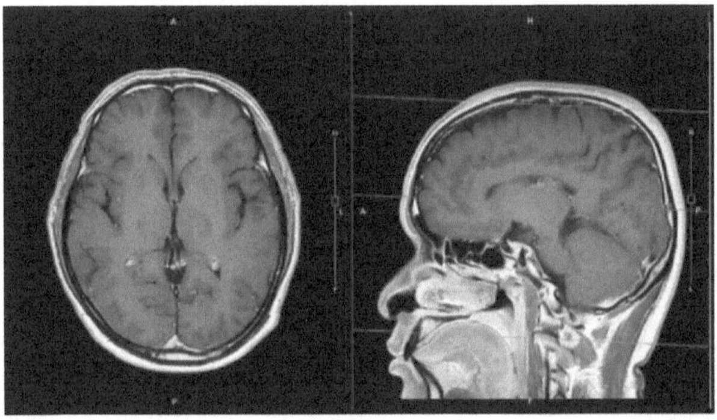

Figure 14.6 Meningioma and pituitary brain tumor detection.

14.7 CONCLUSION

Brain tumors offer a serious health risk, and early detection is critical in preserving patients' lives. Current manual identification procedures based on MRI images are time-consuming and inaccurate, potentially delaying therapy. To solve this, modern image processing techniques paired with deep learning models such as Convolutional Neural Networks (CNNs) present a viable answer. CNNs, a form of neural network, can automatically and accurately detect the existence and size of brain tumors in medical pictures. The use of such automated technologies can considerably enhance the speed and accuracy of tumor identification, improving diagnosis and treatment outcomes and, ultimately, saving more lives. The exceptional version detects brain tumors with 88.699 percent accuracy at the test set, 0.881 f1 rating on the check set, 91 percent accuracy on the validation set and 0.91 f1 score at the validation set. Therefore, we will conclude that the proposed device presents an accuracy of 91.42 percent, outcomes are precise and balanced. The feature enhancement of research is data augmentation. 3D CNN integration and U-Net segmentation can all help enhance tumor detection and localization accuracy. Increasing explainability using Grad-CAM and multimodal MRI inputs improves the model's reliability and clinical value.

REFERENCES

[1] Hossain, T., Shishir, F.S., Ashraf, M., Al Nasim, M.A., Shah, F.M.: Brain tumor 10 detection using convolutional neural network. In: 2019 1st International Conference on Advances in Science, Engineering and Robotics Technology (ICASERT), pp. 1–6 (2019). IEEE. DOI: 10.1109/ICASERT.2019.8934576

[2] Singh, R.: Cerebellum: Its anatomy, functions and diseases. In: Neurodegenerative Diseases-Molecular Mechanisms and Current Therapeutic Approaches. IntechOpen (2020).

[3] Seetha, J., Raja, S.S.: Brain tumor classification using convolutional neural networks. *Biomedical & Pharmacology Journal* **11**(3), 1457 (2018). DOI: 10.13005/bpj/1511

[4] Windisch, P., Weber, P., F¨urweger, C., Ehret, F., Kufeld, M., Zwahlen, D., Muacevic, A.: Implementation of model explainability for a basic brain tumor detection using convolutional neural networks on MRI slices. *Neuroradiology* **62**, 1515–1518 (2020). DOI: 10.1007/s00234-020-02447-9

[5] Santos, D., Santos, E.: Brain tumor detection using deep learning. medRxiv, 2022–01 (2022).

[6] Dahab, D.A., Ghoniemy, S.S., Selim, G.M., *et al.*: Automated brain tumor detection and identification using image processing and probabilistic neural network techniques. *International Journal of Image Processing and Visual Communication* 1–8 (2012).

[7] Xu, Y., Jia, Z., Wang, L.-B., Ai, Y., Zhang, F., Lai, M., Chang, E.I., *et al.*: Large scale tissue histopathology image classification, segmentation, and visualization via deep convolutional activation features. *BMC Bioinformatics* **18**(1), 1–17 (2017). DOI: 10.1186/s12859-017-1559-1

[8] Macchia, R.J., Termine, J.E., Buchen, C.D.: Raymond v. damadian, md: magnetic resonance imaging and the controversy of the 2003 nobel prize in physiology or medicine. *Journal of Urology* **178**(3), 783–785 (2007). DOI: 10.1016/j.juro.2007.05.089

[9] Villarraga-G´omez, H., Herazo, E.L., Smith, S.T.: X-ray computed tomography: From medical imaging to dimensional metrology. *Precision Engineering* **60**, 544–569 (2019). DOI: 10.1016/j.precisioneng.2019.03.007

[10] Ugale, V.D., Pawar, S.S., Pawar, S.: Brain tumour detection using image processing. In: 2022 IEEE 11th International Conference on Communication Systems and Network Technologies (CSNT), pp. 667–672 (2022). IEEE . DOI: 10.1109/CSNT54456.2022.9787333

[11] Shedbalkar, J., Prabhushetty, K., Inchalc, A.: A comparative analysis of filters for noise reduction and smoothening of brain mri images. In: 2021 6th International Conference for Convergence in Technology (I2CT), pp. 1–6 (2021). IEEE. DOI: 10.1109/I2CT51068.2021.9417854

[12] Vocaturo, E., Zumpano, E., Veltri, P.: Image pre-processing in computer vision systems for melanoma detection. In: 2018 IEEE International Conference on Bioinformatics and Biomedicine (BIBM), pp. 2117–2124 (2018). IEEE. DOI: 10.1109/BIBM.2018.8621431

[13] Chudasama, D., Patel, T., Joshi, S., Prajapati, G.I.: Image segmentation using morphological operations. *International Journal of Computer Applications* **117**(18), (2015).

[14] He, L., Ren, X., Gao, Q., Zhao, X., Yao, B., Chao, Y.: The connected-component labeling problem: A review of state-of-the-art algorithms. *Pattern Recognition* **70**, 25–43 (2017). DOI: 10.1016/j.patcog.2017.05.023

[15] Honavar, M., Janota, I., Polkey, C.E.: Histological heterogeneity of dysembryoplastic neuroepithelial tumour: identification and differential diagnosis in a series of 74 cases. *Histopathology* **34**(4), 342–356 (1999). DOI: 10.1046/j.1365-2559.1999.00636.x

[16] Nex, F., Duarte, D., Tonolo, F.G., Kerle, N.: Structural building damage detection with deep learning: Assessment of a state-of-the-art CNN in operational conditions. *Remote Sensing* **11**(23), 2765 (2019). DOI: 10.3390/rs11232765

[17] Cope, B., *et al.*: Implementation of 2d convolution on fpga, gpu and cpu. *Imperial College Report*, 2–5 (2006).

[18] Miller, K.D., Ostrom, Q.T., Kruchko, C., Patil, N., Tihan, T., Cioffi, G., Fuchs, H.E., Waite, K.A., Jemal, A., Siegel, R.L., *et al.*: Brain and other central nervous system tumor statistics, 2021. *CA: A Cancer Journal for Clinicians* **71**(5), 381–406 (2021). DOI: 10.3322/caac.21664

[19] Theckedath, D., Sedamkar, R.: Detecting affect states using vgg16, resnet50 and se-resnet50 networks. *SN Computer Science* **1**, 1–7 (2020). DOI: 10.1007/s42979-020-00500-7

[20] Tajidini, F., Mehri, R.: A survey of using deep learning algorithms for the covid-19 (sars-cov-2) pandemic: A review. In: Conference: 9th National Congress of Electrical and Computer Engineering of Iran (2022).

[21] García, S., Luengo, J., Herrera, F.: *Data Preprocessing in Data Mining.* Vol. 72. Springer Nature (2015).

[22] Reddy, C.K.K., Daduvy, A., Mohana, R.M., Assiri, B., Shauib, M., Alam, S., and Sheneamer, A.: Enhancing Precision Agriculture and Land Cover Classification: A Self –Attention 3D Convolutional Neural Network Approach for Hyperspectral Image Analysis. *IEEE Access*, June 2024. DOI: 10.1109/ACCESS.2024.3420089

[23] Reddy, C.K.K., Rangarajan, A., Rangarajan, D., Shuaib, M., Jeribi, F., and Alam, S., A Transfer Learning Approach: Early Prediction of Alzheimer's

Disease on US Healthy Aging Dataset. *MDPI Mathematics* (July 2024), 2204. https://doi.org/10.3390/math12142204

[24] Reddy, C.K.K., Reddy, P.A., Janapati, H., Assiri, B., Shuaib, M., Alam, S., and Sheneamer, A.: A Fine-tuned Vision Transformer Based Enhanced Multi-class Brain Tumor Classification Using MRI Scan Imagery. *Frontiers in Oncology* (July 2024). DOI: 10.3389/fonc.2024.1400341

[25] Sreelatha, G., Reddy, C.K.K., Mohd Hanafiah, M., Madana Mohana R.: Hybrid electro search beetle optimization based task scheduling and game theory SOA based resource allocation in multi cloud computing. Wiley Journal of Software: Practice and Experience (September 2024). DOI: https://doi.org/10.1002/spe.3370

[26] Kattenborn, T., Leitloff, J., Schiefer, F., Hinz, S.: Review on convolutional neural networks (CNN) in vegetation remote sensing. *ISPRS Journal of Photogrammetry and Remote Sensing* 173, 24–49 (2021). DOI: 10.1016/j.isprsjprs.2020.12.010

Index

Note: Figures are indicated by *italics*. Tables are indicated by **bold**.